Deborah K. Mayer, RN, CRNP
Formerly Head Nurse
Biological Response Modifiers
    Clinical Oncology Research Unit
National Cancer Institute
Frederick, Maryland

Joan Martin Moore, RN, MN
Head Nurse/Clinical Nurse Specialist
Medical Oncology Clinic
Yale-New Haven Hospital
New Haven, Connecticut

Marion E. Morra, MA
Assistant Director
Yale Comprehensive Cancer Center
New Haven, Connecticut

Linda Celentano Norton, RN, MSN
Assistant Professor and Coordinator of Pulmonary Specialty
Yale University School of Nursing
New Haven, Connecticut

Mary E. Ropka, RN, MS
Doctoral Candidate
University of Virginia
Charlottesville, Virginia

Judith A. Spross, RN, MS, CS
Clinical Nurse Specialist
Cancer Nursing Service Clinical Center
National Institutes of Health
Bethesda, Maryland

Glee I. Wahlquist, RN, PhD
Professor and Chairperson
Department of Nursing
Sacred Heart University
Fairfield, Connecticut

Hilary Ann Wood, SRN, SCM, RN
Director
Cancer Treatment Center
Bethesda Hospital, Inc.
Cincinnati, Ohio

FOREWORD

This book is an obvious, timely, and substantial contribution to cancer nursing. In addition, it is a major contribution to nurses from cancer nursing. It is a telling commentary on the positive development of cancer nursing as a specialty that not only is there an urgent need for a ready reference book of this nature, but there also are qualified nurses to write it.

The list of contributing authors is most impressive. These are names well known in cancer nursing. While primarily clinicians, the contributors are also educators, administrators, and researchers. As authors, their commonality is *involvement* in an emerging, exciting, and complex specialty. It could easily be said that a resource book of this nature was a long time coming. It could just as easily be said that its appearance is overdue. My prevailing feeling, however, is that perhaps this book could not have come until now because the experiential knowledge base was still being amassed.

The authors write about what they do. It comes as no surprise that Susan Fisher writes about sexuality, Mary Ropka about nutrition, and Susan Hubbard about the principles of clinical research. This is what they have been speaking and writing about all along. Now, they share their expertise in a concise, up-to-date manner. We learn from the experience of great clinicians. Judy Spross uses the collective experiences of caring for a variety of patient populations as a basis for writing about the protective mechanisms of bone marrow. Jean Jenkin's role in NCI clinical trials forms a foundation for her writing. Such different settings may not be a regular part of the workaday world of many nurses caring for persons with cancer, but they will profit from the variety and collective wealth of experience the authors represent.

There is value to the ongoing refinement of cancer nursing in the book's framework, the ANA/ONS Outcome Standards for Cancer Nursing Practice. That the Standards have moved from their initial formulation to this point of sophisticated application and utility is no small accomplishment. Those who were part of the endless hours of debate about the Standards should feel some sense of pride that the original Standards continue to serve the specialty well. The testing of the Standards over time gives evidence that their originators were well grounded in the practical and common concerns of cancer nursing care. For those nurses seeking to extend the implementation of the Standards toward promoting standardization of care, an abundance of information exists between these covers. The value to the specialty, then, lies in the progress that is documented in developing the knowledge base to meet the Standards.

The value to nurses seems so obvious. This bright red tome will be a ready reference to the practicing clinician. Whether identifying parameters for assessment, rechecking aspects for care planning, or determining if the outcomes of implementation require further planning, this volume sits ready with the answers. Unless, of course, it is already in use!

One of the most remarkable features of the book is the material on oncologic emergencies. This is the most inclusive nursing presentation on this topic presented in one place. This will be of real value to the busy practitioner; one place to identify what to look for and what to do about it. It is exciting as well to see attention paid to aspects of care frequently neglected in the nursing literature — sleep, mobility, and ventilation.

This is an affordable, well-organized resource whose cross-referencing will be appreciated and whose thorough index will be consulted frequently. The editors have obviously given this book a lot of thought. Their insight should serve us well.

Each book published in cancer nursing is a milestone in its own right as it is a measure of where we are in the refinement of care for a population of patients presenting complex and changing needs. This book is a milestone. This is a book specifically designed through its tables, illustrations, and appendices to provide timely information in a succinct and useful way. This is a book whose content is organized the way busy nurses think and act when planning and providing care. Here is a book that will be welcomed and used, and used, and used. Hooray!

Susan B. Baird, RN, MPH
Editor-in-Chief
Oncology Nursing Forum

PREFACE

The knowledge required by nurses to provide effective care for people with cancer and their families has broadened considerably over the past decade. Advances in supportive and curative treatment for cancer achieved by intensive research efforts have made sophisticated care accessible to patients in nearly every sphere of health care. Therefore, nurses in these areas are often required to make decisions about nursing care that must reflect a knowledge of both the disease and the treatment plan.

The purpose of this text is to provide information about cancer care to nurses who must deal with adults demonstrating any one of hundreds of tumor types. To achieve this goal, the book uses a framework of common problem areas encountered by the oncology patient population. In 1979, the Oncology Nursing Society Clinical Practice Committee developed *Outcome Standards for Cancer Nursing Practice* in which ten high-incidence problem areas are defined in terms of positive outcomes from nursing care. Chapters 4 through 13 identify these problem areas, state the standard of care, and describe specific nursing management used to help patients achieve these positive outcomes. This problem-oriented approach, which makes this text usable by nurses practicing in any care setting, is designed to avoid the fragmentation that results from the more common disease-oriented approach to nursing care. By focusing on common problem areas, care for a particular problem (such as constipation) may be performed in a uniform fashion for patients with different tumor types, and thus can be more easily incorporated into a total plan of care.

In addition to the chapters focusing on the outcome standards, the first three chapters of the text describe the principles necessary to understand the behavior of cancer and the rationale for treatment. Chapters 14, 15, and 16 describe the care of patients experiencing any one of fourteen selected obstructive, metabolic, or infiltrative oncologic emergencies. These fourteen were selected because they occur *often* in persons with cancer (e.g., bowel obstruction, hypercalcemia), or because, though rare, they occur *particularly* in persons with cancer (e.g., tumor lysis syndrome, carotid artery erosion). Emergencies such as hyperglycemia or renal failure, which occur more often in the general population, are not included.

Finally, the last two chapters of the book focus on the management of patients receiving special forms of therapy: intravenous or intra-arterial chemotherapy, implanted infusion pumps, and radiation implants, to name a few. Throughout the text, management plans are written in the form of preventive and/or supportive nursing protocols.

The appendices provide information about specific tumor types, staging systems, and available resources. In addition, Appendix A provides a master table correlating tumor type with likely sites of metastases, while Appendix B correlates tumor type with potential oncologic emergency. Coupled with the detailed index and the extensive cross-referencing used throughout the text, these appendices will enable the nurse to rapidly locate related information throughout the book.

A special acknowledgement is due to the Oncology Nursing Society and to the American Nurses' Association, Inc., which kindly gave permission to reprint the Oncology Nursing Society Clinical Practice Committee's *Outcome Standards for Cancer Nursing Practice* that appear at the beginning of Chapters 4 through 13.

It is our hope that this text will promote a standardized approach to the nursing care of persons with cancer, and that it will help the nurse to move logically toward problem prediction, identification, and effective management.

BLJ and JG

ABBREVIATIONS AND SYMBOLS

ADL	activities of daily living
bid	2 times a day
BP	blood pressure
BUN	blood urea nitrogen
CAT	computerized axial tomography
CBC	complete blood count
CNS	central nervous system
CSF	cerebrospinal fluid
dl	deciliter
DNA	deoxyribonucleic acid
D5W	5% dextrose in water
ECG	electrocardiogram
EEG	electroencephalogram
g	gram
GI	gastrointestinal
GU	genitourinary
Hb	hemoglobin
Hct	hematocrit
IM	intramuscular(ly)
IV	intravenous(ly)
kg	kilogram
m	meter
mEq	milliequivalent
mg	milligram
ml	milliliter
mm	millimeter
mM	millimole
mOsm	milliosmole
μg	microgram
μm	micrometer
NPO	nothing by mouth
PO	oral(ly)
prn	as needed
q	every
q 4 hr, etc.	every 4 hours, etc.
qid	4 times a day
R	roentgen
RBC	red blood cell
RNA	ribonucleic acid
SC	subcutaneous(ly)
tid	3 times a day
U	units
WBC	white blood cell

CHAPTER 1

THE BEHAVIOR OF MALIGNANCIES

Michele Girard Donehower

An understanding of the biologic principles involved in the development and spread of neoplasia and of their therapeutic implications is important for persons involved in the care of oncology patients. A strong foundation in the principles of cancer biology facilitates understanding of cancer-related literature, interaction with other health care personnel, and interpretation or reinforcement of explanations to patients. Expansion of a nurse's knowledge of cancer biology will enhance his or her capabilities as both clinician and educator.

This chapter will focus on the nature and characteristics of cancer, the principles of cellular kinetics, the stimuli that may initiate malignant transformation, and the pathogenesis of the metastatic process.

THE NATURE OF CANCER

Proliferative growth patterns

Although the term cancer encompasses a variety of diseases, a common feature of the underlying cellular defect is the loss of control of cell proliferation and differentiation. Neoplastic cells are not subject to the usual restrictions on cell growth and proliferation imposed by the host. Because spurts of cell growth are characteristic of various tissues throughout the life cycle, it is necessary to differentiate malignant neoplastic growth from other forms of cellular proliferation. The spectrum of proliferative growth patterns ranges from benign to increasingly malignant.

Hyperplasia can be defined as an increase in the number of cells of a certain type in a tissue. Although hyperplasia can be a characteristic of neoplasia, it also occurs commonly as a normal physiologic response during episodes of rapid growth and development (such as the prenatal and adolescent periods). It is also a common feature of bone marrow cells and epithelial cells of the GI mucosa. **Metaplasia** occurs when a stimulus initiates a change in the differentiation of a stem cell and results in the replacement of one normal adult cell type with another. Vitamin deficiency and various chemical agents can induce these changes.

Dysplasia is a disturbance in the usual distinct histologic pattern of a group of cells within a tissue. Microscopically, cells within tissues are readily characterized by their intracellular features and their relationship to one another in the architecture of the tissue. Both the cell-to-cell regularity and the arrangement of cells within a tissue may be altered in this type of proliferation. This pattern can be an early characteristic of neoplasms or can result from chronic inflammation. The difference between dysplasia and **anaplasia** is a matter of degree. Anaplastic cells lack any normal characteristics of cellular differentiation and are associated almost exclusively with neoplasia.

Neoplasia is a proliferative abnormality characterized by an autonomous uncontrolled growth pattern. Neoplasms are classified as either benign or malignant. Table 1–1 summarizes the differences between these forms of neoplasia.

Characteristics of cancer cells

Malignant cells possess certain unique cellular and kinetic characteristics. Several major features that have been observed are loss of proliferative control, loss of the capacity to differentiate, altered biochemical properties, chromosomal instability, and increased tendency to metastasize.

Loss of proliferative control. This is a characteristic of all neoplastic cells. Normally, the stimulus for initiating cellular proliferation is the need for cell renewal or replacement. Cell production ceases when the stimulus for proliferation has been removed, resulting in a balance between cell loss and cell production. In cancer cells, the host's normal control mechanisms are unable to stop proliferation once a stimulus has initiated the process. Little is known about the nature of the signal that the cell receives and what intracellular events ensue to trigger proliferative activity. Identifying this signal in normal cells would provide critical information to understanding and controlling neoplastic growth.

Loss of capacity to differentiate. The process by which a stem cell diversifies and acquires completely individual morphologic characteristics is called differentiation. Stem cells within a tissue are committed to become a designated cell type. For example, stem cells

TABLE 1-1

Characteristics of Benign and Malignant Neoplasms

Benign	Malignant
Encapsulated	Nonencapsulated
Noninvasive	Invasive
Highly differentiated	Poorly differentiated
Mitoses rare	Mitoses relatively common
Slow growth	Rapid growth
Little or no anaplasia	Anaplastic to varying degrees
No metastases	Metastases

Reprinted with permission from Pitot, H. C. Fundamentals of Oncology. Marcel Dekker, Inc., New York. 1981. Second edition. p. 23.

within the liver or lung mature and are easily identifiable as to the tissue of origin. Cells that have undergone a malignant transformation vary in their retention of the tissue's morphologic characteristics. The degree to which a malignant cell bears a resemblance to its tissue of origin is characterized by its degree of differentiation. Cells that retain many of the identifiable tissue characteristics are termed well-differentiated. As tumor cells lose these identifying features, they become increasingly undifferentiated, or anaplastic. After a cell has undergone the initial neoplastic transformation, it may continue to evolve histologically toward a more anaplastic state. The concept of differentiation assumes greater significance when treatment effectiveness and metastatic potential of neoplastic cells are under consideration. The more undifferentiated the tumor cell, the more malignant the tumor is considered to be. Tumors that contain poorly differentiated neoplastic cells are frequently associated with a graver prognosis, even though they may demonstrate initial responsiveness to antineoplastic treatments.

Altered biochemical properties. Many cancer cells differ from normal cells in that they exhibit biochemical aberrations that indicate either a loss or a gain of properties. Because of the lack of differentiation of neoplastic cells, certain biochemical properties may be missing because the cell exists in an immature or embryonic form. Or, cells may gain new properties because of changes in enzyme patterns or alterations in DNA. Small cell carcinomas of the lung exemplify this characteristic with their ability to produce a variety of hormones. Although not all cancers display such properties, these biochemical alterations may — in the instances in which they are found — provide the basis for the design of therapies that can exploit them. Progress in this area is likely to come slowly, because the biochemical abnormalities of various tumor types are of a widely diverse nature, and no single treatment approach based on this rationale could be expected to be effective against all cancer cell types.

Chromosomal instability.   The chromosomal instability of cancer cells provides a sharp contrast to the extremely stable chromosomal structure of normal cells. Cancer cells exhibit a much higher incidence of mutations than normal cells. This genetic unpredictability results in the emergence of new, more malignant variants as cancer cells proliferate. These mutations within a tumor population during therapy can result in the creation of a surviving subpopulation of malignant cells that are maximally refractory to therapy.

Capacity to metastasize.   This property is unique to cancer cells; however, not all cancer cells are equally capable of metastasizing. Variants of an original tumor cell tend to become increasingly malignant with each mutation, and a correlation exists between the degree of malignancy of a cell and its metastatic capacity. Other changes that occur in cells to increase their metastatic potential are discussed below.

CELL KINETICS AND TUMOR GROWTH

Cell cycle

It is necessary to understand the behavior of normal cells in the cell cycle in order to compare and contrast them with the activity of a neoplastic cell. In addition, knowledge of the kinetics of cellular reproduction aids in understanding the scientific basis and rationale of cytotoxic therapy. All living cells progress through four major phases of development to reproduce themselves. These phases, collectively known as the cell cycle, are depicted in Figure 1–1. The four phases of the cell cycle are G_1, S, G_2, and M.

The G_1 phase is a period of decreased metabolic activity. During this period, the cell carries out its designated physiologic functions and synthesizes proteins needed for maintenance of the cell. This phase is primarily a stage of readiness, in which cells prepare for entry into the S phase.

Certain cells do not remain in the G_1 pool but enter a state where they become temporarily or permanently quiescent. The term G_0 has been designated to describe those cells not active in the cell cycle. This category includes cells that will never divide (such as brain cells) and cells that are dormant but capable of being stimulated to reenter the cell cycle in times of physiologic need (such as hepatocytes).

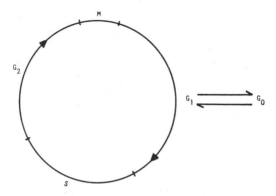

Figure 1-1. Phases of the cell cycle. (*See* text for discussion.)

Cells in G_1 or G_0 receive an intracellular stimulus, or signal, which prompts the cell to enter the active part of the cell cycle, ultimately leading to the replication of genetic material and division of the cell.

The **S** phase is that portion of the cell cycle in which DNA is synthesized. Normal cellular replication is dependent on the orderly synthesis of genetic material. Structural damage or disarray of the DNA molecule during its reproduction can ultimately result in cell death. Cells are most vulnerable to damage in this phase, and it is thought that many cell-cycle-specific chemotherapeutic agents exert their cytotoxic effects during this period.

Another period of relative hypoactivity, G_2, immediately follows the S phase. Cells entering this stage contain the duplicated genetic material synthesized in the S phase. Although some RNA and protein production occurs during G_2, cells in this stage are basically awaiting entry into the mitotic phase, in which cell division occurs.

The **M** phase, or mitosis, is that portion of the cell cycle in which the actual division of the cell occurs. This period is further subdivided into four stages: prophase, metaphase, anaphase, and telophase. During these stages, The parent cell segregates the duplicated chromosomes and divides into two daughter cells. After mitosis, the two new cells either pass through the cell cycle again or enter a resting state in G_1 or G_0.

The durations of M, S, and G_2 are relatively constant, while the length of G_1 is highly variable and determines the overall length of the cell cycle. Rapidly dividing cells are able to complete the cell cycle faster by reducing the length of G_1. Renewing cells and neoplastic cells are examples of this type of cell population.

Cancer cells divide more frequently than normal cells, although they do not pass through the phases of the cell cycle at a faster rate, and a larger fraction of cells within a tumor are dividing at any given time compared with cells within most normal tissues.

Tumor growth concepts

Cells of normal tissues can be divided into three major categories of proliferative activity: static, expanding, and renewing. Normal cells of **static** tissues, such as brain, do not retain the capacity to divide after the postembryonic period. Because of their inability to divide, cells of this type that are damaged or destroyed during the life-span of an individual cannot be replaced. **Expanding** tissues in the body temporarily cease proliferating when they reach their normal adult size, but they are capable of reentering the cell cycle and dividing in times of physiologic need. The liver, kidneys, and endocrine glands contain cells with the potential to repair or replace damaged cells. **Renewing** cell populations have the highest degree of proliferative activity. Cells in this category have a finite life-span and continuously replace dying cells. Blood cells, epithelial cells of the GI mucosa, and germ cells are examples of renewing cell populations. They most closely resemble actively proliferating cancer cells in their degree of activity within the cell cycle.

Tumors, similarly, contain mixtures of actively proliferating, temporarily dormant, and permanently nondividing cells. These three different populations of tumor cells vary in their degree of responsiveness to cytotoxic therapy. Within a tumor mass, there are cells that are incapable of further cell division. As the mass increases in size, some cells are pushed away from the vascular supply. Because of this distance, these cells receive inadequate regional nutrition, leading to necrosis. These cells add only mass to the tumor and are of little concern for treatment purposes.

Another subpopulation of tumor cells is temporarily quiescent and spends an extended period of time suspended in G_1 or G_0. These cells are partially or completely insensitive to the effects of many cytotoxic drugs. Attempts to synchronize entry of these cells into the active part of the cell cycle by administering an activating drug may aid in increasing the number of chemotherapy-sensitive malignant cells.

A third subpopulation of cancer cells consists of those that remain actively proliferating. These are the target of most treatment interventions, because they are extremely sensitive to the effects of chemotherapy.

As tumors grow, they exhibit varying rates of growth. Initially, there is a lag stage. Growth is slow until the tumor becomes vascularized. For growth to continue, the tumor must be penetrated by blood vessels. A period of exponential growth follows vascularization. The tumor cells undergo a series of doublings as they increase in size. Cell growth continues at the periphery of the tumor mass with the center becoming increasingly dormant and ultimately necrosing. Finally, the tumor reaches a critical mass when cell death approximates new cell formation, and a plateau phase is reached. By the time a tumor has grown to a size where it can be clinically detected, it has probably already reached the plateau phase and growth has slowed.

Doubling time is the term used for the time that is required for a mass to double its volume. A mass must reach a size of ≥ 1 cm to reach the lower limit of sensitivity for most clinical methods of detection. In general, a tumor must undergo ~ 30 doublings before it becomes palpable. The doubling times of various tumors have been examined in *in vitro* systems and vary greatly. The actual growth rate in humans is difficult to ascertain because of the number of variables that influence doubling times. For example, *in vivo*, tumor growth may be retarded by hormonal and immunologic factors. Information about doubling times of tumors can be applied to clinical situations to predict what therapeutic responses may occur. In general, rapidly growing tumors have been more responsive to chemotherapy than slow-growing cancers, such as adenocarcinoma of the colon.

Because not all cells within a tumor are dividing simultaneously, growth fraction is an important variable in the determination of a tumor's doubling time. Growth fraction refers to the portion of a tumor mass that is actively proliferating. Tumors with larger growth fractions expand their tumor masses more rapidly. Growth fractions have been estimated at 100% in some germ-cell tumors and as low as 10% in slow-growing adenocarcinomas. Drug responsiveness has been directly correlated with the growth fraction of tumors.

As tumors grow, they tend to undergo an evolution in their histologic patterns. This concept, referred to as tumor progression, is the change in a neoplasm from a very low degree of malignancy, or preneoplastic state, to a rapidly growing, virulent neoplasm. It can be characterized by changes in the growth rate, invasive potential, metastatic frequency, morphologic traits, and responsiveness to therapy. Progression is thought to occur as a result of the natural selection of a cell type that is rapidly growing or metabolizing at a faster rate than other cells in the neoplasm. This then becomes the dominant cell type. In addition, cancer treatments themselves may facilitate tumor progression through their mutagenic effects and hasten the appearance of more malignant variants. Certain lymphomas commonly undergo progression to a more malignant cell type.

The concept of heterogeneity is one that is closely related to the concept of tumor progression. The origin of most neoplasms is thought to be monoclonal. Yet, though originating from a single cell, tumors are not composed of cells with identical cellular characteristics. As the tumor mass grows, the single malignant cell gives rise to a number of clones that differ in their characteristics from the original cell. This diversity of cells within a primary tumor is established early in its development.

The change in the cell composition within a tumor is caused by the growth properties inherent in malignant cells. As previously discussed, malignant cells are more likely to mutate because of their genetic instability. Such mutation results in the emergence of clones with varying growth traits and malignant characteristics. Cells within a neoplasm can be heterogeneous in a number of characteristics: immunogenicity, growth rate, metabolic characteristics, hormone receptors, metastatic potential, radiosensitivity, and susceptibility to cytotoxic drugs. Tumor cells may be heterogeneous in one or many of these traits.

The concept of heterogeneity has far-reaching therapeutic implications. Cells with varying degrees of responsiveness to treatment exist within a primary tumor. Because of this heterogeneous composition, treatments cannnot be consistent in their cytotoxic effects and probably allow cells refractory to therapy to survive and metastasize. A goal of cancer therapy is to design treatments that will succeed despite a tumor's heterogeneity.

CARCINOGENESIS

Although a number of theories have been proposed, no single unifying hypothesis has been offered to explain carcinogenesis, and the exact cause of most human cancers remains unknown. Neoplastic transformation is thought to be a multistep process, and researchers have been successful in identifying risk factors and agents that may act as cofactors in this process.

It has been generally accepted that neoplastic transformation results from some genetic alteration in the cell, which in turn deregulates the control of cell proliferation. The controversy has centered around the question of what stimuli induce the necessary transformation in the DNA of a cell. Genetic, environmental, and viral factors have all been implicated as components of carcinogenesis.

The importance of targeting potential causative factors lies in being able to identify populations at high risk for developing specific cancers and to eliminate, whenever possible, causative factors from the environment. Understanding the mechanisms by which these factors can induce transformation may provide clues about potential interventions that can inhibit the transformation from a normal to a malignant cell.

Viral factors

Viruses have been associated with specific cancers in humans in only a small number of cases. Although evidence of viral-induced cancers in animal systems has existed for many years, the connection between viruses and cancers in humans has been a fairly recent development. The most exciting hypothesis to evolve in this area has been the oncogene theory of carcinogenesis.

It has been proposed that known animal tumor viruses with the capacity to code for the neoplastic transformation of a normal cell may be transmitted into a human cell and become integrated into the host cell's chromosomes. These viral gene sequences, or oncogenes, then direct DNA synthesis in the host cell and become a part of the genetic information transferred to cells of subsequent generations. In many cases, no trace of the preexisting virus remains after the host's chromosomal structure has been transformed. Proteins, coded for by this aberrant DNA, are believed to initiate the neoplastic change in the host cell, although in most cases these gene products have not been identified.

Introduction of the oncogene into the host DNA does not automatically result in the transformation of the cell and the development of a tumor. The transmission of the viral oncogene may be only one step leading to the expression of cancer. The oncogene may remain dormant until it is activated, or derepressed. The events or agents that "turn on" the oncogene remain unknown, but environmental influences and the immunocompetence of the host may play a role in the transformation. In addition, the heterogeneity of tumor viruses as well as of host cells is thought to affect their susceptibility to transformation by oncogenes.

Recent technical advances in the area of molecular biology have enabled researchers to identify some of the viral gene sequences in the chromosomes of humans with various malignant diseases. Table 1–2 lists the viruses that are suspected as factors in the development of tumors in man. To date, these viruses have not been implicated as the direct cause of any human cancer but appear to be cofactors in the presence of other risk factors.

Genetic factors

Because the cells of nearly all human malignant solid tumors contain chromosomal abnormalities, the role of preexisting genetic

TABLE 1-2

Viruses Implicated in the Etiology of Human Cancers

Virus	Disease
Known	
Human T-cell leukemia-lymphoma (HTLV)	Leukemia, lymphoma
Suspected	
Epstein-Barr (EBV)	Burkitt's lymphoma, nasopharyngeal carcinoma
Hepatitis B	Hepatocellular carcinoma
Herpes simplex type II (HSV II)	Cervical carcinoma
Papilloma	Cervical carcinoma, bowel carcinoma
Cytomegalovirus (CMV)	Cervical carcinoma, Kaposi's sarcoma

determinants in the causation of cancer has been a difficult one to define, and the genetic component of carcinogenesis has been difficult to separate from other environmental factors.

Most chromosomal disorders that increase the susceptibility to developing cancer involve extra chromosomes, loss of chromosomes, or translocation of specific arms or areas of the chromosomes within the gene structure. Patients with these types of chromosomal abnormalities are at a much higher risk than the general population for the development of specific neoplasms.

In only a small proportion of cancers is the presence of the genetic factor alone sufficient to induce tumors. In most cases, hereditary neoplasia results from a complication of an inherited defect that predisposes the patient to cancer upon exposure to specific environmental influences.

Certain tumors and tumor syndromes are transmitted hereditarily in a pattern of Mendelian dominance. The development of a tumor at a single site may be the only manifestation of a syndrome or it may be accompanied by the development of multiple tumor sites and other congenital abnormalities. For example, familial medullary carcinoma of the thyroid may occur by itself or in combination with other benign and malignant neoplasms such as neurofibromas, mucosal neuromas, or pheochromocytomas. Mendelian dominant diseases are often characterized by onset at an early age and site multiplicity (e.g., bilateral development of tumors in paired organs). Retinoblastoma occurs bilaterally much more commonly in children with a family history of the disease than in those cases that arise sporadically.

Patients with Mendelian recessive diseases, such as Bloom's and Fanconi's syndromes, have genetically transmitted defects in the chromosome structure that result in chromosomal fragility. These defects increase the sensitivity of chromosomes to damage by various other environmental factors. In xeroderma pigmentosum, there is an enzyme deficiency that impedes repair of DNA in skin damaged by ultraviolet light. This unrepaired damage to genetic material results in the development of multiple skin cancers of various histologies.

Some inheritable premalignant conditions may be in the form of a severe intrinsic immunologic deficiency that may contribute to the increased risk of developing cancer. Patients with these syndromes are most prone to develop malignancies of the lymphatic tissues; however, other sites, such as brain and stomach, may also be affected. These syndromes include ataxia-telangiectasia, the Wiskott-Aldrich syndrome, and "late onset" or "common variable" immunodeficiency. Each disorder has defects of both cellular and humoral immunity.

Risks among relatives of patients with certain cancers have been shown to be statistically higher than in comparable control families or in the general population. Again, the influences of environmental factors have been difficult to separate from a possible genetic etiologic component, but in general, these familial patterns appear to reflect a genetically transmitted susceptibility to neoplasia that raises the empiric risk for various cancers anywhere from 3- to 30-fold. One of the most important of these predilections is the exaggerated risk of breast cancer in women whose mothers or sisters have developed the disease.

Environmental and life-style factors

Chemical carcinogenesis.   During recent years, an increasing number of chemicals have been identified as possible carcinogens. A variety of industrial and medicinal compounds, food additives, tobacco smoke, and other naturally occurring substances have been determined to be carcinogenic in animals or humans.

It has been proposed that many chemical carcinogens achieve their effect through the multistage process of initiation and promotion. An **initiator** is an agent capable of permanently and irreversibly altering the DNA structure within a cell. The resulting conversion of normal cells to latent tumor cells can occur after a single exposure to the agent. Although initiation is most often associated with chemical compounds, radiation and viruses are examples of physical and biologic agents that may exert their carcinogenic effect in this fashion.

Promotors are thought to alter the genetic expression, or degree of differentiation, of a cell. Repeated, frequent application of or exposure to a promotor is necessary to stimulate latent tumor cells to form tumors and complete the neoplastic transformation. The effects of promoting agents are transitory and potentially reversible. Hormones and growth-stimulating factors are examples of agents that can function as promotors.

Both initiation and promotion are necessary for the complete transformation of the cell, but the sequence of these events is of critical importance. A cell must first be transformed by an initiating agent before further neoplastic changes can occur. The change induced by an initiator is permanent and results in the cell being forever susceptible to further neoplastic transformation by a promotor. In experimental systems, tumors can be induced even when there is a prolonged interval between the change produced by exposure to an initiating agent and the application of a promotor. Promoting agents can elicit neoplasia only if preceded by the appropriate initiating effects. A single exposure to the promotor and/or prolonged intervals between exposures will not result in actual tumor development in animal systems.

Some classes of chemicals can act either as initiators or promotors, or can be considered complete carcinogens that have the capacity both to initiate and to promote. An agent's ability to act as a complete carcinogen may be dose related or vary with other environmental influences.

Radiation carcinogenesis. It has long been recognized that radiation is a carcinogen. Both ionizing and electromagnetic radiation (ultraviolet light, x-rays) have been shown to cause neoplastic transformation in experimental models and humans. The actual risk of cancer is thought to be associated with the degree of damage caused to the DNA molecule. Damage to a single chain of the double helix, such as that caused by ultraviolet light and x-rays, has a higher potential for repair, and consequently, a lower risk of tumor development. Ionizing radiation commonly causes breaks in both chains of the DNA molecule, resulting in a mutation and a higher likelihood of developing cancer.

Several factors have hindered the evaluation of the carcinogenic effects of radiation in humans. Examining the dose-incidence data in these populations has been complicated by the difficulty in separating the effects of radiation dose on cancer risk from those other factors that may contribute to the development of neoplasia; however, the probability that a single, short-term exposure to radiation causes a neoplastic transformation in human cells is highly remote. A multistep process, similar to that in chemical carcinogenesis and influenced by genetic and environmental factors, is thought to be involved. Figure 1–2 illustrates the complex interaction of factors and events that may be involved in radiation carcinogenesis.

The long latency period between exposure and tumor development has also complicated the evaluation of radiation as a carcinogen, but several types of human neoplasms have been associated with prior exposure to radiation. Skin cancer, leukemias, lymphomas, osteosarcoma, and tumors of the thyroid, breast, and lung have all been observed to occur at varying lengths of time after exposure to radiation.

Dietary carcinogenesis. The study of nutritional carcinogenesis is a relatively new area of investigation, and researching the problem of diet as a factor in tumor induction is a difficult process. To date, epidemiologic and animal studies have provided the bulk of available information. High levels of dietary fat, nitrosamines, coffee, and deficiencies of certain micronutrients within the diet have been associated with the development of cancers in humans.

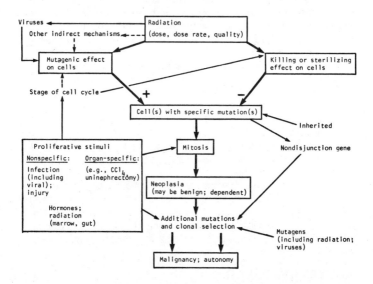

Figure 1–2. Theoretical framework for radiation carcinogenesis. *From* Cole, L. J., and P. C. Nowell. Radiation carcinogenesis: the sequence of events. *Science* (December 1965). p. 1785.

Ingestion of **dietary fat** causes an increase in the secretion of bile, and the metabolites of bile acids may act as tumor-promoting agents in colonic cancer. Cells that have first been initiated by some other agent or an intrinsic genetic defect may be transformed with repeated exposure to consistently high levels of these metabolites. In addition, increased fat intake can modify the endocrine status of the host by increasing the synthesis of hormones. This may affect the induction of cancer in endocrine-dependent sites. Recent studies have correlated an increased incidence of cancers of the breast, colon, and prostate with high levels of dietary fat intake.

Nitrites are found in cured, smoked, and pickled foods. The formation of **nitrosamine compounds** known to be carcinogenic in animals may possibly occur by an endogenous reaction of ingested nitrites with other dietary components. Yet, intake of elements known to be carcinogenic does not necessarily lead to development of cancer in humans. Cells may be initiated by a nitrosamine compound, but unless other promoting factors are present, neoplastic expression of the cell will not occur.

Although the mutagenicity of **coffee** has been reported by several investigators, data regarding the association between coffee intake and colonic and pancreatic cancers have been conflicting. This area requires further investigation, with particular attention to other dietary and environmental factors that may influence the role of coffee as a cancer-causing agent.

Dietary **deficiencies of vitamins and other trace elements** have been linked with the development of head and neck cancers. These findings have prompted investigations of the anticarcinogenic potential of various micronutrients. It is proposed that supplementation of elements within the diet, such as vitamins A and C, riboflavin, and selenium, may exert a protective effect within the host by inhibiting initiation or promotion of cells at selected target organs. The role of these dietary components as anticarcinogens is theoretical and remains to be proven in humans.

Although the results of some studies indicate that certain nutritional factors, preservatives, and methods of food preparation may contribute to the etiology of some cancers, the evidence concerning the role of dietary factors is circumstantial and requires further investigation before substantiated recommendations for dietary policies can be made.

ROUTES OF SPREAD

The ability of a malignant cell to metastasize and invade non-adjacent tissues is its most virulent property, because metastatic lesions, not primary tumors, account for the majority of deaths related to cancer. Knowledge of the pathogenesis and patterns of metastasis allows the nurse to understand the rationale behind the design of effective therapies for preventing or controlling the spread of disease, appreciate the clinical implications of current research findings, and interpret clinical changes in patients with disseminated disease.

The spread of neoplastic cells from a primary tumor occurs via two major mechanisms: direct spread to contiguous areas or metastatic spread to nonadjacent tissues. Direct spread occurs as a result of direct invasion, serosal seeding, or surgical instrumentation. Metastatic lesions develop at distant sites after cells enter the hematogenous or lymphatic channels. Clinically, dissemination of tumor cells may not be limited to one mechanism, because spread via one route may facilitate entry into another system. For example, direct invasion may be a starting point for the further distant metastasis of a primary tumor, because invasion and extension into local tissues can lead to the penetration of body cavities and provide access to the vascular and/or lymphatic channels. In addition, although the lymphatic and vascular systems are separate channels, they have anatomic connections throughout the body that allow disseminating tumor cells to pass freely between the lymphatics and blood vessels.

Direct spread

Direct invasion occurs when cells from the primary tumor penetrate and destroy adjacent tissues within the host. Although little is actually known about the mechanisms of direct invasion, several factors are thought to be involved in this process. Some tumor cells secrete a substance called tumor angiogenesis factor, which stimulates new capillary formation. Once vascularized, the primary tumor growth rate increases, and the ability to invade local tissue is enhanced. Mechanical pressure and rate of tumor growth may also contribute to local infiltration. Rapid tumor growth can create an intratumor pressure that forces fingerlike projections of tumor cells into neighboring tissues. Cell motility has also been implicated as a factor in tumor cell dispersion, but *in vitro* studies have been inconclusive in supporting this mechanism.

Tumor-secreted enzymes may also play a role in the destruction of normal tissue barriers, thereby allowing invasion of tumor cells. The penetration of the basement membrane that exists between parenchymal cells and connective tissue is necessary before tumor cells can invade adjacent tissue and enter the capillary system. A strong correlation has been established between the invasive and metastatic capabilities of tumor cells and the intracellular levels of specific enzymes. For example, because type IV collagen is the major structural protein of these membranes, tumor cells with high levels of collagenase IV are better able to destroy and invade this tissue.

When tumor cells spread locally into host tissue and effectively penetrate body cavities, these cells can embolize and attach to the serosal surfaces of viscera within the cavity. Serosal seeding is a common occurrence with lung and ovarian tumors. Although these cells may implant on the surface of organs within the pleural and peritoneal cavity, infiltration into the parenchyma of the organ is uncommon. Treatment directed to the metastatic implants on serosal surfaces within the peritoneal cavity has been the focus of recent clinical investigations into the use of chemotherapy instilled into the peritoneal cavity.

Surgical instrumentation may also provide a pathway for the spread of malignant cells. Contamination of new tissue planes can occur during the course of a surgical diagnostic biopsy, thoracentesis, or paracentesis. For example, tumor cells from a pleural effusion can be seeded by the needle used during a thoracentesis when it is withdrawn. Reports of malignant skin nodules developing after such a procedure are not uncommon. In addition, manipulation of the primary tumor during surgery theoretically may cause a release of cells into the circulation, posing an increased threat of the development of metastatic foci. Any of these invasive procedures must be considered as a potential mechanism for the local dissemination of malignant cells.

Hematogenous spread

Spread of disease via the hematogenous route is a complex process, requiring specific tumor/host interactions for a metastasis to develop. By itself, entry of malignant cells into the bloodstream is insufficient for establishing a metastatic focus. In fact, <1% of all tumor cells entering the circulation are able to survive transport to a distant organ site and develop as a metastatic lesion. *In vitro* experiments have demonstrated that a sequence of activities and specific tumor/host interactions are required for a tumor cell to establish itself successfully as a metastatic implant (Fig. 1–3).

The first steps in the pathogenesis of a metastasis are the growth and local invasion of host tissue and penetration of the walls of the local blood vessels. It is thought that the tumor mass must reach a "critical size" before it is able to shed cells into the circulation. The correlation of actual tumor size with the incidence of metastasis seems to vary. Certain tumors will predictably shed cells into the circulation when they reach a certain size; others, such as breast cancer, have been found to metastasize even when the primary tumor is quite small.

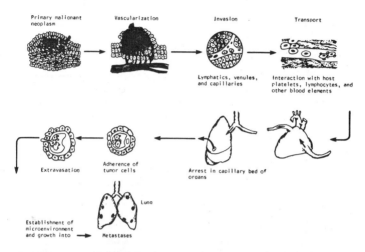

Figure 1-3. The pathogenesis of a metastasis. *Reprinted with permission from* Fidler, I. J. Tumor heterogeneity and the biology of cancer invasion and metastasis. *Cancer Research* (September 1978). p. 2652.

Release of tumor angiogenesis factor from the growing primary tumor induces growth of new capillary sprouts into the primary tumor site to supply nutrients necessary for further growth. This neovascularization within the primary tumor then provides ready access to the general circulation. Penetration of these new blood vessels by tumor cells is not difficult, because vascularized tumors often contain defective-walled vessels caused by reduced oxygenation and necrosis within the tumor. These offer little resistance to infiltration by malignant cells.

Once the vessel has been penetrated, tumor cells either move passively through the bloodstream or remain at the site of invasion, where they proliferate and shed tumor emboli into the circulation. Detachment from the primary tumor can occur as a result of several factors. Because of a lack of cohesiveness, malignant cells are more likely to separate from the primary tumor and enter the main circulation. Cells with a high mitotic index (rate of growth), such as cancer cells, are thought to be less adhesive than those with slower growth rates. In addition, enzymes on the cell's surface may play a role in loosening cells from the primary tumor.

After entering the circulation, these tumor cells aggregate with platelets, lymphocytes, or other tumor cells and form a fibrin-platelet clot, which helps protect them from the hostile host environment and facilitates their adherence to the capillary walls of the target organ. These aggregates of cells are more successful than lone tumor cells in adhering to the endothelium of the target organ's vessels.

Once implanted into the vessel wall of the affected organ, the tumor cell must exit the circulation of the organ and penetrate the organ tissue in order to proliferate. The tumor cell is thought to damage the intact endothelium of the blood vessel in some way, and the cell invades the organ tissue itself.

The last major step in the metastatic process is the vascularization of the new tumor implant. Without adequate blood supply, the cells remain dormant and harmless, receiving only enough diffused nutrition to maintain their viability. New blood vessels, again induced by the release of tumor angiogenesis factor, are required for the continued growth of the newly established metastasis.

Lymphatic spread

Lymphatic spread occurs when malignant cells penetrate a lymph vessel. This allows development not only of a focus within the affected lymph node but spread throughout the lymphatics, and subsequently, the vascular system. Relatively little is known about the mechanisms and/or control of lymphatic spread. It was originally thought that anatomic location was the major determinant in the spread of tumor cells to the locally draining lymphatics, but it has been observed in some instances that metastatic tumor cells may bypass local lymph nodes and seed in more distant nodes in the lymphatic chain.

Actually, several factors may be involved in determining where tumor cells first seed within this system. Initially, regional lymph nodes may exert a barrier effect and impede the passage of tumor cells into the lymphatics. In addition, there is an initial immunologic response to the presence of tumor cells that occurs in the regional lymph nodes and is characterized by the release of immunocompetent cells. It is unknown whether this early immunologic response has any effect on the ultimate progression of disease. At some point, the local lymph nodes lose their ability to filter and destroy tumor cells, and they become infiltrated with malignant cells. The cause of this transformation in their capabilities is unclear. Tumor growth itself may reduce the efficacy of filtration. In addition, chronic inflammation within the node or fibrosis resulting from radiation can alter the barrier effect of these lymph nodes. The presence of malignant cells in the lymph nodes may also occur as a result of some overall change in the host's immunocompetence. When the barrier effect of the lymph nodes changes as a result of these factors, passage of neoplastic cells throughout the lymphatic system is unhindered.

Patterns of lymphatic spread have been observed with many tumors. It has been theorized that cells of certain tumors may have a site predilection for lymph nodes that is comparable to the organ specificity demonstrated by metastatic tumor cells within the vascular compartment.

Patterns of metastasis

Recent experimental studies have supported clinical observations that certain tumors consistently metastasize to particular organs. Although lung, liver, bone, and brain are the commonest sites of metastasis, many tumors have been observed to have unique patterns of metastasis that may include not only these common target organs but some more unusual sites as well. The usual sites of metastasis for some common tumors are listed in Appendix A.

The preferential distribution of metastasis is not random and is probably related to tumor cell characteristics that promote growth in some organs and not in others. Certain properties on the surfaces of tumor cells are probably responsible for the organ specificity of metastatic cells. Cell-surface glycoproteins may create organ-homing tendencies that allow neoplastic cells to migrate to specific organs and attach themselves to tissues. In addition, it is thought that, although tumor cells may lodge in the capillary beds of multiple organs, certain microenvironmental characteristics determine whether tumor growth will be supported.

Specific and predictable patterns of lymphatic and/or hematogenous spread have been identified clinically for many tumors. For example, testicular tumors generally favor the lymphatics as an initial route of spread. Once entry into the lymphatic channels has occurred, vascular spread follows, and the lungs are the most common distant target organ for this particular tumor. Knowledge of the expected tissue distribution of metastasis is important to the clinician who must accurately stage the patient at the time of diagnosis, plan appropriate therapy, and monitor progress. Only through knowledge of the natural history of an individual tumor can the specific routes and sites of metastasis be anticipated.

Bibliography

1. Cole, L. J., and P. C. Nowell. Radiation carcinogenesis: The sequence of events. *Science* (December 1965). 1782–1786.

    Good discussion of the mechanisms and interrelated factors of radiation-induced neoplasia.

2. del Regato, J. A. Pathways of metastatic spread of malignant tumors. *Seminars in Oncology* (March 1977). 33–38.
   Reviews the routes of spread and preferential patterns of metastasis for various tumors.

3. Fidler, I. J. Tumor heterogeneity and the biology of cancer invasion and metastasis. *Cancer Research* (September 1978). 2651–2660.
   Reviews the steps in the metastatic process and discusses the concept of heterogeneity as it relates to metastasis.

4. Gallo, R. C. The virus-cancer story. *Hospital Practice* (June 1983). 79–89.
   Good overview of the role of viruses in the etiology of cancer.

5. Harnden, D. G. The genetic component in oncologic diseases. *In* Symington, T., and R. L. Carter, editors. Scientific Foundations of Oncology. Year Book Medical Publishers, Inc., Chicago. 1976.
   Discusses the role of heredity in the predisposition to and development of neoplastic disease.

6. Hill, B. T. Cancer chemotherapy: the relevance of certain concepts of cell cycle kinetics. *Biochimica et Biophysica Acta* (December 11, 1978). 389–417.
   Review of cell cycle kinetics and concepts of tumor growth with discussion of the clinical implications for designing cancer therapies.

7. Krontiris, T. G. The emerging genetics of human cancer. *The New England Journal of Medicine* (August 18, 1983). 404–409.
   Summarizes recent research on cell transformation and discusses clinical and research implications of the "oncogene theory."

8. Lowenthal, J. P., editor. Nutrition in cancer causation and prevention. *Cancer Research* (May 1983, supplement). 2385s–2519s.
   Proceedings of a workshop covering the epidemiologic and biochemical aspects of dietary carcinogenesis and the role of diet in the prevention of cancer.

9. Ruddon, R. W. Cancer Biology. Oxford University Press, New York. 1981.
   Good comprehensive resource on the basic mechanisms of carcinogenesis and the etiology and pathophysiology of human cancer. Excellent primary reference.

10. Sugarbaker, E. V. Some characteristics of metastasis in man. *American Journal of Pathology* (December 1979). 623–632.
    Brief discussion of the clinical characteristics of metastasis.

CHAPTER 2

CANCER TREATMENT

Susan Molloy Hubbard

It is a striking fact that cancer is the disease that people fear most. The word is often used in our society as a metaphor for death. This is paradoxical because cancer is now one of the more curable chronic diseases when the principles of cancer surgery, radiation therapy, and chemotherapy are applied in a well-integrated, multidisciplinary treatment approach. Current estimates of the relative 5-yr survival rate for all patients with "serious" cancers in the USA have risen from 45% in 1980 to 50% in 1983, and the chance of surviving 20 yr for those who survive 5 yr is 85%. This 50% figure does not include the 400,000 patients who develop superficial cancer of the skin or in situ cancer of the uterine cervix annually who are curable with local forms of surgery or radiotherapy. If these easily cured cancers were included in the estimate of serious cancers, 58% of cancer patients would be long-term survivors. Moreover, these estimates do not reflect the improvements in survival that will undoubtedly be realized when the impact of current advances in treatment becomes widely observed.

Whereas the rate of cancer mortality is falling in all individuals under age 55, the most dramatic increases in survival have occurred in children. When the expected death rate from cancer in 1950 is compared with the expected number of deaths in 1980 for individuals <15 yr of age in the USA, cancer mortality has fallen 80% for Hodgkin's disease, 68% for kidney cancer, 50% for leukemia, 50% for sarcoma, 32% for non-Hodgkin's lymphoma, and 31% for all other cancers. These declines indicate that the advances in cancer treatment that are being developed at research centers are being applied widely throughout the country.

The reason that the likelihood of complete cure and prolonged survival for cancer patients is steadily improving is that fundamental changes have occurred in our understanding of the biology of cancer, and this information has proven to have practical applications. This chapter will discuss the development of modern cancer therapy and the basic biologic principles that contribute to the selection of a particular therapeutic approach for an individual cancer patient.

A key consideration in the treatment of cancer is the therapeutic intent. When cure is the goal, the initial management of the patient is often the most critical period and can determine the ultimate outcome. The development of an individualized treatment plan for a patient must take into consideration the following factors: (1) the biology and natural history of the cancer, (2) the extent of disease dissemination (including specific sites of involvement); and (3) the potential of surgery, radiotherapy, chemotherapy, and immunotherapy to eradicate all viable cancer cells. Surgery and radiotherapy alone are generally curative in cancers that are truly localized, and they play a major role in palliation when the neoplasm has disseminated throughout the body.

Cancer chemotherapy can be curative even when widespread disease is present, because drugs can, at least theoretically, destroy cancer cells in all parts of the body. Modern treatment programs are designed to maximize the curative potential of each modality by using it to exploit the different biologic characteristics of each cancer. Today, surgery and radiotherapy are often integrated with chemotherapy to preserve bodily function and to prevent distant metastases. For example, excisional biopsy and high-dose irradiation can be used for the treatment of small lesions in women with breast cancer, and limb-sparing surgery can be combined with high-dose irradiation in patients with soft-tissue sarcomas.

Diagnosis and staging

A surgical biopsy to accurately determine the pathologic diagnosis of a cancer is critical to the selection of therapy. Subclassification according to further histologic examination is also important for many cancers. Histologic grading and biochemical characterization may be required to accurately pinpoint the diagnosis and malignant characteristics of a specific tumor. In general, knowledge about the extent to which the cancer has spread is essential in order to plan effective treatment. An accurate diagnostic evaluation may require a myriad of laboratory tests and procedures. While time-consuming and sometimes uncomfortable, these staging procedures are essential to determining what (if any) additional treatment should be given following diagnosis and removal of the primary tumor (*see* Table 4–6).

The diagnostic evaluation should be based on the biologic characteristics of the cancer, specifically the most common patterns of dissemination to regional and distant sites. Therefore, specific staging procedures employed for a specific patient are tailored to the pathologic diagnosis. In developing a staging plan, the side effects of a given procedure are carefully balanced against the need for the information that can be obtained. Only when the test results will affect the selection of treatment should staging procedures be performed.

Patients should expect to undergo some of the staging procedures, such as chest and abdominal x-rays or CAT scans, regularly during the course of treatment and at the end of therapy, because these procedures yield information vital to monitoring the effects of therapy on the cancer. Some of these tests will be used to determine the extent of tumor regression with treatment, while others will be used to measure the severity of toxic effects that are associated with treatment, such as myelosuppression. Again, while inconvenient or uncomfortable, these tests are absolutely essential to determine whether disease has disappeared after treatment and whether normal tissues have recovered from any untoward effects of treatment.

Once the cancer has been staged (see Appendix C), a decision can be made about the need for further treatment. Besides the type of cancer and its stage, there are many factors that both the patient and physician must consider together to develop a treatment plan, including the biologic characteristics of the tumor, particularly its growth rate. If the patient's general health is good, however, a decision to administer the most rigorous course of treatment is wisest if it offers the patient the possibility of a prolonged remission of disease or total cure with a normal life expectancy. If, on the other hand, the patient has serious health problems or the cancer is known to be very indolent, administration of aggressive treatment may be inadvisable. If so, the treatment should be aimed at palliation of symptoms to improve quality of life.

SURGERY

Although cancer was described as early as 1600 B.C., the ability to cure it is a relatively recent achievement. Before 1900, few patients with serious cancers survived for long periods after the development of the disease. Around the turn of the century, ether became available for general anesthesia and the principles of antisepsis were introduced, making the development of cancer surgery possible. The first commonly used surgical procedure for treating cancer was the radical mastectomy, a procedure developed in the early 1900s by a surgeon named Halsted. He based this operation on the belief that cancer spread by directly invading tissues surrounding the tumor and designed an extensive surgical procedure that removed the entire breast and all the tissues surrounding it. In women whose cancer was truly localized to the breast, this operation was (and still is) curative. As modern anesthesia, antibiotics, and blood-component therapy were incorporated into surgical practice and surgical techniques were refined, the cure rate with surgery in truly localized cancers began to increase steadily.

By 1930, with surgery and radiotherapy available to treat localized forms of cancer, between 20 and 25% of cancer patients were curable. By 1950, with further refinements of surgical techniques and the development of even more powerful and sophisticated x-ray equipment, approximately 33% of all cancer patients were curable. During the 1950s, the rate of improvement began to level off, however, and it became clear that new approaches to treatment were needed if cure rates were to continue to improve. Around this time, scientists studying the biology of cancer began to realize that the major cause of treatment failure with surgery and radiotherapy was the shedding of viable cancer cells into the bloodstream and lymphatic system and that this phenomenon could occur before the cancer was detectable clinically.

The knowledge that microscopic metastases were often present at the time the cancer was diagnosed and were the reason that recurrent disease appeared after apparently curative procedures explained why progress against cancer had leveled off in the 1950s and gave investigators the critical piece of information necessary to understand why these treatments were not always effective in patients who appeared to have truly localized cancer. Therefore, it is helpful to think of cancer as having three separate and biologically important compartments, as expressed in the TNM (for Tumor, Node, Metastases) classification developed by the International Union Against Cancer (UICC) and summarized in Appendix C.

Curative surgery

When a cancer is localized, or contained within the T compartment, surgery is curative if it is anatomically possible to resect the entire tumor mass. The extent of curative surgery depends not only on the site of the primary lesion and the volume, but also on the nature and degree of direct invasion of surrounding tissues or structures. Therefore, radical surgery is useful in the management of localized, bulky tumor masses and in tumors that recur locally. Patients should, however, understand the nature, degree, and permanence of the mutilation involved as well as the possible complications.

Treatment failures in truly localized cancers (T compartment) are related to inability to resect all cancer cells because the primary lesion is inaccessible or because resection would unduly compromise a vital structure. When a cancer spreads, regional lymph nodes (the N compartment) are often the first site of involvement. If regional lymph nodes are the only site of metastasis, a more extensive surgical procedure may produce cure. The use of radical mastectomy was an attempt to prevent local recurrences by resecting the entire breast and all regional lymph nodes.

Regional (N compartment) failures often occur when involved lymph nodes are not removed during the surgical procedure. The role of surgical resection of regional lymph node metastases is both diagnostic and, less frequently, therapeutic. In some instances, radical lymphadenectomy can be curative. In most cancers(breast carcinoma, malignant melanoma, and colorectal carcinoma), lymph node dissection provides important staging information but, if lymph nodes are positive, surgery is rarely curative because of the strong association between nodal metastases and later relapse in distant sites. When radical surgical techniques fail to cure patients, the cause of treatment failure is the dissemination of clinically undetectable cancer cells (M compartment) beyond the surgical field. These occult metastases are eventually manifested as recurrent, or metastatic, disease.

Palliative surgery

Palliative surgical procedures are often employed to relieve symptoms. Obstructive symptoms produced by tumor masses can be successfully managed with surgical intervention. Small-bowel and ureteral obstruction are not uncommon in the clinical course of ovarian cancer or other pelvic cancers. Although surgical bypass and decompression have no intrinsic therapeutic effect, they may provide considerable relief, improve performance status, and facilitate definitive treatment with radiation or chemotherapy.

Surgery also has a role in the management of bulky metastatic cancer. Surgical procedures that remove bulky tumor masses can enhance the effectiveness of treatment with radiotherapy or chemotherapy. Surgery has also been valuable when removal of a solitary life-threatening metastasis, such as a single brain lesion, is necessary. Finally, neurosurgical procedures can provide pain relief for individuals whose pain cannot be controlled with analgesics and narcotics.

Nursing management

Preoperative care. Nursing care in the preoperative period should focus on the reduction of surgical mortality and education of patients about the postoperative period. Major deficiencies, such as negative nitrogen balance and severe anemia, must be preoperatively corrected with high-protein diets or total parenteral nutrition and blood transfusion to decrease the risk of surgical mortality. In addition, the nurse should assess patients for potential problems that can complicate wound healing, nutrition, and physical rehabilitation. Patients should be educated about the immediate postoperative period, taught deep-breathing techniques, and given a general description of what may be expected after the operative procedure. This is particularly important if the surgery is disfiguring, alters normal body function, or affects sexual identity.

Postoperative care. In the immediate postoperative period, priority should be given to the prevention of complications at the site of the surgical wound. If skin flaps have been raised and/or free skin or other tissues transferred, it is essential to maintain tissue viability by assuring that drainage tubes sutured into the wound are effective in removing blood, plasma, or air. Intact skin coverage is necessary to prevent infection, fistula formation, wound breakdown, and flap necrosis. The potential for hematoma or frank bleeding in the surgical wound must be recognized. The potential for postoperative complications in patients who have had radical head and neck explorations is especially great. Chyle leakage, wound breakdown, and carotid artery rupture may necessitate emergency nursing interventions. Pressure dressings over amputation sites require frequent inspection for drainage and circulation. Intake and output records must be designed to reflect the status of each separate drainage site.

Anticipation of complications is critical, as is early intervention. Among the most important considerations are: (1) maintenance of vital physiologic functions; protection of operative sites; (2) accurate monitoring, interpretation, and documentation of pertinent observations about changes in condition; (3) prevention of infection through aseptic management of surgical sites; (4) maintenance of respiratory function; (5) passive exercises and assistance in early ambulation; (6) management of pain with analgesics; (7) maintenance of nutrition; (8) physical and psychosocial rehabilitation; and (9) preparation of patients for radiation or chemotherapy where required. Discussions of these areas of care are included in subsequent chapters.

Compromise of host defense mechanisms in the cancer patient increases the likelihood of development of a nosocomial infection in the postoperative period. Length of hospitalization, stage of disease, and the number of invasive procedures that have been performed before surgery often affect the incidence of infection. Since the most frequent source of sepsis from nosocomial infection is the urinary tract, it is important to avoid postoperative bladder catheterization whenever possible. If indwelling catheters are necessary, sterile, closed-catheter drainage systems minimize infectious complications. Since poor respiratory ventilation accounts for a significant incidence of infectious complications, deep breathing exercises and early ambulatory activity should be encouraged (*see* Chapter 13).

When a bowel enterostomy is made for primary control of a pelvic tumor, patients must adjust to permanent changes in bowel or bladder function (see Chapter 11). Control of a colostomy varies with the level of surgical intervention and individual patient needs. Diet, irrigation, and medication can often be synchronized to achieve control. Education by a committed primary nurse or a specially trained enterostomal therapist must include detailed information and opportunities for practice sessions prior to discharge from the hospital. Sharing information with a spouse or family member is often the most important contribution that a nurse can make to the patient's physical and emotional adjustments. When family members know what to expect, they can often modify life in the home to facilitate long-term rehabilitation. Often this understanding can be best approached with visual teaching aids. Nurses should also be prepared to discuss sexual concerns as they arise with patients and should be aware of current developments in reconstructive surgery (i.e., long bone replacement, penile implant, mammoplasty, vaginoplasty) in order to guide and counsel patients in this regard (see Chapter 12).

RADIATION THERAPY

Radiation is a phenomenon that occurs naturally throughout the universe and is a normal component of the human environment. It was not recognized, however, until 1895, when Wilhelm Konrad Roentgen discovered x-rays (rays of unknown origin). X-rays can penetrate material that is opaque to normal light, produce fluorescence of certain materials, and blacken silver emulsion on a photographic plate. These properties are invaluable in radiology, where they are utilized to produce diagnostic x-rays. X-rays are emitted when electrons within an atom are excited, accelerate to high speed, and release energy. The absorption of the energy carried and released by the rays produces ionization, which in turn produces the effects of radiation. Ionization causes physical and chemical changes in living cells, altering cellular structure and function. Radiotherapy is used to exploit the lethal qualities of this energy to kill cancer cells.

The nursing care of cancer patients undergoing radiation therapy involves education about the purpose, method of administration, prevention of complications, and the management of unavoidable local or systemic toxicity. In order to fulfill these responsibilities, the nurse must have knowledge of the physical and biologic principles of radiotherapy, the relationship between radiosensitivity and tissue tolerance, the onset and character of commonly encountered side effects, and the measures that should be initiated to ameliorate toxicity.

It is imperative that the nurse understand the therapeutic intent and whether radiation therapy will be administered alone or in combination with surgery and/or systemic chemotherapy.

Two types of radiation are employed in the treatment of cancer: **electromagnetic rays** or **waves** (x-rays and gamma rays) and **particulate radiation** (electrons, protons, neutrons, alpha particles, beta particles, and pi-mesons). The common characteristic of all radiation energies is the capacity to ionize atoms within the tissues they penetrate.

The various types of ionizing radiation differ in wavelength, frequency, and velocity (electromagnetic radiation) or in the size and charge of the particle (particulate radiation). Radiation energy is measured in electron volts (eV). Low energy is measured in thousands of electron volts (keV). High energy is measured in millions of electron volts (MeV). The depth to which these particles can penetrate is a function of the energy with which they are propelled and the mass of the particle.

Ionizing radiation can be classified into three categories, each with a different power of penetration. **Alpha** particles are relatively large, positively charged particles that can be stopped by a few sheets of paper or a few centimeters of air. **Beta** particles are smaller, negatively charged electrons that have greater penetrating power but can be stopped by a few millimeters of material with the density of water or aluminum. **Gamma rays** and **x-rays** are electromagnetic quanta of energy that have diffusion characteristics similar to those of light. They can penetrate water and tissue but cannot penetrate lead, which has a high density. Gamma radiation can occur in nature from radioactive elements, such as radium, or can be artificially created. X-rays are physically and biologically similar to gamma rays except that they are artificially produced by bombarding a nonradioactive element with accelerated electrons in a vacuum.

Radioisotopes from radium or manufactured radionuclides are frequently used in **interstitial** or **intracavitary** administration of radiation. **Radioactive implants** permit the delivery of high doses of radiation to localized areas in specific tissues. The rationale for using radioactive implants is that the dose of radiation decreases rapidly as the distance from the source increases. The use of internal radiation is discussed in Chapter 18. The precautions that must be taken to protect others from radiation depend on the type of radiation used (alpha, beta, or gamma) because the duration of radioactivity, or the half-life, varies considerably. External beam equipment is designed to deliver gamma rays, x-rays, or electrons.

Different types of equipment are used to generate suitable radiation for the external treatment of various cancers. Radiation equipment that generates low-level energy, ranging from 40 to 140 keV, is employed for the treatment of superficial lesions of the skin. At this voltage, the radiation particles generated can penetrate only short distances before all their energy is released and absorbed. Tissues beyond a specific distance receive little or no radiation damage.

More powerful equipment is used to generate radiation energy ranging from 200 to 300 keV (orthovoltage radiation) when deeper penetration is required. Because greater tissue penetration is achieved, treatment of deeper areas, such as breast tissue, is possible. The maximum dose of radiation still occurs at the skin surface with this type of equipment, however. Erythema and desquamation of skin appear rapidly, even at moderate doses of radiation. The degree of skin toxicity encountered with orthovoltage radiation is dependent on the anatomic site, as well as on the total dose of radiation. In areas such as the groin and axilla, where skin is moist and in apposition to other skin surfaces, skin reactions are often severe and limit the dose that can be given. The patient or the source of the radiation must be rotated so as to deliver the total dose from different entry ports and decrease the severe skin toxicity that would result from using a single field to administer the therapeutic dose of radiation.

Until the 1950s, orthovoltage equipment was the most powerful available, and therefore skin toxicity was commonly a serious problem faced by irradiated patients. In the 1950s, more powerful megavoltage equipment became available. These units generate more penetrating radiation, which does not produce its maximum dose at the skin surface. The maximum dose is delivered to a specific depth that is determined by the radiation energy generated by the unit. Because the dose to skin is often only 30% of the maximum dose, there has been a significant decrease in skin toxicity with these units. The **cobalt-60 unit**, which emits radiation of 3 MeV, is the most common megavoltage unit in use today. Even more powerful linear accelerators that produce either electron or x-ray beams in the range of 4 to 18 MeV are now available, however. In addition to depth of penetration and excellent skin sparing, megavoltage radiation has an additional characteristic that makes it desirable in cancer therapy. The high-energy transfer reduces radiation scatter to normal tissues. This decreases both the incidence and severity of radiation sickness, which is related to the volume of body tissue that receives significant amounts of radiation. Linear accelerators also deliver 200 to 1,000 rads/minute, which minimizes patient discomfort because treatment times are short.

The impact of megavoltage radiation on survival in cancer patients with a variety of different tumors has been dramatic and is demonstrated in Table 2-1, which compares overall survival achieved with megavoltage radiation to that achievable with kilovoltage equipment.

Biologic effects of ionizing radiation

The mechanism by which ionizing radiation exerts its biologic effect is a complicated process consisting of many interactions. Basically, what happens is that a quantity of energy collides with an orbital electron in an atom of tissue, knocking it out of position and producing an ion — an electrically charged particle — which in turn ionizes, or excites, neighboring atoms in surrounding tissue. As a result of this energy transfer, charged particles and other ionizing agents are formed within the cell. These products interact with cellular DNA and damage the DNA molecule by causing breakage in one or both strands. The damage to DNA causes faulty transcription of genetic information, defective DNA repair, metabolic abnormalities, acceleration of the aging process of the cell, and mutations, and loss of the ability to divide and reproduce, as well. While cells in all phases of the cell cycle can be damaged by radiation (*see* Fig. 1-1), the lethal effect of radiation may not be apparent until after cell division occurs. In some instances,

TABLE 2-1

Improvements in Survival with the Development of Megavoltage Radiation

Cancer type	1955 (kilovoltage)	1970 (megavoltage)
	%	%
Testis, seminoma	65–70	90–95
Retinoblastoma	30–40	80–85
Hodgkin's disease	30–35	70–75
Testis, embryonal	20–25	55–70
Cervix	35–45	55–65
Prostate	5–15	55–60
Ovary	15–20	50–60
Nasopharynx	20–25	45–50
Tonsil	25–30	40–50
Bladder	0–5	25–35

Adapted from Kramer, S. Definitive radiation therapy. *Ca — A Cancer Journal for Clinicians* (September-October 1976). p. 272.

irradiated cells can successfully undergo five or six cell divisions before the lethal effects of the radiation kill the cells and their progeny. Radiation exposure is clinically measured in terms of the radiation absorbed dose, the dose of radiation absorbed by the tissue, or *rad*.

The sensitivity of cells to the biologic effects of ionizing radiation is highly dependent on the presence of oxygen. Killing hypoxic cells requires a dose of radiation 2 to 3 times higher than that required to achieve the same therapeutic effect in well-oxygenated cells. For this reason, the total dose of radiation therapy is delivered in fractions. As each fractionated dose of radiation causes tumor shrinkage, cells that were hypoxic are brought closer to the vascular supply. This increases the level of oxygenation and thus the effect of each successive radiation treatment. Radiation therapy is generally administered in fractionated doses of 150 to 300 rads/day, 5 days/wk. Fractionation of radiation over time is also designed to allow maximal repair of sublethal damage to normal cells. Therefore, the dosage of radiation administered to a patient is stated with reference to the daily fraction administered and the total time course (i.e., 4,000 rads at 200 rads/day for 5 days/wk over 4 wk).

Tumor sensitivity.   Tumors can be defined as radiosensitive or radioresistant. Tumor cells and normal cells that are undergoing cell division are more sensitive to radiation. Also, radiosensitivity of malignant tumor cells is usually commensurate with the radiosensitivity of their cell of origin. Epithelial cells, hair follicles, hematopoietic cells, and germinal cells are highly radiosensitive. For clinical purposes, a radiosensitive tumor is defined as one that can be eradicated by a dose of radiation that permits recovery of normal cells in irradiated tissues. Virtually all cancer cells can be destroyed by radiation. The dose required to kill in some types of cancer cells is so high, however, that normal cells in the radiation fields are also irreversibly damaged. Such cancers are designated radioresistant.

Certain chemicals may have the capacity to sensitize hypoxic, and therefore radioresistant, tumor cells to the cytotoxic effects of radiation exposure. These substances are referred to as radiosensitizers. Such drugs mimic the sensitizing effects of oxygen. They may also enter into hypoxic cells and release cytotoxic substances. Interestingly, some of these agents were originally developed as antibacterial agents for anaerobic organisms because of their ability to diffuse and penetrate deeply into tissues likely to contain hypoxic cells. There is evidence that some of these drugs can achieve concentrations that are equivalent to concentrations achieved in the circulation.

An attempt is being made to develop chemicals that can provide protection of normal tissues from radiation-induced damage but afford no protection to malignant tissue. These are called radioprotective agents. Development of effective radiosensitizers and radioprotectors could make many tumors now considered radioresistant amenable to control with radiotherapy.

Curative radiation therapy

Cancers that are curable with radiotherapy are generally those that are radiosensitive and tend to remain relatively localized. The pattern of metastasis should also be predictable and, in general, limited to regional nodes relatively close to the primary lesion. Cancers such as stages I and II Hodgkin's disease, localized lymphocytic and histiocytic lymphomas, cancer of the uterine cervix, seminomas of the testis, and a variety of localized head and neck cancers are highly curable with irradiation. Radiotherapy is also administered when a localized tumor is inoperable because of its anatomic location, when a tumor is operable but not completely resectable, when nodal metastases are suspected, when the goal of therapeutic surgery is to avoid an extensive, mutilating procedure (e.g., the administration of breast irradiation following excisional biopsy instead of radical mastectomy). Preoperative radiation may increase the curative potential of surgery and permit the use of less extensive surgery in rectal cancer and in head and neck tumors. When administered preoperatively, relatively low doses of radiation are employed to kill tumor cells so that the integrity of normal tissue will not be severely compromised. Prophylactic radiotherapy is also used successfully to treat the brain and spinal cord before clinical evidence of disease has developed. This is a standard part of the curative therapy in acute lymphocytic leukemia of childhood.

Palliative radiation therapy

Radiotherapy is frequently useful for local palliation of uncontrolled symptomatic metastases, especially in lymph nodes, soft tissue, and bone. Indications for palliative radiation include pain, threatened ulceration, compression of vital structures such as the brain, spinal cord, or superior vena cava, and the presence of bony metastases that are likely to fracture, especially in weight-bearing bones such as the femur or a vertebra. Generally, patients in these situations have widespread disease and require systemic treatment to achieve true tumor control. Treatment schedules should be planned, when possible, so that they do not compromise the delivery of systemic therapy.

Nursing management

External radiation therapy requires isolation of patients during the administration of therapy. Therefore, patients often experience substantial anxiety about the actual treatment procedure. Patients should be informed that treatment is painless and whenever possible the patient should be oriented to the radiotherapy equipment that will be used. Facts about treatment techniques that will be employed should be reiterated and supplemented often. Although the radiotherapist will inform the patient about procedures that are used to establish treatment portals, shield normal tissues, and maintain the body in position during therapy, the nurse should review this information in detail with the patient and family and supplement it as required.

Knowledge about normal tissue tolerance in the radiation field can enable the nurse to anticipate the onset and severity of side effects. Since side effects rarely occur in the first 2 wk, the nurse has time to prepare patients and assist them to initiate self-care. Self-care measures taught by the nurse should be simple, easily carried out, and logical in relation to anticipated toxicities. Education of patients in self-care can decrease unnecessary morbidity and also provide concrete evidence to patients that they have an important and active role to play in their treatment. Thoughtful pretreatment planning should take into account problems related to child care, employment, finances, and transportation that need to be worked out in advance. Radiation-induced toxicity is either **localized**, affecting only the tissues within the radiation field, or **generalized**, which is commonly known as radiation sickness. Detailed discussions of the nursing management of clinical problems encountered by persons receiving radiotherapy follows in Chapters 7 through 13. These include skin toxicity, xerostomia and stomatitis, bone marrow depression, anorexia and nausea/vomiting, diarrhea, and urinary dysfunction.

The late complications of radiation therapy, which are summarized in Table 2-2, may appear several years after the completion of treatment. Most late complications reflect diminished vascular supply and increased fibrosis in heavily irradiated areas. Unlike acute radiation reactions, these complications are often chronic and not always amenable to treatment. Fortunately, severe complications, such as radionecrosis, are not common. The most common late effects include stenosis, diffuse fibrosis, fistulas, and ulceration. Nursing care is symptomatic and based on the degree of functional impairment. Since the reproductive organs are highly sensitive to the effects of radiation, and temporary or permanent sterility is produced, the effects of radiotherapy on reproductive capacity must be explained to patients of childbearing age who are likely to be cured of their disease. Exposure of mature sperm to ionizing radiation can produce germ-line mutations. Therefore it is generally recommended that men refrain from fathering children for two years after treatment.

TABLE 2–2

Late Effects of Radiation Therapy on Normal Tissue

Organ system	Reaction
Skin	Fibrosis, atrophy, telangiectasia, and tanning over irradiated areas. Acute "recall phenomenon" may occur after the administration of certain antineoplastic drugs such as dactinomycin.
GI epithelium: oral cavity	Fibrosis; telangiectasia. Decreased taste acuity or the loss of taste sensation. Dental caries.
esophagus	Fibrosis.
stomach	Infarction; fibrosis; necrosis.
intestines	Infarction; fibrosis; necrosis; chronic enteritis.
Salivary gland	Decreased taste acuity. Xerostomia. Dental caries.
GU epithelium: kidneys	Vascular occlusion; renal failure.
bladder	Fibrosis. Bladder contracture. Urinary frequency.
Blood and bone marrow	Anemia, leukemia.
Hair follicle	Premature baldness.
Lungs	Pulmonary fibrosis.
Heart	Fibrosis. Myocarditis or pericarditis is rare.
Brain and spinal cord	Paralysis. Vascular obliteration leading to infarction and occlusion.
Eyes	Cataracts.
Thyroid	Clinical hypothyroidism. Thyroid cancer.
Bone and cartilage: child	Arrest of growth, shortening of bone.
adult	No response.
Germ cells	Temporary or permanent sterility. Premature menopause in women. (Fertility may return to normal depending on the dose of irradiation administered to the gametes and age.)

CHEMOTHERAPY

By the early 1950s, scientists discovered that drugs could selectively kill the microorganisms that caused malaria and tuberculosis. This discovery led to the successful development of broad-spectrum antibiotics and the modern management of infectious disease and also stimulated research to develop drugs that would selectively kill cancer cells in like manner. The discovery of the anticancer effects of two chemicals, nitrogen mustard and methotrexate, provided the impetus needed to stimulate the development of cancer drugs on a systematic basis.

The anticancer effects of nitrogen mustard were discovered during World War II after an explosion of mustard gases in Naples, Italy. Physicians observed that, as an aftermath of this explosion, many of the soldiers exposed to these gases died with atrophy of the lymph glands and bone marrow hypoplasia. Because of these observations, a similar chemical, nitrogen mustard, was administered to patients with widely disseminated lymphomas, and transient but impressive antitumor responses were observed. In 1947, research on folic acid, a form of vitamin B, led to the discovery of the antitumor activity of methotrexate in acute leukemia. The breakthrough followed the observation that in patients with acute leukemia, folic acid accelerated the production of abnormal WBCs by the bone marrow. Administration of folic acid antagonists, which inhibited the metabolic effects of folic acid, proved to be cytotoxic to leukemic cells, and methotrexate was identified as the most useful compound. In the mid-1950s, methotrexate was also tested in women with widely disseminated choriocarcinoma, a rare but inevitably fatal cancer of the placenta. Much to the surprise of skeptics, the administration of methotrexate as a single agent produced complete cures in a significant fraction of women with pulmonary metastases. Chemotherapy is now the primary treatment modality used to cure twelve disseminated cancers:
1. Acute lymphocytic leukemia in children.
2. Acute myelogenous leukemia.
3. Burkitt's lymphoma.
4. Choriocarcinoma.
5. Diffuse histiocytic lymphoma.
6. Embryonal rhabdomyosarcoma.
7. Ewing's sarcoma.
8. Hodgkin's disease.
9. Nodular mixed lymphoma.
10. Ovarian carcinoma.
11. Testicular carcinoma.
12. Wilms' tumor.

In the past 25 yr over 50 drugs with significant antitumor activity have been identified, and at least 30 are now commercially available. Six major categories have been identified: alkylating agents including the nitrosoureas, antimetabolites, antibiotics, plant alkaloids, immunologic stimulants, and steroid hormones. There are also miscellaneous agents that are not easily classified. Tables 2-3, 2-4, 2-5, 2-6, 2-7, and 2-8 list chemotherapeutic agents by class, Table 2-9 lists agents that modulate the immune system, and Table 2-10 lists classes of hormonally active agents. The tables present data on dosage, schedule, and major toxicities.

Alkylating agents. Alkylating agents (*see* Table 2-3) are drugs that kill cells by interfering with the structure of DNA. The alkyl groups attach to DNA, causing misreading of the DNA code, breaks in the DNA molecule, and cross-linking of the DNA strands. Because synthesis of other cellular components continues, growth becomes unbalanced and cell death results. Alkylating agents are effective in killing cells in all phases of the cell cycle. Therefore, their antitumor activity is *not* cell-cycle-specific. They do, however, produce a greater antitumor effect in rapidly dividing cells.

Nitrosoureas. A number of structurally related nitrosourea compounds that act on a variety of neoplasms have been developed (*see* Table 2-4). Their antitumor activity is thought to be similar to that of alkylating agents. Some are useful both PO and parenterally. Others are available in only one formulation. They are effective in brain tumors because of their lipid solubility, which permits them to cross the blood-brain barrier after systemic administration. The most impressive toxicity of this class is delayed and cumulative myelosuppression, which develops 3 to 4 wk after administration. As a result, the interval between each treatment is usually 6 wk.

Antimetabolites. An antimetabolite (*see* Table 2-5) is a chemical analogue of an essential metabolite, so closely resembling it that the drug enters the essential metabolic pathways. An antimetabolite is a fraudulent substrate for essential biochemical reactions and interferes with or blocks normal biosynthesis of nucleic acids necessary for synthesis of DNA and RNA. Because the antitumor activity of antimetabolites is exerted, or expressed, when cells are in the synthetic phase of the cell cycle (S phase), they are considered cell-cycle-specific (*see* Fig. 1-1). Antimetabolites can be subdivided into purine, pyrimidine, and folic acid antagonists.

Antitumor antibiotics. Anticancer antibiotics (*see* Table 2-6) are a heterogeneous group of compounds produced by various bacterial and fungal organisms. Most antibiotics are *not* cell-cycle-specific. In general, antibiotics interfere with DNA synthesis by binding with DNA at various points and preventing RNA synthesis.

Plant alkaloids.   Certain antitumor agents (*see* Table 2–7) are prepared from plants. The two most established compounds are vincristine and vinblastine; they are both derived from the periwinkle plant. These agents cause metaphase arrest by inhibiting spindle formation during cell mitosis, as well as causing inhibition of DNA and protein synthesis. Although the two have very similar structures, mechanisms of action, and metabolism, the dosage, toxicity, and antitumor spectrum of each are different. Vincristine produces little bone marrow toxicity, whereas myelosuppression is the major side effect of vinblastine. Neurotoxicity, which is probably related to the agent's binding to spindle proteins, is the major toxicity with vincristine administration, whereas it is minimal with the use of vinblastine. Because their antitumor activity is exerted during mitosis, they are also considered cell-cycle-specific (*see* Fig. 1–1).

Miscellaneous agents.   L-asparaginase (*see* Table 2–8) is the only enzyme to be used successfully in cancer chemotherapy. It is prepared from various sources, including guinea pig serum, yeast, and *Escherichia coli* bacteria. The enzyme converts L-asparagine, an essential amino acid involved in protein synthesis, to L-aspartic acid. Many leukemia and some lymphoma cells require exogenous L-asparagine stored in body tissues, while normal tissues can independently synthesize this amino acid. Resistance to this drug may be related to an increased production of cellular L-asparagine synthetase, which converts L-aspartic acid to L-asparagine. L-asparaginase is effective in inducing remission of acute lymphoblastic leukemia. Its major life-threatening toxicity is anaphylaxis. Myelosuppression is rare, but hemolytic anemia, liver dysfunction, severe nausea, and coagulation abnormalities are not uncommon. Acute pancreatitis and hypoglycemia (related to depressed serum-insulin levels) also occur and are dose-related.

There are a variety of other drugs that cannot be classified in any of the groups listed above and whose mechanism of action is unknown. The toxicity of many is well documented, however, and should be understood by nurses administering them in cancer treatment.

Immune stimulants and immunotherapy.   Immunocompetence of the host may be an important surveillance mechanism that prevents the development of neoplasms. Theoretically, the body should recognize as foreign the tumor-specific or tumor-associated antigens produced on the surface of the cancer cell. Once the host has recognized this foreign antigen, the immune system attempts to destroy the abnormal cells. Experimental evidence suggests that a normal immune response may continually be killing abnormal cells as they are formed before they can develop into clinical cancer. It is unclear whether a failure in immune surveillance is always involved in tumor

TABLE 2–3
Alkylating Agents

Drug	Dose, route, and schedule	Acute side effects	Myelosuppression (1 [mild] to to 4 [severe])
Mechlorethamine hydrochloride, HN$_2$, nitrogen mustard (Mustargen)	0.4 mg/kg IV q 3–4 wk 6 mg/m^2 day 1 and day 8 q 4 wk	Severe N/V in ½–2 hr, lasting 2–12 hr. Metallic taste. Fever, diarrhea, chills in 1 hr. Anorexia lasting several days.	4
	0.2–0.4 mg/kg intracavitary	Fever, chills, malaise, mild N/V.	0–1
	10 mg/m^2 in 50 ml aqueous solution 3 times/wk, then q wk topically		0–1
	10 mg/m^2 ointment in Aquaphor base q day		1
Cyclophosphamide CYT (Cytoxan, Endoxan)	500–1,500 mg/m^2 IV q 3–4 wk 60–120 mg/m^2 PO q day continuous Dose titration based on WBC	Dose-related N/V in 3–12 hr, can last 8–10 hr. Anorexia common. Dizziness, sinus congestion can occur with rapid infusion of high doses.	3
Ifosfamide (IFEX, Holoxan) [NSC 109724]‡	1,200 mg/m^2 IV 5 days q 3 wk 4 g/m^2 IV q 3 wk	Dose related N/V in 2–10 hr; often persists several days.	3
L-phenylalanine mustard, L-PAM, melphalan (Alkeran)	0.2 mg/kg PO q day × 5 days q 4–6 wk 0.05–0.1 mg/kg PO continuous Dose titration based on WBC	Chronic nausea/ anorexia can occur.	3
Chlorambucil (Leukeran)	0.05–0.2 mg/kg PO q day continuous Dose titration based on WBC	Well-tolerated at standard doses.	3
Busulfan (Myleran)	0.05–0.2 mg/kg PO q day continuous Dose titration based on WBC	Well-tolerated.	3

Hematologic nadir	Comments
Biphasic, occurring at 7–10 days and 24–30 days	BMD. Potent tissue vesicant. Give only in established IV line. Sodium thiosulfate may decrease tissue damage if extravasated. Chemical thrombophlebitis and venous discoloration common. Add 100 mg IV hydrocortisone sodium succinate (Solu-Cortef) to infusion to decrease thrombophlebitis. Allergic and anaphylactic reactions rare. Maculopapular rash, alopecia, and tinnitus also occur. Avoid direct eye contact.
	Pain common, secondary to intense inflammatory reaction. Turn patient immediately to maximize drug distribution.
	Gloves should be worn during application. Aqueous solution is applied topically and intralesionally in mycosis fungoides. Hypersensitivity reactions frequently occur with topical use. Desensitization is generally effective. Hyperpigmentation, urticaria, and pruritus occur.
	Ointment greatly simplifies application and appears to increase absorption into the skin. Associated with a lower incidence of hypersensitivity reactions. Decreases dry-skin problems created by aqueous preparation.
7–14 days	BMD. Vigorous hydration with oral or IV fluids (>3 liter/day) to maintain adequate urine output to decrease risk of hemorrhagic cystitis. Discontinue if dysuria or hematuria develop. Barbiturates and phenytoin may increase toxic effects by affecting activation by hepatic microsomal enzymes. Inappropriate antidiuretic hormone secretion can occur at doses >50 mg/kg. Alopecia with regrowth during treatment in 50%. Daily oral cyclophosphamide may be taken in divided doses with meals. Do not administer IV preparation unless all crystals are dissolved. New lyophilized powder now available. May be given as slow bolus. Interstitial pneumonitis after prolonged continuous administration. Potentiation of anthracycline cardiotoxicity reported.
7–14 days	Mild BMD. Hemorrhagic cystitis. Fluid intake must be at least 2 liters/day to maintain urine output. Administration of N-acetyl-cysteine protects bladder from toxicity. Ascorbic acid also may reduce bladder toxicity. Alopecia. Nephrotoxicity, lethargy, and confusion at high doses. Transient hepatotoxicity. Chemical thrombophlebitis. Hepatic microsomal enzyme activation affected by phenytoin and barbiturates.
Biphasic, occurring at 7–10 days and 24–30 days	Well tolerated. Little alopecia. Take on empty stomach. Occasional dermatitis and stomatitis. IV preparation investigational; serious hypersensitivity reactions have been reported with IV use. Pulmonary fibrosis seen after prolonged administration. Delayed and cumulative BMD may occur.
7–14 days	BMD. Occasional dermatitis. Hepatotoxicity rare. Oral absorption reliable. Barbiturates may increase toxicity secondary to induction of hepatic drug activation. Pulmonary fibrosis can occur after prolonged use. GI distress only at high dosages. Total cumulative dose: 2 g.
10–30 days	Cumulative and prolonged BMD. Reliable absorption. Prolonged use associated with pulmonary fibrosis. Gynecomastia. Adrenal insufficiency. Hyperpigmentation. Pregnancy has occurred during therapy. Effective contraception is required. Total cumulative dose: 600 mg.

Drug	Dose, route, and schedule	Acute side effects	Myelosuppression (1 [mild] to to 4 [severe])
Triethylene-thiophosphoramide, TSPA (Thiotepa)	0.2 mg/kg IV or IM q day × 5 q 3–4 wk	Well-tolerated.	3
	0.5 mg/kg IV or IM q 1–4 wk		
	1–10 mg/m^2 IT		0
	10–60 mg q 3–4 wk for intracavitary use and intravesicular bladder instillation	Local irritation. Dysuria; urgency.	1
Cisplatin, CDDP (Platinol)	60–120 mg/m^2 IV q 3–4 wk	Severe N/V in 1 hr, lasting 6–24 hr. Anaphylactic reactions; convulsions.	1
	15–20 mg/m^2 IV q day × 5 days 3–4 wk		
	90 mg/m^2 IP in 2 liters dialysate q 3 wk (investigational)	N/V; abdominal discomfort. Sterile ascites.	
CBDCA cyclobutane dicarboxylate platinum, JM8 [NSC 241240]‡	200–400 mg/m^2 IV q 4 wk	Mild N/V.	2
Aziridinyl-benzoquinone, AZQ [NSC 182986]‡	6–8 mg/m^2 × 5 days q 4 wk	Mild N/V.	2

BMD, bone marrow depression; IP, intraperitoneal(ly); IT, intrathecal(ly); KCl, potassium chloride; NS, normal saline; N/V, nausea or vomiting.
‡ Indicates National Service Center number, an early designation.

initiation. It is known, however, that persons with immunodeficiency diseases and those whose immune system is suppressed for prolonged periods (as after renal transplants) have an increased incidence of cancer. There does exist evidence that a competent immune system is involved in controlling the growth of cancer.

Immunotherapeutic agents (*see* Table 2–9) are optimally effective when maximal tumor cell removal or destruction is achieved with

Hematologic nadir	Comments
10–28 days	BMD. Can be given IM or SC or instilled into bladder. Poor oral absorption. Allergic reactions and dermatitis. Dose reductions are required for patients with existing hepatic, renal, or bone marrow dysfunction. Myelosuppressive effects potentiated by prior radiation and other alkylating agents. Paresthesias reported after IT administration.
	Pain, N/V, dizziness, headache can occur with intracavitary instillation. Leukopenia can occur after bladder instillation.
7–14 days	Renal toxicity. Administration of CDDP with 250 ml hypertonic (3%) saline and extensive hydration with NS and KCl can protect against renal damage. IV hydration and diuresis with furosemide and/or mannitol is also used to reduce renal toxicity. Anaphylactic reactions with tachycardia, hypotension, erythema, wheezing, and facial edema. Treat with antihistamines and hydrocortisone sodium succinate (Solu-Cortef); then pretreat with same for future doses. Check creatinine clearance, BUN, electrolytes. Peripheral neuropathy, ophthalmic toxicity. Magnesium wasting requiring magnesium sulfate replacement (IM/PO) to manage neuromuscular irritability. Neurologic toxicity is dose-limiting in high doses (40 mg/m^2 × 5 days).
	Nephrotoxicity dose-limiting at 90 mg/m^2. Administration of mannitol and sodium thiosulfate (7.5 g/m^2 loading dose and 2.13 g/m^2 q 12 hr) permits IP administration of CDDP at 270 mg/m^2 without nephrotoxicity and toxicity; N/V is dose-limiting. Dwell time 4 hr. Strict catheter asepsis is essential. Fullness and abdominal discomfort commonly seen secondary to increased intra-abdominal pressure.
7–14 days	Myelosuppression without renal toxicity. Mild neurologic toxicity in patients previously treated with cisplatin. No ototoxicity.
14–21 days	Cumulative BMD, especially thrombocytopenia. Penetrates CSF. Do not administer unless solution is clear. Dissolution of particles in IV preparation is extremely slow. Stomatitis, diarrhea, anorexia.

surgery, radiation, or chemotherapy. The basic rationale for immunotherapy is that certain biologically active substances can stimulate the host immune system to destroy the last residual cancer cells, thereby producing a permanent cure. Since radiation and chemotherapy produce immunosuppression, patients must be evaluated for immunocompetence before the institution of immunotherapy.

Immunotherapy can be classified as passive or active, specific, or nonspecific. An example of passive immunotherapy is the transfer of sera containing antibodies to the client with cancer. Active

TABLE 2-4
Nitrosoureas

Drug	Dose, route, and schedule	Acute side effects	Myelosuppression (1 [mild] to 4 [severe])
Carmustine, BCNU (BiCNU)	150–200 mg/m² IV q 4–6 wk Total cumulative dose: 1,200–1,500 mg/m²	Severe N/V in 2–4 hr. Local pain, flushing.	4
Lomustine, CCNU (CeeNU)	100–130 mg/m² PO q 4–6 wk	Moderate-severe N/V in 2–6 hr. Diarrhea, anorexia.	4
Semustine, Methyl CCNU, MCCNU [NSC 95441]‡	150–200 mg/m² PO q 4–6 wk	Moderate-severe N/V in 1–4 hr. Anorexia.	4
Chlorozotocin, DCNU (CZT) [NSC 178248]‡	150 mg/m² IV q 6 wk 40 mg/m² q day × 5 days IV q 6 wk	Mild N/V.	1
Streptozotocin, streptozocin (Zanosar)	500 mg/m² IV q day × 5 days q 3–4 wk or 1,500 mg/m² IV q wk	Moderate-severe N/V in 1–4 hr. Anorexia. Reactive hypoglycemia secondary to insulin release. Burning and local pain.	1

BMD, bone marrow depression; N/V, nausea or vomiting.
‡ Indicates National Service Center number, an early designation.

immunotherapy involves the stimulation of the host's immune system and can be nonspecific or specific in nature. Active, nonspecific immunotherapy involves the use of substances that augment cellular and hormonal immunity. Active, specific immunotherapy involves immunization with tumor cells or tumor extracts. Vaccines are prepared from the patient's own tumor cells or from a similar tumor, in an attempt to produce cytotoxic antitumor antibodies that can destroy the tumor.

At present, cancer centers throughout the country are conducting clinical trials with an antiviral protein called interferon. This natural substance is produced by body cells; the interferons derived from lymphocytes and fibroblasts are the ones being the most closely studied. Antitumor effects have been noted with the use of this substance in patients with a variety of malignancies.

Hematologic nadir	Comments
4–6 wk	Marked facial flushing and venous spasm secondary to alcohol diluent. Increase volume and decrease rate of infusion to decrease pain. Chemical thrombophlebitis often occurs in several days. Delayed and cumulative BMD. Tissue vesicant. Pulmonary fibrosis and renal damage seen with prolonged use. Hepatotoxicity in 20% of cases. Must be refrigerated and protected from light. Avoid direct contact with skin and eyes. Enters CSF. Venous discoloration.
4–6 wk	Delayed and cumulative BMD. N/V may be reduced if taken at bedtime with antiemetics. GI absorption in 30–60 min. Alopecia. Stomatitis. Renal toxicity with prolonged use. Hepatotoxicity unusual. Enters CSF. Anorexia often lasts several days. Pulmonary toxicity with prolonged use.
4–6 wk	Delayed and cumulative BMD. Take on empty stomach at bedtime. GI absorption in 30–60 min. Stomatitis. Renal failure can occur after prolonged administration. Persistent anorexia. Pulmonary fibrosis can also occur after prolonged use.
4–6 wk	Mild BMD with prominent thrombocytopenia. Diabetes with ketoacidosis. Transient hepatotoxicity. Interstitial pulmonary fibrosis. Chemical thrombophlebitis. Renal toxicity can occur as with other nitrosoureas.
7–14 days	Mild BMD. Administer with 1–2 liters hydration to prevent nephrotoxicity. Check for glycosuria, proteinuria, and hypophosphatemia prior to each dose. Teach patients about symptoms of hypoglycemia and management of insulin shock. Slow infusion to decrease local venous burning. Diarrhea and abdominal cramps can occur. Tissue vesicant. Transient, mild hepatotoxicity. Mild anemia. Protect from light. Myelosuppression has occurred with prolonged use.

Steroid hormones.   **Adrenal corticosteroids** (*see* Table 2–10) can be administered in large nonphysiologic doses to alter the hormonal balance and to modify the growth of neoplasms. Prednisone is the most commonly used steroid hormone. The mechanism of action of corticosteroids is not clearly understood. It is thought that they may interfere at the cell membrane and inhibit RNA synthesis of protein. They are known to inhibit mitosis and to have the capacity to destroy lymphocytic elements. Corticosteroids are active in a variety of neoplasms and are commonly used in combination chemotherapy because of their lack of bone marrow toxicity. They are potent immunosuppressive agents, however. Because steroids also are anti-inflammatory drugs, they are useful in the management of cerebral edema; however, their anti-inflammatory properties have the disadvantage of disguising the cardinal signs and symptoms of infection.

Research into the mechanism of hormonal action has revealed that steroid-binding receptor glycoproteins exist in hormonally dependent

TABLE 2–5
Antimetabolites

Drug	Dose, route, and schedule	Acute side effects	Myelosuppression (1 [mild] to to 4 [severe])
Arabinosylcytosine, cytarabine, ARA-C (Cytosar)	100 mg/m^2 q 12 hr IV or SC × 7–21 days	Dose and schedule dependent N/V.	4
	100 mg/m^2 continuous IV infusion × 10 days		4
	20–30 mg/m^2 IT		0
5-Fluorouracil, 5-FU (Adrucil, Efudex [topical])	7.5–12 mg/kg IV × 5 days, then 12–15 mg/kg q wk	Dose and schedule dependent N/V.	3
	IP administration at concentrations up to 4 mM in 2 liters dialysate × 8 exchanges q 2 wk (investigational)	Abdominal discomfort.	+/−
Methotrexate, MTX, amethopterin (Folex, Mexate)	20–80 mg/m^2 IV, IM, PO	Mild-moderate nausea.	3
	10–15 mg/m^2 IT q wk	Chemical arachnoiditis, vomiting, fever, headache.	
	high-dose MTX 1–10 g/m^2 plus leucovorin rescue (*see below*)	Mild-moderate N/V.	+/− (unusual)
Folinic acid, citrovorum factor, CF, calcium leucovorin, leucovorin	15–25 mg q 3–6 hr IV or PO × 8–12 doses Begin 2–6 hr after end of MTX infusion		0
Hydroxyurea (Hydrea)	25 mg/kg PO q day continuous	Minimal N/V. Anorexia.	3
	100 mg/kg IV q day × 3 days		

Hematologic nadir	Comments
7–14 days	Marked BMD. Less N/V with slow infusions. Anorexia and mild oral ulcerations common. Flulike syndrome with fever and headache. Stomatitis. Diarrhea. Arthralgias. Use with caution if hepatic dysfunction exists. Rash; sensitivity to sunlight; use of sunscreens recommended. Continuous infusions of 3 g/m^2 q 12 hr $\times$ 5 days used to induce bone marrow aplasia. Systemic toxicity from IT use uncommon; neurotoxicity with IT use common. Should be reconstituted in Elliott's B solution for IT use.
7–14 days	Dose-related BMD. Promote oral hygiene. Stomatitis is often preceded by sore mouth and tongue. Pharyngitis, diarrhea, and proctitis may be severe. Interrupt therapy when GI toxicity appears. GI toxicity often immediately precedes serious myelotoxicity. Diffuse hair thinning, nail cracking and loss occur. Increased toxicity post adrenalectomy. Decreased myelotoxicity with intra-arterial use. Conjunctival irritation. Cerebellar ataxia, visual disturbances. Oral absorption erratic. Topical 5-FU (Efudex) in malignant keratoses. Sensitivity to sunlight. Use of sunscreen is recommended. Hyperpigmentation. Dermatitis. Dwell time 4 hr/exchange. Fullness, mild abdominal discomfort common secondary to increased intra-abdominal pressure. Strict catheter asepsis is critical. Chemical peritonitis at high concentrations (5 mM). Addition of 50 mEq $NaHCO_3$ increases drug solubility. High portal vein concentrations suggest that IP route may be used to deliver 5-FU levels to the liver.
7–14 days	BMD. Renal impairment delays excretion and increases systemic toxicity. Renal function must be checked prior to each dose. GI ulceration can develop along all of GI tract, requiring discontinuation of therapy. Pulmonary toxicity and serious hepatotoxicity can occur with prolonged administration. Dilute preservative-free MTX powder in Elliott's B solution for IT use. Omit systemic MTX dose when giving IT dose. MTX levels in CSF should be monitored carefully. MTX is protein-bound. Avoid sulfonamides, aspirin, tetracycline, phenytoin, and chloral hydrate, which displace MTX from plasma proteins. Acute, reversible MTX pneumonitis occurs with prolonged administration. Stop MTX and treat with steroids. Maintain urinary pH > 6.5–7.0 and high urinary output to prevent precipitation of MTX in renal tubules. Adjust urinary pH with IV $NaHCO_3$ to maintain urine alkalinity. Check pH q 3–6 hr during therapy. Check BUN, creatinine, LFTs prior to each dose. Use only preservative-free MTX. Continue CF until plasma MTX $< 10^{-8}$ molar (0.45 $\mu g/100$ ml). Allergic sensitization occurs but is unusual. Otherwise free of side effects.
1–7 days	BMD. GI toxicity only at high doses > 70 mg/kg. Pretreat patients with allopurinol because rapid fall in leukemic cells occurs. Renal toxicity. Rash. Neurologic toxicity.

Drug	Dose, route, and schedule	Acute side effects	Myelosuppression (1 [mild] to to 4 [severe])
6-Mercaptopurine, 6-MP (Purinethol)	1–2.5 mg/kg PO q day (IV preparation investigational) Dose titration based on WBC	Nausea, anorexia, fever.	2
6-Thioguanine, thioguanine (Tabloid)	1–3 mg/kg PO q day with dose titration as required 100 mg/m^2 IV × 5 days	Well-tolerated.	2
5-Azacytidine [NSC 102816]‡	150–300 mg/m^2 IV q 3–5 days	Dose and schedule-dependent N/V and profound diarrhea, fever, and hypotension with rapid infusions.	4

BMD, bone marrow depression; CF, citrovorum factor; IP, intraperitoneal(ly); IT, intrathecal(ly); LFT, liver function test; NaHCO$_3$, sodium bicarbonate; N/V, nausea or vomiting.
‡ Indicates National Service Center number, an early designation.

or responsive tissues. Binding of hormones to these receptor sites can alter the synthesis of RNA and protein in target tissues. Receptors for estrogens, androgens, progesterones, and corticosteroids have been identified in the cytoplasm of cells and probably explain their antitumor activity. Unresponsiveness to hormonal therapy is now thought to be related primarily to the absence of these steroid-binding receptor proteins in tumor tissue.

Tissues that are normally dependent on or responsive to endogenous physiologic hormones are often responsive to **endocrine manipulation** when the tissues develop neoplasms. Frequently this hormonal dependence can be exploited as therapy. Carcinomas of the breast, endometrium, and prostate, and thyroid neoplasms are often responsive to endocrine manipulation.

Surgical management of breast cancer has historically used endocrine ablation to achieve regression of the disease. Castration (oophorectomy and orchiectomy) has been used successfully to produce tumor regression in breast cancer and in prostate cancer. Failure to respond to castration is thought to be related to the absence of steroid-binding receptor proteins.

Exogenous estrogen and androgen therapy produce tumor regression in hormone-responsive metastatic cancers. Progestins, which are compounds related to progesterone, can also be useful in the treatment

Hematologic nadir	Comments
5 days–6 wk	BMD. 6-MP dose reduction to 25–33% if allopurinol is given concurrently. Allopurinol inhibits 6-MP degradation by xanthine oxidase. Hepatic or renal dysfunction requires dose reduction. Monitor for hepatotoxicity and stomatitis at high doses. Cholestatic jaundice. When combined with doxorubicin, risk of hepatotoxicity may be increased. Pulmonary toxicity with prolonged use.
7–28 days	BMD. Reduce dose if stomatitis/diarrhea develop. Full dose can be given with allopurinol. Monitor for hepatotoxicity. Administer oral dose on an empty stomach to facilitate complete absorption. Myelosuppression is more severe after IV administration.
7–14 days	BMD. Continuous 24-hr infusions, given as 4 6-hr infusions. Must be used in 6 hr, unstable after reconstitution. Ringer's lactate solution provides optimal pH and stability. Can be given SC but is painful and causes brown skin discoloration. Stomatitis. Hypophosphatemia. Pruritic rash. Neurologic toxicity (weakness, lethargy) reported but rare. Hepatotoxicity rare but serious complication.

of metastatic carcinomas. With the use of progestinal agents, remissions in endometrial cancer may last several years, especially in those women who have experienced a long disease-free interval between primary resection and recurrent disease or who have well-differentiated tumors (*see* Table 2–10).

The growth of some papillary thyroid adenocarcinomas may be controlled by thyroid hormones, which act by inhibiting the secretion of thyroid-stimulating hormone (TSH) by the pituitary. Control with thyroxine is limited to tumors responding to the normal TSH feedback mechanism.

Combination chemotherapy

Treatment of advanced cancer, where the tumor burden is large, is frequently most successful with combination chemotherapy. Potentially curative dosages of a single agent may be so high that life-threatening or fatal toxicity precludes its use. Furthermore, repeated administration of tolerable dosages over prolonged time periods can result in the development of resistant tumor-cell lines. Various mechanisms for resistance to chemotherapeutic agents have been proposed, including rapid repair of drug-induced DNA damage (alkylating agents), development of alternate metabolic pathways (antimetabolites), inadequate uptake of the drug by tumor cells (methotrexate), inadequate drug activation (antimetabolites), and increased inactivation of drugs (arabinosylcytosine).

TABLE 2–6
Antitumor Antibiotics

Drug	Dose, route, and schedule	Acute side effects	Myelosuppression (1 [mild] to to 4 [severe])
Dactinomycin, actinomycin-D (Cosmegen)	0.015 mg/kg IV × 5 days q 3–4 wk	Moderate-severe N/V in 2–5 hr, lasting 12–24 hr.	4
Bleomycin sulfate (Blenoxane)	5–15 U/m^2 IV, IM, or SC (or intralesional) q wk	Mild N/V. Anorexia. Chills and fever to 103–105°F. Anaphylactic and hypotensive reactions (may be delayed).	0
Doxorubicin hydrochloride (Adriamycin, ADM)	30–75 mg/m^2 IV q 3–4 wk	Dose-related N/V. Local pain in small veins. Allergic and hyper-sensitivity reactions.	4
	30–60 mg/m^2 intravesicular bladder instillation	Dysuria, urgency.	
	IP 40 mg in 2 liters dialysate without heparin (investigational)	Abdominal discomfort. N/V.	
Daunomycin hydrochloride, daunorubicin, DNR (Cerubidine)	30–60 mg/m^2 IV × 3 days q 3–4 wk	Moderate-severe N/V. Local pain in small veins. Allergic reactions.	4
Mithramycin	0.025–0.05 mg/kg IV q other day to toxicity	Moderate-severe N/V 6 hr lasting 12–14 hr. Fever.	3
	0.025 mg/kg IV for tumor-related hypercalcemia		0
Mitomycin-C (Mutamycin)	2 mg/m^2 IV q day × 5 days 15–20 mg/m^2 IV q 6–8 wk	Mild-moderate N/V in 1–2 hr lasting 2–3 days. Fever.	4
	20–60 mg (1 mg/ml) intravesicular bladder instillation	Bladder irritation. Dysuria, urgency.	

Hematologic nadir	Comments
7–14 days	Marked BMD. Use preservative-free diluent to prevent drug precipitation. Dosage calculated in *micrograms*. Tissue vesicant. Administer as slow bolus in established IV line. Oral ulcerations. N/V tends to decrease with daily use. Prolonged anorexia common. Severe radiation recall reactions with necrosis can occur. Acneiform rash, alopecia, hyperpigmentation. Stomatitis, glossitis, diarrhea, proctitis.
	Little BMD. Powder is diluted in NS or sterile water. Anaphylactic reactions noted in lymphoma. Test doses of 1–2 U are recommended; then observe 2–4 hr. Total cumulative dose should not exceed 400 U because of risk of pulmonary fibrosis. Acetaminophen and antihistamines can decrease febrile reactions. Reduce dose if creatinine is >1.5 mg/dl. Stomatitis, alopecia, hyperpigmentation, erythema of skin. Cutaneous toxicity may be severe and require cessation of therapy. Fatigue and anorexia may be prolonged and severe. Fever can produce severe dehydration; encourage vigorous hydration.
10–14 days	BMD. Tissue vesicant. Hypersensitivity reactions can occur. Dose reduction of 50–75% with hepatic dysfunction (bilirubin >1.5). Cardiotoxicity — limit total dose to 550 mg/m^2. Red urine. Local venous spasm with pain, erythema, urticaria, and pruritus along vein. Recall reactions in irradiated sites. Complete alopecia. Stomatitis; proctitis. Bladder instillations associated with urgency, local irritation, and chemical cystitis. Incompatible with heparin and 5-FU; do *not* mix together. IP administration associated with mild myelosuppression. Sterile ascites and pain.
10–14 days	BMD. Tissue vesicant. Cardiotoxicity; limit total dose to 550 mg/m^2. Dose reduction with hepatic dysfunction. Red urine. Stomatitis and diarrhea unusual. Alopecia common. Incompatible with heparin; do *not* mix together.
10–14 days	BMD, especially thrombocytopenia. Hemorrhagic diathesis. Coagulation abnormalities and hemorrhage often preceded by flushing and epistaxis. CNS toxicity with neuromuscular excitability, severe headache. Dermatitis, proteinuria, azotemia, and electrolyte abnormalities (decreased levels of PO$_4$, K, Mg, Ca). Tissue vesicant. Unstable in acidic solution. Dilute with sterile water. Discontinue drug if abnormal LFT/RFT results develop. Renal toxicity may be cumulative. Value in the medical management of patients with hypercalcemia.
21–28 days	Delayed and cumulative BMD. Tissue vesicant; chemical phlebitis. Hepatic activation and metabolism. Stomatitis, diarrhea. Delayed renal toxicity reported. Malaise, anorexia, weight loss common, even in responders. Pulmonary and cardiac activity reported.
	Palmar rash that often resolves with oral antihistamines and/or topical steroids. Dysuria, urgency.

BMD, bone marrow depression; Ca, calcium; IP, intraperitoneal(ly); K, potassium; LFT, liver function test; Mg, magnesium; NS, normal saline; N/V, nausea or vomiting; PO$_4$, phosphate; RFT, renal function test.

TABLE 2–7
Plant Alkaloids

Drug	Dose, route, and schedule	Acute side effects	Myelosuppression (1 [mild] to 4 [severe])
Vincristine sulfate, VCR (Oncovin)	0.5–2 mg/m^2 IV q wk	N/V unusual.	0–1
Vinblastine sulfate, VLB (Velban)	6 mg/m^2 IV q wk 0.1–0.4 mg/kg IV q wk 1.5–2 mg/m^2/day × 5 q 4 wk	N/V unusual.	4
Etoposide, VP16–213, epipodophyllo-toxin (Vepesid) [NSC 14150]‡	200–250 mg/m^2 IV q wk 50–60 mg/m^2 IV q wk 50–60 mg/m^2 IV q day × 5 q 4 wk 125–140 mg/m^2 IV 3 times/wk q 4 wk	Mild N/V. Headache. Hypotension. Fever, chills. Anaphylaxis. Bronchospasm.	3 3
Teniposide, VM26, thenylidene [NSC 122819]‡	20–30 mg/m^2 IV q day × 5 days q 3 wk 67–100 mg/m^2 IV q wk	Fever. Hypotension. Bronchospasm. Anaphylaxis with cardiovascular collapse.	3
Vindesine, desacetyl vinblastine amide (Eldisine)	2–3 mg/m^2 IV q wk	Occasional N/V or diarrhea.	3

ADH, antidiuretic hormone; BMD, bone marrow depression; DTRs, deep tendon reflexes; NS, normal saline; N/V, nausea or vomiting.
‡Indicates National Service Center number, an early designation.

The development of resistance to single drugs has stimulated the development of treatment programs using drug combinations to circumvent the mechanisms of resistance and to reduce the tumor cell population to a number that can be destroyed by the host's own defense mechanism. Effective drug combinations also cause multiple lesions in cancer cells and produce a greater antitumor effect than would be achieved by giving each of the drugs in sequence. In addition, effective combinations decrease the cancer cell's ability to repair damage and

Hematologic nadir	Comments
	Mild BMD. Tissue vesicant. Biliary excretion. Decrease dose with hepatic dysfunction. Peripheral neuropathy, paresthesias, and loss of DTRs. Increased neurotoxicity in elderly and immobile patients. Abdominal pain, constipation, paralytic ileus. Use of stool softeners recommended. Bladder atony. Vocal cord paresis. Hyponatremia and syndrome of inappropriate ADH secretion. Jaw pain.
5–10 days	Dose-related BMD. Dose reduction if hepatic dysfunction exists. Stomatitis. Neurotoxicity at high doses (>20 mg). Corneal ulceration if splashed into the eye. Alopecia.
7–10 days	BMD. Tissue vesicant. Chemical phlebitis. Unstable in D5W. May precipitate in NS after 30 min. Use quickly; give only clear solutions. Severe hypotension with rapid infusion. Infuse over ½ hr, checking BP often. Stop drug if hypersensitivity reactions develop. Keep infusing NS. Treat with antihistamines and epinephrine. Alopecia. Headache. Peripheral neuropathy. Oral formulation causes GI toxicity, N/V, diarrhea.
7–10 days	BMD. Tissue vesicant. Chemical thrombophlebitis common. Infuse slowly over 15–30 min. If hypersensitivity reaction develops, stop drug and treat with epinephrine and antihistamines. Keep infusing NS or D5W. Compatible with both dextrose and saline solutions. Alopecia.
	BMD. Do not administer with other vinca alkaloids. Great potential for cumulative neurotoxicity if given with other vinca alkaloids. Neurotoxicity is dose-limiting. Loss of DTRs and paresthesias common. Proximal muscle weakness. Severe jaw pain. Abdominal cramping; diarrhea. Paralytic ileus occurs but is rare. Hoarseness. Mild stomatitis. Tissue vesicant.

delay or prevent the development of resistance. Use of drugs in combination with surgery and radiotherapy enables the physician to maximize the anticancer effects of each of these modalities while minimizing the toxic side effects of treatment on normal tissues.

Adjuvant chemotherapy after what appears to be curative surgery or radiotherapy is now used to augment the curative potential of these modalities in patients who have a high risk of recurrence. Prophylactic adjuvant therapy is used in an attempt to completely eradicate occult residual disease. Because occult disease cannot be identified or measured, only treatment programs with proven efficacy should be employed. Furthermore, the absence of measurable disease necessi-

TABLE 2-8
Miscellaneous Agents

Drug	Dose, route, and schedule	Acute side effects	Myelosuppression (1 [mild] to to 4 [severe])
L-asparaginase (Elspar)	1,000–20,000 U/m^2 q 10–14 days	Anaphylaxis. Moderate-severe N/V. Fever, chills. Urticaria. Malaise.	0–1
Acridinyl anisidide, M-AMSA, AMSA [NSC 249992]‡	90–120 mg/m^2 IV q 4 wk 25–40 mg/m^2 IV q day × 3 days q 3 wk	Severe pain and burning in vein. Moderate-severe N/V.	3
Hexamethylmelamine, HXM, HMM [NSC 13875]‡	6–12 mg/kg PO q day × 14–21 days or continuous	Moderate-severe N/V.	1
Dacarbazine, DTIC, imidazole carboximide (DTIC-Dome)	150–250 mg/m^2 IV q day × 5 days q 4 wk	Moderate-severe N/V in 1–3 hr. Local pain.	3
Mitotane, 0, P′-DDD (Lysodren)	2–10 g PO q day continuous	Severe N/V. Anorexia.	0
Procarbazine, methylhydrazine hydrochloride (Matulane)	100–200 mg/m^2 PO × 14 days or continuous	Moderate-severe N/V that subsides with daily use. Flulike syndrome that decreases over time.	3
Mitoxantrone hydrochloride, DHAD (Novantrone)	10–14 mg/m^2 IV q 3 wk	Mild N/V.	3
Methyl-GAG MGBG, mitoguazone [NSC 32946]‡	260–600 mg/m^2 IV q wk 3–4 mg/kg deep IM q wk	Hypotension. N/V. Dizziness, weakness, and malaise. Persistent anorexia.	1

BMD, bone marrow depression; MAO, monoamine oxidase; N/V, nausea or vomiting.
‡ Indicates National Service Center number, an early designation.

Hematologic nadir	Comments
	Give over 30 min. Anaphylaxis precautions. Desensitization and skin testing may have value in preventing hypersensitivity reactions. Prophylactic antihistamines may control reactions. Risk increases with repeated use. Malaise, anorexia. Hepatotoxicity common within 2 wk. Hyperglycemia. Coagulation abnormalities. CNS abnormalities; lethargy. Pancreatitis. Azotemia. Use only clear solutions.
7–14 days	BMD. Tissue vesicant; chemical thrombophlebitis. Increase diluent to 500 ml and decrease rate to decrease venous spasm and pain. Do not infuse in <1 hr. Unstable in chloride solutions. Administer in 500 ml D5W over 1 hr. Dose reductions if hepatic dysfunction exists. Renal toxicity. Diarrhea, stomatitis. Paresthesias. Orange urine; yellow skin discoloration.
21–28 days	GI toxicity may be dose-limiting at high doses. Neurotoxicity with peripheral neuropathies, agitation; confusion; hallucinations; petit mal seizures. May exacerbate vincristine-related neuropathy. Rash. Hematologic toxicity is generally mild.
10–14 days	Flulike syndrome with fever, myalgia, and malaise lasting 7–10 days. Facial flushing and paresthesias. Tissue vesicant. Protect from light. Change in color from yellow to pink denotes drug decomposition. Metabolic activation by liver. Precipitation with hydrocortisone sodium succinate (Solu-Cortef). Potentiates allopurinol activity. Mild BMD. Alopecia. Decrease rate of infusion to decrease pain from venous spasm.
	CNS toxicity with lethargy, vertigo, visual disturbance. Acute adrenal insufficiency. Allergic rash. Sensitivity to sunlight.
14–28 days	BMD. Dose reductions for patients with compromised renal function. Sympathomimetics, tricyclic antidepressants, other MAO inhibitors, and foods rich in tyramine can cause acute hypertensive crisis. Advise patients to avoid alcohol — can cause disulfiramlike reaction. Barbiturates, phenothiazines, antihistamines may increase CNS-depressive effects. Hypersensitivity reactions with fever, rash, urticaria, and angioedema. CNS abnormalities, depression. nightmares, mania, psychosis. Postural hypotension. Interstitial pneumonitis/pulmonary fibrosis.
7–14 days	BMD with platelet sparing. Alopecia. Little GI toxicity. Cardiac arrythmias in some doxorubicin-treated patients. No renal, hepatic, or cardiac toxicity reported to date. Bluish discoloration in vein used for infusion; greenish urine.
7–14 days	Toxicity is dose- and schedule-dependent. Little BMD. Severe mucositis with 5-day infusions. Anorexia and weight loss common. Hypotension with rapid infusions; give as 30-min infusion. Deep IM injections can be given if venous access is difficult; however, IM injections are associated with severe dizziness and a transient feeling of burning that spreads from the face to the entire body. Vasculitis. Skin ulcers. Neuropathy. Chemical thrombophlebitis. Delayed hypoglycemia.

TABLE 2-9

Biological Response Modifiers

Agent	Mechanisms of action‡	Administration	Side effects	Nursing implications
BCG (bacillus Calmette-Guérin) Pasteur, Tice, Glaxo, Trudeau, Phipps strains differ in ratio of live to dead organisms and storage. Freeze-dried preparations activated by specific diluent.	A	Intradermal near major lymph node drainage sites Scarification	Flaring recall at old sites, itching, fever, malaise. Scarring is permanent.	Acute observation of responses and accurate documentation. Acetaminophen 2 tablets q 4–6 hr for symptomatic relief of fever and malaise. Cold compresses and talc to relieve itching. Topical lidocaine if itching severe. Regional lymphadenitis must be differentiated from tumor metastases with patient and family. Delay swimming and bathing until crust formation has occurred.
		Intracavitary instillation Abdominal paracentesis Pleural thoracentesis Bladder instillation via urethral catheter	Fever, chills.	Turn patient side to side to distribute BCG in cavity. Patient usually quite ill. Supportive measures. Observation as above.
		Intralesional: MD injects usually (for melanotic lesions)	Local draining, abscess at injection sites.	Aspirin and acetaminophen prn for fever, lymphadenitis.
		Oral	Nausea	
MER (methanol extraction residue of BCG) nonviable.	A	Rotating intradermal sites	Flaring recall at old sites. Lesions are painful, draining. Ulcers can be 0.5 cm deep.	Choose skin sites carefully. Deep and persistent scarring. Soothe local areas with cool wet soaks. Analgesia prescription prn.

	‡			
C-parvum (Corynebacterium parvum) nonviable.	A	SC abdominal wall and/or IV solution over 30 min	12- to 48-hr fever, chills, nausea, headache. Abdominal sites often painful. Can abscess if not kept in subcutaneous tissue.	Supportive measures as above.
Levamisole	R	Oral	Nausea, vomiting.	Administer with food, antiemetic.
Thymosin	R	SC	Systemic itching.	Administer antipruritic.
Poly IC/Poly LYS interferon inducement [NSC 301463]§	E	IV	Nausea, vomiting.	Symptomatic treatment.
Interferons	E	IM	Fever, chills, fatigue, headache, weakness, nausea, vomiting, diarrhea, anorexia, bone marrow depression.	Supportive measures.
Human tumor antigens	E	In Phase I and II studies; side effects and toxicity data unknown.	Fever, chills, fatigue, weakness, nausea, vomiting anorexia have been reported.	
Tumor cell surface antigens	E			
Monoclonal antibodies	E			
Interleukin	E			
Transfer factor	E			

MD, physician.
‡A, immunoaugmenting agent; E, immunoenhancement agent; R, immunorestorative agent.
§Indicates National Service Center number, an early designation.

TABLE 2–10

Hormonally Active Chemotherapeutic Agents

Drug (brand name)	Dose, route and schedule when used as a single agent	Side effects
Androgens		
Fluoxymesterone (Halotestin)	10–30 mg/day PO	Cholestatic jaundice. Dosage reductions required for hepatic dysfunction. Increased appetite and weight gain; anorexia and N/V at high doses. Hypercalcemia in immobile patients, especially those with bone metastases. Masculinization, hirsutism, acne, patchy alopecia, voice change. Decreased libido. Sodium and fluid retention. Monitor weight; low-salt diet.
Calusterone (Methosarb)	40 mg qid PO or 0.3 mg/kg/day PO	Injectable products are poorly soluble, oil-based esters, resulting in slow release and prolonged biologic activity. Patients may become sensitized to oil carriers.
Testolactone (Teslac)	250 mg qid PO or 100 mg IM 3 times/wk	
Testosterone propionate (Oreton)	50–100 mg IM 3 times/wk	
Testosterone enanthate (Delatestryl)	600–1,200 mg IM q wk	
Dromostanolone propionate (Drolban)	100 mg IM 3 times/wk	

Estrogens

Drug	Dose	
Diethylstilbestrol, DES, stilbestrol (Stilbium)	1–15 mg PO q day (prostate cancer 1–3 mg PO q day)	Rapid rise in serum calcium in patients with bone metastases. Sodium and fluid retention with hypertension leading to CHF and thromboembolic complications. Monitor weight; low-salt diet. Feminization, gynecomastia, endometrial hypertrophy, uterine bleeding, areolar hyperpigmentation. Urinary frequency. Sensitization to oil carrier. Natural and synthetic compounds vary with regard to onset of activity, bioavailability, and duration of activity. Chlorotrianisene is extremely fat soluble, and considerable fat storage occurs, accounting for delayed onset and prolonged duration. Individual products should be chosen selectively, based on such properties. N/V resembling morning sickness at high doses. N/V often subsides with continued treatment.
Diethylstilbestrol diphosphate (Stilphostrol, Honvol)	500–1,000 mg IV × 5 day then 250–100 mg IV q wk	
Chlorotrianisene (TACE)	12–25 mg PO tid	
Conjugated equine estrogenic compound (Premarin)	1–10 mg PO tid	
Ethinyl estradiol (Estinyl)	0.5–1.0 mg PO tid	

Antiestrogenic compounds

Drug	Dose	
Tamoxifen citrate (Nolvadex)	10–80 mg PO q day	Induction of ovulation and lactation; hot flashes. Transient "flare" in skin, soft tissue, and bone metastases. Hypercalcemia. Mild leukopenia and thrombocytopenia. Mild estrogenic activity seen; vaginal discharge, bleeding, and pruritus. Corneal opacity and retinopathies with prolonged high doses >240 mg/day >1 yr.

Drug (brand name)	Dose, route and schedule when used as a single agent	Side effects
Progestins		
Hydroxyprogesterone caproate (Delalutin)	1.0–2.5 g IM 2 times/wk	Generally well-tolerated. Minimal fluid retention. Alopecia. Occasional hypercalcemia in patients with bone metastases. Cholestastic jaundice. Use with care in patients with hepatic dysfunction. Thromboembolic phenomena. Patients may become sensitized to oil carrier. Natural progestins are rapidly inactivated. Slow-release formulations administered IM.
Medroxyprogesterone acetate		
Provera [PO]	20–200 mg PO q day	
Depo-provera [IM]	200–800 mg IM 2 times/wk	
Megestrol acetate (Megace)	40–300 mg PO q day	
Adrenocortical steroids		
Prednisone (Deltasone)	40–60 mg/m² PO q day	Agents vary with respect to mineral corticoid potency (sodium and fluid retention); intermittent administration can increase the risk of serious toxicity. Adrenalectomized patients must increase steroids in stress, infection, trauma. Oral preparations irritate GI mucosa; administered with antacids.
Prednisolone (Delta-Cortef)	40–60 mg/m² IM q day	
Methylprednisolone (Medrol) Sodium m. succinate (Solu-Medrol) M. acetate (Depo-Medrol)	10–25 mg IV or IM	Prolonged use may produce immunosuppression; GI ulceration and hemorrhage; hyperglycemia, diabetes, hyperlipidemia, weight gain; sodium and fluid retention, hypertension, edema, potassium wasting; emotional lability, euphoria, psychosis; muscle wasting; osteoporosis, aseptic necrosis of bones; glaucoma, cataracts; cushingoid appearance, acne; secondary amenorrhea, growth failure. Suppression of pituitary-adrenal axis upon long-term withdrawal

Drug	Dose	Toxicity
Hydrocortisone (Cortef) H. sodium succinate (Solu-Cortef)	100–500 mg IV or IM q day	
Dexamethasone (Decadron)	0.5–16 mg PO, IV, or IM q day	
Chemical adrenalectomy Aminoglutethimide (Cytadren, Elipten)	750–2,000 mg PO q day	Skin rash within 5–7 days lasting 8 days. Lethargy; somnolence. Addisonian characteristics; secretion of aldosterone with postural hypotension and hyponatremia. Hypothyroidism. Virilization. Mild nausea, vertigo, nystagmus. BMD rare.

BMD, bone marrow depression; CHF, congestive heart failure; N/V, nausea or vomiting.

tates the use of randomized controlled trials to document improvement in disease-free survival rates. Because systemic treatment with chemotherapy cannot be administered to patients without risk, the potential benefits and risks of such programs must be carefully weighed. Use of adjuvant programs that effectively eradicate residual cancer cells has great potential for changing the primary surgical management of many tumors, permitting use of less extensive and less disfiguring surgical techniques.

Nursing management

Acute and chronic side effects occur with the use of most chemotherapeutic agents. Unique toxicities specific to individual drugs have been summarized in Tables 2-3 to 2-10. Patients who are educated about potential toxicities can actively participate in their therapy to reduce or prevent complications related to treatment. The ability of patients to become involved in the management of their disease is, to a great degree, dependent on the quality of their interactions with their physicians and nurses. The demonstration of professional competence and knowledge, as well as the generation of mutual trust, fosters the development of a therapeutic relationship, which also facilitates effective patient education about treatment-related morbidity. Nurses should remember to present information about specific neoplasms, available therapeutic options, and side effects associated with treatment in terms of probabilities rather than in absolutes. While it is important to prepare patients for difficult realities that may lie ahead, it is also important to provide hope.

GI side effects. Nausea and vomiting are the most commonly encountered complications of antineoplastic agents. Symptoms may appear shortly after administration or may be delayed by 8 to 12 hr and persist for periods ≤24 hr, with gradual resolution of symptoms. While they may occur as separate problems, nausea and vomiting frequently appear as a clinical syndrome associated with physiologic changes such as dizziness, pallor, tachycardia, and diaphoresis. The incidence and severity of symptoms are known to be dose-related with some, but not all, agents. Induction of symptoms may be related to: (1) direct irritation of the GI tract (such as is caused by ipecac); (2) stimulation of a chemoreceptor trigger zone in the medulla oblongata that is sensitive to certain blood-borne compounds; (3) a central effect on the vomiting zone, a motor and reflex center in the floor of the fourth ventricle that regulates and coordinates the sequence of events during emesis; (4) anticipatory anxiety; or (5) a combination of factors. Symptoms can often be ameliorated with the prophylactic and regular use of phenothiazines and/or sedatives. These agents have a variety of actions including depression of the vomiting center and blocking the effect of drugs on the chemoreceptor trigger zone. Patients should be encouraged to use antiemetics liberally and advised about the timing, scheduling, and side effects of antiemetics so that maximum relief can be achieved. Current research in the management of nausea and vomiting includes studies on diversion and relaxation techniques to reduce symptomatology and on new antiemetic preparations as well. Delta-9-tetrahydrocannabinol (THC), the major active ingredient of marijuana, has been employed with some success in clinical settings where conventional antiemetics have failed.

Anorexia may occur in conjunction with nausea and vomiting, or it may be related to physiologic changes induced by tumor (such as GI obstruction by tumor, or loss or distortion of taste). Anorexia may also stem from emotional disturbances, especially depression and anxiety. Selection of appropriate therapeutic measures should be based on identification of a probable etiology. Intervention may include nutritional counseling, dietary modification, nutritional supplements, and/or the use of IV parenteral nutrition to prevent severe nutritional deficiencies.

Diarrhea may occur as a result of GI mucosal irritation secondary to a toxic effect of the drug on the bowel. Antidiarrheal agents are often useful. When significant diarrhea occurs, hydration must be increased, especially when drugs that are nephrotoxic or are eliminated in urine have been administered. Constipation is generally related to a direct effect of the drug on the nerve supply of the bowel, causing hypomotility. Prophylactic use of laxatives is warranted with vincristine, the most common etiologic agent.

Cutaneous and mucosal toxicity. Mucositis, or stomatitis, is a serious and potentially life-threatening complication that is generally seen with antimetabolites and antitumor antibiotics. Mucositis occurs when renewal of the epithelial cells lining the GI tract is inhibited by chemotherapeutic agents. Toxicity is manifested as erythema, pain, and ulceration of the mucosa of some or all of the entire GI tract. Ulcerations of the bowel are associated with watery diarrhea and, with more severe toxicity, bleeding. Dose reductions and/or interruptions in therapy are often necessary. Local analgesics, debridement, and topical antibacterial and antifungal therapy can prevent superinfection with opportunistic organisms (*see* Chapter 9C).

Alopecia is a common complication of chemotherapy that, while not serious, has a profound psychologic impact on patients. A number of studies now suggest that hair loss may be decreased or prevented with techniques that produce scalp hypothermia. If alopecia is a major concern to the patient, the use of these techniques may prove beneficial. For those patients who are not suitable for such interventions, the provision of wigs, empathy, and reassurance that regrowth of hair often occurs during therapy is often helpful (*see* Chapter 9C).

Macular or pustular rashes, desquamation, and epidermolysis may also occur as a direct effect of the drug on the skin or as an immunologically mediated allergic reaction. Areas of previous irradiation are particularly susceptible to dermatologic toxicity. Dose reductions, interruption, or cessation of therapy may be necessitated by severe toxicity.

The cytotoxic action of chemotherapeutic agents can cause hyperpigmentation and retardation of nail growth. Patients should be reassured that these side effects of therapy are not related to disease progression.

Hyperuricemia can occur after the administration of chemotherapeutic agents when there is rapid lysis of tumor cells (*see* Chapter 15B). High serum-uric-acid levels result from the breakdown of nucleoproteins in these cells. At high concentrations, uric acid precipitates in the renal tubules and can cause serious or irreversible kidney failure. Allopurinol prevents the formation of uric acid and should be given prophylactically with hydration prior to the initiation of chemotherapy when rapid cell lysis is thought possible. This is particularly important in patients with acute leukemia and lymphoma, where the use of chemotherapy can produce rapid and dramatic reductions in tumor volume. As noted in Table 2–5, the dose of 6-mercaptopurine should be decreased when allopurinol is given.

Hematologic toxicity. Myelosuppression is the most common dose-limiting toxicity that is associated with chemotherapeutic drugs. Severe leukopenia may result in life-threatening or fatal complications. Bone marrow suppression is manifested as anemia, thrombocytopenia, and leukopenia and can sometimes be managed with blood component therapy (*see* Chapter 9A).

Immunosuppression. In addition to having a direct effect on normal hematopoiesis, many commonly used chemotherapeutic agents are potent immunosuppressants. Impairment of the host's immune system increases the risk of infectious complications. Return of normal immune function may take as long as 1 to 2 yr after the cessation of all therapy. At present, chemotherapeutic programs are designed to provide intensive therapy that alternates with rest periods on a regular schedule to enhance immunologic recovery.

Long-term effects of chemotherapy

Reproductive capacity. Cancer chemotherapeutic agents can affect testicular and ovarian function and, therefore, a potential long-term complication of successful therapy is potential sterility. While gonadal and reproductive capacity may return after the completion of treatments, patients who are in their reproductive years must be informed that irreversible sterility is a potential complication in men and women. Chemotherapy may cause sublethal chromosomal damage to male or female gametes, so the risk of fetal abnormalities after therapy is real, although it is poorly defined to date. It is important to remember that while chemotherapy *may* cause infertility, methods of contraception should be discussed, because many agents are teratogenic and pregnancy should be avoided during therapy. Long-term storage of spermatozoa in special facilities may be considered in young males planning future families.

Hepatic, pulmonary, and renal effects. Prolonged administration of chemotherapeutic agents may reversibly or permanently damage the liver, lung, and kidney. The incidence and severity of such effects are not fully documented at present. The potential for such toxicity must, however, be considered when the decisions about the duration of therapy are made, especially in patients receiving adjuvant therapy for undetectable residual cancer. Prolonged administration of both methotrexate and 6-mercaptopurine is associated with chronic hepatotoxicity. Toxicity can include hepatic fibrosis, jaundice, and ascites. Prolonged treatments with busulfan, methotrexate, and carmustine have been linked to the development of diffuse interstitial and intra-alveolar pulmonary infiltrates. These infiltrates may gradually resolve when therapy is terminated and steroids are administered or may result in progressive deterioration in pulmonary function despite discontinuation of the agent. Treatment with high-dose methotrexate, cisplatin, and the other nitrosoureas is associated with renal toxicity. The incidence of permanent renal damage and renal failure after cessation of therapy with these agents is not yet documented.

Alkylating agents, antimetabolites, antitumor antibiotics, and procarbazine used as single agents, with irradiation, or with drug combinations can produce cytogenetic aberrations, suggesting that these drugs have the potential for causing cancer as well as treating it. A relationship between cancer and immunodeficiency has also been established in animals and in patients with congenital immunodeficiency syndromes (e.g., Wiskott-Aldrich syndrome, ataxia telangiectasia), in patients with acquired immune deficiency syndrome (AIDS), and in renal transplant recipients who are being treated with highly potent immunosuppressive drugs to prevent organ rejection. It is thought that drug-induced immunosuppression may permit cells damaged by drugs or radiation to proliferate and become clinically manifest as a second neoplasm. Although this circumstance is disturbing, it is important to remember that the vast majority of patients cured with chemotherapy would have died without drug treatment. Therefore, the risks of a second cancer must be balanced against the benefits to each patient in terms of quality of life and prolongation of survival. Because the greater and more prolonged use of antitumor agents will place a greater number of patients at risk of developing drug-induced second neoplasms, it has become increasingly important for nurses to understand the risk: benefit ratio thoroughly, to follow their patients carefully for any evidence of a second cancer, and to ensure that patients are informed about this potential complication.

While many advanced malignancies are now curable with drugs, with or without irradiation, the solid neoplasms of later life, particularly adenocarcinomas originating in the GI tract and lung, remain a formidable therapeutic challenge. For patients with these cancers, the potential toxicities and risks of aggressive therapy must be carefully weighed and presented when discussing the potential benefits of therapy. The goal of cancer treatment should always be based on the potential for cure and a careful assessment of the side effects. At times, less intensive treatment or supportive care, consisting of pain control and psychologic support, may be the wisest therapeutic choice. While supportive care may not affect the ultimate outcome, it can often allow the patient extended periods of functional and pain-free life. It is essential, therefore, for nurses to be attuned to the psychologic needs of patients as they care for their patients' physical needs and to maintain a concerned and supportive attitude in their relationships. There is no single, simple cure-all for cancer—and probably never will be. We have learned that each cancer is, in actuality, many different diseases, and each cancer must be approached as a unique entity. We have made great strides in curing many cancers, now that we understand that systemic therapy with drugs can be used to eradicate undetected cancer cells left behind after surgery or radiation therapy. There is great reason for continued optimism, given the current research efforts to improve effective therapies already available and to prevent and/or manage untoward side effects of treatment.

Bibliography

1. Becker, T. M. Cancer Chemotherapy: A Manual for Nurses. Little, Brown & Co., Boston. 1981.

   In table format, provides information about most chemotherapy drugs in use today: drug names, class, pharmacologic information, method of administration, base-line studies to monitor, indications for use, side effects, and nursing care.

2. Chabner, B. Pharmacologic Principles of Cancer Treatment. W. B. Saunders Co., Philadelphia. 1982.

    A sophisticated and comprehensive presentation of the pharmacology and pharmacokinetics of chemotherapy agents. Excellent for nurses involved in clinical trials of investigational drugs.

3. Clinical Practice and Education Committees. Cancer Chemotherapy Guidelines and Recommendations for Nursing Education and Practice. Oncology Nursing Society, Pittsburgh. 1984.

    A useful pamphlet for nurses involved in administering chemotherapy and in teaching chemotherapy administration courses. Includes guidelines for drug preparation, administration, and disposal.

4. DeVita, V. T., S. Hellman, and S. A. Rosenberg, editors. Cancer: Principles and Practice of Oncology. J. B. Lippincott, Philadelphia. 1982.

    A 2,000-page textbook edited by three acknowledged leaders in oncology. Presents the state of the art of basic scientific principles guiding the study, diagnosis, and treatment of cancer, as well as the practice of treating the many forms of cancer and its complications.

5. Dorr, R. T., and W. L. Fritz. Cancer Chemotherapy Handbook. Elsevier North-Holland, Inc., New York. 1980.

    Provides a detailed discussion of the pharmacology of antineoplastic agents by class, and "drug data sheets" for each individual agent. Includes brief sections on organ toxicity as well as ethical and legal implications.

6. Levine, A. S., editor. Cancer in the Young. Masson Publishing USA, Inc., New York. 1982.

    A comprehensive textbook for physicians covering pediatric tumors. Included are discussions of cancer biology, diagnosis, antitumor and supportive treatments, and descriptions of specific pediatric cancers.

7. Marino, L. B., editor. Cancer Nursing. C. V. Mosby Co., St. Louis. 1981.

    A comprehensive textbook for nurses. Includes introductory chapters describing cancer biology and research principles, discussions of specific tumor types with representative case examples, and content related to rehabilitation of the cancer patient.

CHAPTER 3

PRINCIPLES OF CLINICAL RESEARCH

Susan Molloy Hubbard

Oncology has emerged as an important area of clinical specialization over the last two decades, largely because of the success of clinical research in identifying chemotherapy as an effective cancer treatment. The complexity of modern treatment regimens and the tremendous need for the education and psychosocial support of patients has created a need for ongoing collaboration between physicians and nurses who share responsibility for the primary care of patients. This chapter will discuss the role of the nurse in cancer research in relation to the principles of clinical research, the phases of clinical investigation, ethical considerations, and the requisite clinical skills.

The role of the clinical research nurse in cancer clinical trials

Historically, the nurse's involvement in the conduct of clinical research was task-oriented and limited to the provision of nursing care to patients participating in clinical trials. This functional approach to research emphasized strict adherence to the physician's orders without stressing the need for knowledgable participation of nurses in the study. Therefore, the involvement of nurses in clinical research was peripheral to the research process.

The role of the nurse in chemotherapy research was one of the first that emphasized active collaboration in research. This expanded role in research developed at certain research centers in the beginning of the 1970s during early clinical trials to evaluate the therapeutic potential of drugs in the treatment of advanced cancer. It has grown as the curative potential of modern cancer chemotherapy has become widely appreciated and applied in the community. The need for skilled nurses who could share responsibility for the safe administration of PO and IV investigational cancer chemotherapy stimulated the development of this new, expanded nursing role. A feature that made this role unique was that the nurse was considered an integral member of the primary research team, rather than a member of the ancillary support staff. As integral members of the research team, these nurses were able to participate in patient-care rounds and conferences that enabled them to learn about the biology of cancer, the natural history of the cancers under investigation, the special needs of the cancer research patient, and the fundamentals of clinical research. Their active involvement in the management of patients participating in clinical trials enabled them to actively participate in clinical research while fostering the incorporation of nursing considerations into research protocols. By assuming major responsibilities for the collection, analysis, and publication of research data, chemotherapy nurses at certain centers developed a role as a coinvestigator in clinical trials. Coincident with this development, oncologists recognized that the nurses' assumption of this role greatly enhanced the quality of clinical trials. A survey of growth over a 6-yr period at one large cancer center has demonstrated that the integration of chemotherapy nurses into a research team permitted the number of outpatient visits for IV chemotherapy to virtually quadruple, as did the number of research protocols. A recent review of growth in oncology nursing as a clinical specialty reports that the membership in the Oncology Nursing Society has grown from 20 nurses in 1976 to 5,500 members in 1983, with 66% of the membership involved in direct patient care, with 43% employed by hospitals.

Because chemotherapy research nurses understood the protocols and the data emanating from the clinical trials, they served as an educational resource for patients, providing information about the investigational regimen and practical information about the management and/or reduction of toxicity of the therapy. Because patients gained a major new source of information about their disease and treatment, their acceptance of the nurse as chemotherapist was excellent, and further evolution of this role was facilitated. The expertise provided by these nurses has enabled the research team to develop new techniques for administering chemotherapy more effectively and has permitted the evaluation of treatment techniques, such as intermittent intraperitoneal dialysis, to move into the ambulatory care setting.

As nurses recognized that clinical research needed to become an integral component of clinical nursing practice, the concept of initiating and collaborating in research achieved greater acceptance as a continuing professional responsibility. In addition to their involvement in the delivery of investigational therapies, nurses conducted clinical research designed to evaluate the efficacy of nursing interventions in dealing with the special nursing-care needs demanded by new treatment approaches, and they initiated clinical studies to evaluate the impact of innovative nursing care on the incidence and severity of disease- and treatment-related morbidity.

Nursing in clinical research

A clinical trial is a research study designed to answer a question that has therapeutic implications for patients. It is literally an experiment, performed at the patient's bedside or in the outpatient clinic rather than in a research laboratory. While a clinical trial does not always produce a definitive answer to the question that has been posed, it should always produce data that are biologically valid and ethically sound. Conduct of a sound clinical trial depends on a clear definition of the research question and a clear description of the scientific data that support the hypothesis, and on the development of a research protocol that captures clinical and laboratory data on all of the biologic variables known to be important. Unlike laboratory research, in which experimental variables can often be precisely manipulated, conditions in clinical research are often not easily controlled. Patients, families, scheduling, transportation, finances, and a myriad of psychosocial conflicts complicate clinical research, requiring cooperation by many members of the health-care team.

The participation of nurses in clinical research can be divided into two major categories: roles in which the nurse's primary emphasis is on the provision of *direct* patient care, and roles in which the nurse's primary emphasis is on the *improvement* of care through research and the safe and effective conduct of clinical trials. Although the focus of each role differs, the responsibilities and concerns of each are complementary and should blend to serve the care needs of the research patient. Staff nurses in both inpatient and outpatient areas concentrate on the delivery of direct patient care. They must approach patient care in a way that reflects an understanding of individual needs and the priorities that must be established to meet those needs. The philosophic and structural foundations of primary nursing support this purpose. The major tenets of primary nursing are that the nurse should provide: (1) advanced knowledge and skills gained from continuing education and experience in areas such as cancer care; (2) individualized care that reflects adaptation of standardized procedures and care plans to the unique circumstances of each patient's situation; (3) continuity of care that is achieved by assumption of primary responsibility for care planning and delivery of care; and (4) care evaluation for specific patients for prolonged time periods, spanning multiple hospital admissions and outpatient visits. In primary nursing, the ultimate responsibility for the nursing care given to a patient does not change with daily assignments or tours of duty; the overall plan of care is formulated by primary nurse on a 24-hr basis and is communicated to other staff members through a detailed nursing-care plan.

Establishing primary nursing care as a system for the care of research patients is analogous to providing each patient with a primary-care physician and represents an essential component of a true multidisciplinary team approach. The primary nurse serves as a focal resource who coordinates the broad spectrum of services that are required to meet the varied physical and emotional needs of specific cancer patients. The clinical research nurse serves the primary nurse as a consultative resource on research issues affecting patient care. Given the fact that the focus of the clinical research nurse is the improvement of patient care through research, specific roles and responsibilities assumed by these nurses may best be discussed by considering the specific phases of clinical investigation used to develop and evaluate new cancer chemotherapeutic agents. Understanding the evaluation process provides a framework for viewing how a nurse can function in each of the four clinical phases of drug development. In each phase, the nurse has assumed important responsibilities that affect the welfare of research patients and the scientific evaluation of a new agent.

The drug development process begins with the identification of a compound with observed or potential antitumor activity. Once identified, the compound is subjected to careful scrutiny for antitumor activity in experimental tumor systems. This screening process permits scientists to narrow the number of compounds to be tested to those that consistently demonstrate antitumor activity in one or more experimental tumor systems. At the conclusion of the screening evaluation, the compound's ability to retard the growth of cancer cells, prolong survival, or produce objective signs of tumor regression is determined. If the test substance demonstrates activity by significantly prolonging the life of the test animal or significantly retarding the growth of cancer cells as contrasted with a control group treated with a biologically inactive substance, the drug is considered a potential candidate for clinical trials. Once its biologic activity is established, the test compound must undergo the second preclinical step in development, which is purification and formulation. During this process, the compound is refined, its chemical structure is identified, and it is formulated so that it can be administered PO or injected. The refined material is then tested in rodents and large animals in an attempt to identify a safe starting dose that is not likely to produce toxicity to normal tissue in patients. Once a safe starting dose can be estimated and acute and chronic side effects in animals are established, an application for approval of use in patients with widespread cancer is made to the Food and Drug Administration.

Phase I trials.   The Phase I trial is the initial phase of clinical investigation and represents the first time that a new treatment is evaluated in cancer patients. While this discussion will focus on the Phase I evaluation of a new drug, a Phase I study may evaluate: (1) a biologic substance, such as interferon, that modifies the immune response; (2) a new treatment schedule using an established drug (e.g., high-dose methotrexate with leucovorin rescue); (3) a new route of drug administration (i.e., intraperitoneal dialysis); and/or (4) new treatment techniques (i.e., whole-body hyperthermia). The goals of the Phase I study are to establish a maximally tolerated dose, to define toxicity to normal tissues, and to determine an optimal dosage and schedule for future clinical trials (Table 3–1). These goals entail identification of major dose-limiting effects and the onset, duration, and degree of reversibility of these toxic effects. Therefore, at the initiation of every Phase I trial, the clinical research nurse must know the available preclinical pharmacologic and toxicologic data that support the scientific rationale for bringing the investigational therapy into clinical trial. Not only do these preclinical data validate the clinical trial, but they also have value in predicting the specific toxic effects that may develop in patients and in serving as an early guide to the selection and escalation of initial dosages. Preclinical toxicologic assays may miss or underestimate important toxicity in humans, however. Therefore, the nurse must possess knowledge of the cancer and the patient's clinical status to be able to discriminate between the effect of the disease process and the side effects of the new treatment. Because Phase I studies are also designed to obtain pharmacokinetic data on human absorption, bioavailability, metabolism, and excretion, the clinical research nurse may coordinate or perform pharmacokinetic studies in patients in Phase I trials.

Most cancer patients considered eligible for Phase I trials have little or no chance of deriving significant benefit from other established forms of treatment. These patients generally have cancers that are known to be unresponsive to current therapeutic modalities or have progressed while receiving conventional therapy. Those patients with extensive prior therapy and progressive disease are often physically and emotionally debilitated and tolerate drug toxicity poorly. Although careful dose escalation procedures are employed in Phase I trials to reduce the risk of serious toxicity, a major concern of the clinical research nurse is the early recognition and management of unusual or unexpected side effects representing acute, delayed, or cumulative

TABLE 3-1

Phases of Clinical Trials for New Cancer Chemotherapeutic Agents

Phase	Research goals	Nursing considerations	Nursing responsibilities
I	Determination of a therapeutic dose (the highest dose with acceptable toxicity) and schedule of administration for further clinical trials. Definition of toxic effects on normal tissue. Generation of data about bioavailability and the clinical pharmacology of the agent.	Ensure patient safety and comfort. Incorporate nursing considerations into treatment protocol. Educate patients about treatment-related benefits and side effects as data base grows. Consider ethical issues surrounding the adequacy of informed consent and the discussion of therapeutic alternatives.	Know available preclinical data on the: scientific rationale for use in humans; mechanism of action; appropriate route(s) of administration; data on absorption, metabolism, and excretion; factors known to alter metabolism; acute, dose-limiting toxicity seen in animals (organs affected, onset, duration, reversibility); chronic, cumulative, or delayed side effects seen in animals. Apply preclinical data to clinical trials in patients: anticipate adverse reactions seen in animals to enable early recognition of toxicity in patients; recognize the potential for unexpected and unpredicted adverse reactions. Develop clinical skills: Provide supportive physical and emotional care: educate patients about their disease and

treatment; develop nursing care plans to minimize disease- and treatment-related morbidity.

Assess patient: Assess objective and subjective clinical changes; review all pertinent clinical studies; discriminate between drug-related effects and disease-related effects.

Document all treatment-related changes in the patient's medical record and flow sheet: record therapeutic effects objectively noted and subjectively reported by patient; record objective and subjective evidence of acute, chronic, delayed, or cumulative side effects on normal tissues; record data on any pharmacologic studies performed.

Participate in decisions concerning dose escalation, schedule manipulation, determination of optimal dose.

Disseminate research results in publications that: recommend dose and schedule for Phase II trials; delineate the onset, duration, severity, and reversibility of all therapeutic effects and toxicity to normal tissues.

Phase	Research goals	Nursing considerations	Nursing responsibilities
II	Identification of antitumor activity in a spectrum of cancers (applicable to single agents and/or new combinations). Exploration of ability to achieve increased response rate with dose and schedule manipulations. Elaboration and extension of Phase I data on toxicity.	Ensure that all patients entered into the trial are eligible and fully able to be evaluated. Fully document all treatment-related benefits and side effects. *See also* Phase I.	Know about the cancer and its natural history, enabling evaluation of response and toxicity. Know about the influence of disease-related abnormalities on drug metabolism and excretion. Use clinical expertise to maximize the impact of tumor regression on quality of life; develop and implement effective interventions to prevent or minimize treatment- or disease-related toxicity; educate patients to maximize personal control and participation in therapy. Document therapeutic and toxic effects in the medical record in an accurate and comprehensive manner. Disseminate research results.

III/IV	Prospective comparison of the investigational therapy against an established form of treatment in previously untreated patients to:	Confirm and extend data on acute and chronic toxicity.	*See* Phase I and Phase II.
	determine the impact of the therapy on disease-free and overall survival; identify any prognostic factors affecting curability (stage, histology, tumor volume, age, hormonal status, etc.); assess the impact of therapy on the quality of life; establish value of regimen as adjuvant therapy in patients who have a high risk of developing recurrence after local therapy; integrate the regimen with other modalities of treatment (surgery or radiotherapy).	Delineate management and educate about long-term complications of the disease and/or therapy. Continue care. Provide rehabilitative support facilitating normalization of life-style. *See also* Phase II.	

toxicity that has not been identified previously. This is especially important because therapeutic efficacy may not be observed during Phase I trials, and significant toxicity may compromise subsequent efforts to achieve palliation of disease. Accurate and detailed documentation of observations by the clinical research nurse are critical to the patient's welfare and constitute a major contribution to the quality of this type of clinical trial.

All disease- and treatment-related effects should be recorded as they evolve in the patient's medical record and summarized on a sheet commonly called a flow sheet (Fig. 3–1). Flow sheets concisely summarize the data on all drugs administered and data on therapeutic response and toxicity. Entries requiring a more detailed description or comment can be numbered and explained in the area designated for comments. A human figure is provided so that significant clinical data can be illustrated in a way that can be used to evaluate changes in clinical parameters. Fluctuations in hematologic and biochemical parameters, diagnostic studies, specific tumor markers, and performance status are easily assessed, as are the rate of response, remission duration, and time to maximal response. Important data can readily be extracted from the flow sheet and computerized to permit rapid analysis of data, thus facilitating the early recognition of important trends during any clinical trial. Clinical research nurses have played a major role in the development and enhancement of these flow sheets.

The probability of obtaining a beneficial response to a new treatment during a Phase I clinical trial is difficult to estimate. Often the optimal dosage and schedule for administration of the new therapy are unknown and, in the interest of patient safety, the initial dosages administered are often well below the therapeutic dose range. Therefore, the identification of *any* evidence of antitumor activity in a Phase I trial represents an important observation. The clinical research team uses a standardized set of criteria to categorize the therapeutic responses throughout each phase of clinical investigation:

Complete remission (CR): Complete regression of all evidence of cancer by every criterion (physical, radiologic, biochemical) *and* a return to normal performance status. All residual symptomatic abnormalities must be related to side effects of therapy. The duration of complete remission must exceed 1 mo (remissions are always expressed in terms of duration).

Partial remission (PR): Objective regression of 50% of all measurable tumor accompanied by subjective improvement. The duration of partial remission should be expressed in months. The appearance of any new lesion or increase in size of residual lesions terminates the partial remission.

Minor responses (MR) or improvement (I): Objective tumor regression of 25 to 50% with subjective improvement. In some studies improvement means that significant subjective improvement has occurred without objective tumor regression or regression of some, but not all, measurable lesion has occurred.

No response (NR): No objective change in the tumor mass is seen or the response represents <25% regression. No significant subjective improvement is seen.

Progression (P): Growth of measurable disease or appearance of new metastases.

It is important to emphasize that the failure to observe objective responses during Phase I trials does not necessarily mean that the treatment will not demonstrate antitumor activity in subsequent clinical trials when an optimal dose and schedule are established and can be used with patients. The absence of objective responses during Phase I clinical trials is *not* a sufficient reason for deleting the investigational agent from further trials. The only reason for not advancing a new antitumor agent or therapeutic approach to Phase II is the presence of unacceptable toxicity to normal tissues.

Phase II trials. Phase II clinical trials are designed to evaluate the new drug or treatment program against number of cancers, employing a dosage and schedule established as safe during Phase I studies. The goals of Phase II trials are to determine a response rate in a statistically measurable number of patients with a specific type or stage of disease and to determine the spectrum of antitumor activity by evaluating the new agent in a broad range of common cancers. Throughout the trials, research nurses must use their knowledge of cancer biology to help them evaluate the effects of the new treatment on the disease process. Nursing responsibilities include physical assessment of patients, documentation of objective and subjective changes in clinical parameters of response and/or progression, and documentation of normal tissue tolerance and drug toxicity through serial laboratory determinations (Table 3-1). To avoid unexpected toxicity, the clinical research nurse should attempt to identify all disease- or treatment-induced abnormalities of normal organ function that may alter the anticipated activation, metabolism, or excretion of systemically administered compounds. The nurse can help to maximize the impact of a therapeutic response on the quality of the patient's life by educating him in ways to minimize or prevent treatment complications. Reduction of avoidable toxicity can ensure that therapeutic benefit will not be lost because of unnecessary treatment delays and also that the administration of subsequent therapies will not be compromised when or if recurrent disease develops.

MEDICAL BRANCH FLOW SHEET

NIH-442-2 (REV. 10-77)

B.S.AREA | Date (Yr:

| PROTOCOL NO. | TUMOR TYPE |
| CLIN. ASSOC. | STUDY CHAIRMAN |

(C) Show Tumors 1,2,3,4,5, and code each with letters:

B = Bone   S = Skin/SC   H = Hepatic
C = CNS   L = Lung   M = Breast
N = Nodes   P = Pleura   O = Other(Specify)

Day on Study or Cycle/Day

THERAPY
- DRUGS
- OTHER
  - Radiotherapy
  - Transfusions
  - Antibiotics

HEMATOLOGY
- WBC/mm^{3}x10^3
- Hgb g% or Hct %
- Platelets/mm^{3}x10^3
- Polys%/Lymphs%
- Bone marrow

CHEMISTRIES
- Uric acid mg%/Urinalysis
- Ca/PO$_4$mg%
- Alk.Phos.
- Bilirub. mg% tot.
- SGPT/SGOT
- alb/Tot.prot g%
- LDH
- BUN/Creat. mg%

Figure 3–1. Flow sheet. EMI is equivalent to CAT.

For results to be scientifically and ethically sound, the number of patients with a specific tumor type fully evaluable at the end of Phase II studies must be sufficient to establish a response rate (or lack of response) with statistical confidence. Therefore, patients entered onto Phase II protocols must be carefully evaluated for eligibility. If the criteria for eligibility are not carefully considered and treatment or follow-up is not properly performed, the clinical trial will fail to generate meaningful data about therapeutic efficacy. This issue is an ethical concern for research nurses because patients who participate in research often do so on the assumption that valid new knowledge will be generated by their participation. An important responsibility of the nurse in clinical research is a commitment to inform the investigator principally responsible for the research protocol of any concerns about patient eligibility and/or protocol violations.

Phase III trials. In Phase III clinical trials the major focus is on the attainment of complete responses. In these studies, a new agent or treatment approach that has demonstrated significant antitumor activity in Phase II studies is compared against a standard or conventional form of treatment (Table 3–1). Phase III trials are disease-oriented trials designed to determine response rate in a specific cancer as well as the duration of complete and partial responses that are achievable. Patients are randomly allocated to one of the treatment groups to prevent the investigators from introducing bias into the selection of therapy. To ensure comparability between treatments, only newly diagnosed, previously untreated patients are generally considered eligible. For such clinical trials to be ethical, the investigational treatment must have sufficient activity to justify randomization with a treatment of known efficacy, and the protocol design must be adequate to definitively compare the two therapies. Thus the clinical protocol must be carefully constructed to ensure that patient eligibility is clearly defined, that there is a sufficient number of patients in each treatment group, and that there is stratification of patients by all known important prognostic variables. Objective criteria for the determination of complete and partial responses and of disease progression must be clearly established. In addition, the period of treatment and follow-up must be adequate to allow meaningful comparisons of overall therapeutic efficacy and toxicity. As participants in such studies, nurses must be able to explain the study design and the rationale for randomization to patients and their families, as well as to other medical and nursing personnel.

Because Phase III trials address issues that relate to remission duration and ultimately cure, they require years of careful follow-up before the therapeutic question can be answered. During this period of posttreatment observation, the nurse's concerns shift from the management of acute nursing care problems to health-care maintenance and from delineation of acute toxicity to the identification of chronic or long-term complications of treatment.

Because the goal of a Phase III trial is to establish the relative therapeutic value of the treatments under investigation, protocol violations must be prevented so that all patients entered into the randomized trial will be fully evaluable. An experienced nurse who follows patients throughout their treatment can ensure that dose and schedule modifications are uniform and that all study measures are evaluated at the specified intervals so that all patients can be evaluated fully. Because many research programs now offer training programs for physicians in oncology, the clinical research nurse often provides the major source of continuity in care and emotional support. In such situations, the nurse's knowledge of the disease process, the clinical protocols, and the patients' individual needs assumes even greater importance because primary physicians may change frequently.

Phase IV trials. In the final phase of clinical investigation, new treatments that are effective in producing complete remissions in patients with advanced cancer are integrated into multimodal therapies for patients with cancers that appear to be localized at the time of diagnosis but are known to have a significant incidence of recurrence after apparently curative surgery or radiation. These clinical trials are commonly known as studies of adjuvant therapy. Because all patients are clinically free of disease when adjuvant therapy is instituted and a certain, albeit unknown, fraction are already cured and do not need the adjuvant treatment, the prevention of treatment-related morbidity and documentation of all long-term complications are especially important, so that a complete assessment of the risk of potential morbidity can be made.

Apprehension and anxiety about treatment failure can become a major psychologic problem in prolonged adjuvant treatment programs. Compliance with an extended course of adjuvant chemotherapy when there is no evidence of disease can often be difficult. If nurses recognize this conflict as a potential problem, they can prepare to assist patients to deal with any ambivalence they feel about taking the treatment and to make adaptations in their life-style that are compatible with a prolonged course of adjuvant therapy. In these situations, patient education must be reinforced with reassurance, encouragement, and support that help patients to reestablish a sense of control over their lives.

Ethical considerations for nurses in clinical research

There are general issues requiring consideration by all nurses and physicians involved in research, because ethical considerations are the foundation of every clinical trial. The balance between the need for better cancer treatment and the needs of a specific individual is crucial to a sound clinical trial. Furthermore, it is essential to differentiate between an individual's human rights and his personal needs. Protection of rights is essential, even when the needs of each individual cannot be completely met. Nurses in the research setting can provide invaluable assistance in ensuring that these rights are protected in clinical trials.

To be ethical, every clinical trial must ask a question of significant scientific and humanitarian value. Moreover, the need for performing the therapeutic experiment must justify the risk of discomfort or harm to study subjects. To ensure this justification, each research protocol must clearly articulate the scientific rationale, the ratio of potential benefits: risks, the safeguards to be used to protect subjects from injury, and very specific information about the proper execution of the study. The components of a research protocol are listed below:

1. Clear statement of the research question and the study objectives.
2. Clear description of scientific data supporting the specific research question to be tested (if a new drug to be evaluated, data on preclinical pharmacology and toxicology should be included).
3. Explicit criteria for eligibility and exclusion of patients.
4. The treatment plan including: randomization scheme, if two or more treatments are being compared; criteria for stratification by important variables.
5. Dose and schedule information: specific details about the dose, schedule, route, timing, and duration of each drug or treatment modality that is to be administered; dose-modification schedules specified by type of tissue toxicity (i.e., bone marrow depression, GI toxicity, neurotoxicity, etc.).
6. Evaluation criteria: description of all parameters to be evaluated for response and/or disease progression; definition of criteria for complete and partial response, stabilization, disease progression, and treatment failure; criteria for evaluation of performance status (Karnofsky rating or other scale).
7. Research parameters to be evaluated, with intervals clearly specified: clinical parameters; laboratory studies; diagnostic examinations (x-rays, radionuclide scans, CAT, etc.).
8. Statistical evaluation section.
9. Informed-consent document.
10. Proof of review and approval by a duly constituted investigational review board.

Nurses involved in clinical research have assumed major responsibilities for ensuring that all of these requirements are met and that any special requirements for nursing care and patient education are incorporated into the protocol during the design of the clinical trial.

Another ethical concern is informed consent. In the USA, informed consent, obtained without coercion, is a legal prerequisite for participation of human subjects in clinical trials. While legal responsibility for obtaining the informed consent rests with the primary physicians, it is a moral responsibility shared by all members of the research team (see Chapter 5). Moreover, each research patient must be adequately informed about the investigational nature of the clinical trial, because personal benefit cannot be guaranteed with assurance.

Because informed consent must be maintained to be valid, it is an ongoing process. Therefore, it is essential to consider the nurse's ethical responsibilities in clinical research within the framework of patient education. At the outset of any educational program, the nurse should assess the nature of the patient's previous health-care experiences, identify exactly what the patient knows, what he thinks that he needs to know or learn, and his level of anxiety. Only by identifying the patient's perceived needs can an educational program be planned that will involve the patient in the learning process. This point is crucial because learning is an active process that requires participation of both teacher and learner.

Education about any therapy should include information about immediate and long-term benefits as well as the adverse effects. By developing educational materials that help patients to understand why certain procedures and treatments will be initiated on their behalf, the nurse can assist patients to become truly informed and to become active participants in the treatment process. In one institution, the staff nurses on the oncology unit have devised a series of booklets that describe each of the diagnostic tests, their discomforts and/or side effects, and why the examinations are needed to plan or evaluate therapy. Each patient receives a booklet when the procedure is proposed. The patient is given time to review the booklet, formulate questions, and discuss the procedure with the nurse prior to giving written consent. Use of these booklets permits nurses to clarify information as needed and to ensure that the patient's consent is truly informed and voluntary.

Clinical skills

The state laws that govern the IV administration of investigational drugs by registered nurses vary because these functions were formerly considered areas of medical practice. To authorize nurses to assume these responsibilities, most states have adopted consensus statements, issued jointly by the state's medical society, nursing association, and hospital association, that describe the legal accountabilities and the liabilities that are shared by the physician and nurse.

Before allowing nurses to assume responsibility for the administration of chemotherapy, most employers require them to demonstrate a sophisticated level of knowledge in a written and practical examination about a variety of cancers, as well as the drugs, their mechanisms of action, normal dose ranges, routes of administration, and physiologic effects. To meet their professional standards, nurses have independently formalized training programs and developed and published standards of practice, educational requirements, quality-assurance programs, and evaluation criteria to ensure that nurses are qualified by knowledge and skills.

Legally, a nurse must have a signed and dated written order from a physician specifying the patient who is to be treated and the way that therapy is to be administered. Nurses are expected to verify the drug and the dosage and can be held negligent for errors in drug administration even if the physician made an error in writing the drug order. Therefore, the patient's record and the treatment protocol should be readily available so the nurse can verify that the drugs and dosages are correct. Since orders for many cancer chemotherapeutic agents are based on the patient's weight or body-surface area, the nurse should also have access to a nomogram to check dose calculations (Fig. 3–2). Calculations of dosage by body-surface area allows greater consistency in dosing, whether individuals are fat or thin.

Since chemotherapeutic agents have serious toxicities, liability is always a concern for the chemotherapy nurse. Should a malpractice suit be brought against a nurse, the following issues would be considered: (1) were the policies or guidelines of the state and/or employer on the IV administration of chemotherapy followed; (2) was the drug administered in a prudent and proper manner in accordance with the physician's orders; (3) was reasonable judgment exercised before and during the infusion (i.e., assessing patients for reactions and the venipuncture site for evidence of infiltration); (4) were appropriate actions undertaken to manage the reaction or extravasation; (5) was the physician informed promptly concerning the nature and severity of the reaction; (6) were the incident, objective findings, and all medical and nursing interventions documented in the medical record; and (7) were subsequent evaluations of the patient performed to assess the need for further medical or nursing intervention.

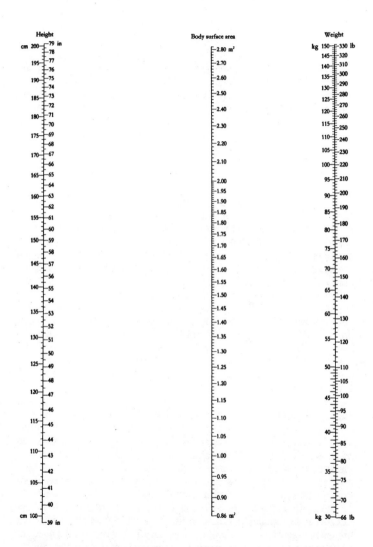

Figure 3–2. Nomogram for the determination of body surface area of adults from height and weight.

In general, a nurse will not be held liable for harm that results to a patient if the action is not deemed beyond the scope of the nurse's role as defined by legal or institutional policies, and if the nurse exercised good clinical judgment throughout the infusion (Table 3–2). If the nurse also consults a physician promptly when a problem occurs, initiates appropriate measures to manage the adverse effects, and documents objective findings and the therapeutic measures that were taken in the medical record, the legal requirements concerning safe and prudent practice will be fulfilled. The need for individual malpractice insurance must be based on a realistic assessment of the coverage provided by the nurse's employer.

Current trends in oncology

As oncology has become an established area of clinical specialization, the demand for sophisticated clinical services has grown. In response to this need, nurses have worked closely with oncologists to design and run well-organized inpatient and outpatient units so that clinical research can be successfully conducted in a diversity of clinical settings. This type of multidisciplinary collaboration has helped to establish the development of a collegial relationship between the nurse and physician as a standard of cancer nursing practice.

Role expansion in oncology nursing has also resulted in the development of adult and pediatric nurse-practitioner programs that provide advanced preparation and skills and enable nurses to assume responsibility for the overall management of selected cancer patients. Under the general supervision of an oncologist, nurse practitioners provide and coordinate the care of patients, within written guidelines, in the areas of chronic and continuing care, rehabilitation, and terminal care. Such nurses also order and administer cancer chemotherapy and manage patients who are receiving these drugs on well-established protocols. Nurse practitioners have also joined oncologists in clinical practice and have developed models for joint practice where roles and responsibilities for all aspects of patient care are shared. To ensure that the quality of care delivered in these and other programs is both consistent and high, new standards of care have been developed, implemented, and evaluated in clinical practice.

Integration of nurses into clinical research teams at research centers has served as a model for collaboration between cancer physicians and nurses in other settings. A variety of settings exists to meet the needs of specific communities for nursing expertise in cancer care and clinical research. Recognition of the importance of nursing's contributions to clinical research is demonstrated by the fact that a number of the national oncology cooperative groups not only support collaboration in medical research but also extend membership to nurses and offer financial support for role development, educational programs, and nurse-initiated research. Indeed, the full potential for nursing role development and expansion in oncology is only just beginning to emerge. Nurses are identifying new practice roles in epidemiology, programs for screening and early detection, continuing care, public education, home care, and the terminal phases of illness.

Dealing with the complications of cancer therapy has always been an area of special concern for the clinical research nurse. In recent years, there has been emphasis on nurse-initiated research, and a number of studies aimed at minimizing or preventing drug-related side effects have been performed.

One area of concern has been the prevention of complications related to the IV administration of chemotherapy. The problem of managing inadvertent extravasation of potent tissue vesicants has generated several descriptive studies evaluating the use of corticosteroids and/or sodium bicarbonate as therapeutic measures to decrease local tissue damage. While controlled studies of the various interventions that have been proposed are needed to establish their efficacy, these descriptive studies suggest that prompt nursing intervention may decrease local tissue damage.

As the use of central venous, intra-arterial, intraperitoneal, and other indwelling catheters and infusion pumps for cancer chemotherapy has become more widespread, nurses have become involved in studies designed to develop and evaluate structured educational programs that will enable patients to maintain these indwelling catheters successfully for prolonged periods without infectious complications and other morbidity. With patient and family education by nurses, many cancer patients who would have otherwise remained hospitalized are now, with indwelling catheters and infusion pumps, managed safely as outpatients and can be given parenteral nutrition, antibiotics, and cancer chemotherapy at home. Concern about the frequent need to remove central venous catheters that have become occluded with blood clots has generated nurse-initiated studies demonstrating that fibrinolytic enzymes can be used safely and effectively as declotting agents, thus preserving many patients from the need for premature catheter removal and reinsertion.

Concern about the psychologic effect of alopecia has stimulated nurses to investigate the prevention of hair loss by decreasing blood flow to the scalp with external compression or vasoconstriction using scalp ischemia or hypothermia. Several studies have indicated that protection can be obtained with both techniques. Important variables affecting the amount of protection that can be achieved can include the

TABLE 3-2

General Procedures for IV Chemotherapy

Factor	Intervention
Patient preparation	Verify patient's identity.
	Check patient's clinical status, hematologic parameters, and blood chemistries for significant abnormalities that would influence drug dosage.
	Verify that drugs and drug dosages are correct.
	Prepare patient for venipuncture and drug administration by: positioning patient for comfort and ease in venipuncture; removing or loosening tight-fitting clothing and jewelry; discussing any special precautions that must be taken, probable side effects, and ways to manage toxic effects of treatment; administering premedications (antiemetics, antihistamines, etc.); preparing and setting aside emergency drugs for unexpected anaphylactic reactions and/or extravasation of potent tissue vesicants.
	Verify identity of drug and correctness of drug dose. Syringes or IV solution bottles should be clearly labeled with the patient's name and identification number.
Drug administration	Apply tourniquet and thoroughly examine arms to identify suitable veins, evaluating each for patency.
	Perform venipuncture using sterile technique, in the most distal portion of a suitable vein. Scalp-vein needles are generally used.
	Infuse nonirritating sterile solution.
	Check area around venipuncture site for evidence of extravasation of infusate into SC tissues and remove needle if there is any evidence of infiltration (blanching, swelling).

	Tape wings of scalp-vein needle securely in place without obscuring area above the site of venipuncture so the site can be monitored for evidence of extravasation during the infusion. Infuse drug as specified in written order, checking throughout the infusion to make sure that the drug is infusing properly.
Drug infusion	Monitor patient during drug administration for: change in vital signs, complaints of pain, shortness of breath, etc.; evidence of extravasation; speed of infusion (if specified in drug order or known to be an important factor). If extravasation occurs, document all pertinent facts in the medical record, notify the physician, and treat the extravasation as indicated with an effective antidote (if the agent is a tissue vesicant).
Postinfusion care	After drug infusion is complete, infuse nonirritating solution for a brief "flush" period to ensure that none of the drug remains in the tubing or needle. Remove IV needle if further hydration and special precautions are not warranted. Instruct patient to apply pressure to site to prevent hematoma formation. Apply Band-Aid or other covering after bleeding has ceased.

Adapted from Knobf, M. K. Intravenous therapy guidelines for oncology practice. *Oncology Nursing Forum* (Spring 1982). p. 30–34.

specific drug and dosage, drug clearance from the plasma, the presence or absence of hepatic metastases, and age. Additional studies by nurses of alopecia have been geared toward assessing the effects of hair loss on body image and social interactions to determine whether supportive nursing interventions can play a role in successful adaptation to hair loss.

Studies to determine whether systematic nursing intervention can decrease the oral complications of chemotherapy have clearly demonstrated that patients who receive systematic programs of oral care, according to well-defined guidelines, develop significantly less stomatitis and fewer infectious complications. Further research to develop effective protocols of oral care that patients find tolerable can make an enormous contribution to cancer care because oral complications often necessitate the interruption of chemotherapy, severely compromise the nutritional and fluid intake of patients, and lead to serious local and systemic infections in immunocompromised and pancytopenic patients.

In an attempt to identify important variables that affect the severity of nausea and vomiting, several nurse investigators have found that a significant proportion of patients experience symptoms during the 24-hr period preceding treatment, indicating that a psychologic component, either conditioned or anticipatory, may play an important role in this syndrome. These findings have confirmed a clinical impression held by many oncology nurses and have served to stimulate research to evaluate adequacy of current antiemetic regimens and the value of relaxation and diversionary techniques in the management of nausea and vomiting. Psychologic research has indicated that these techniques can be used successfully to relieve many physiologic changes associated with severe stress. Use of relaxation and diversionary techniques for pain control, management of nausea, and reduction of anxiety represents an innovative approach by nurses to modify these responses to stressful experiences.

Clinical specialization in cancer research has significantly increased the nurse's involvement in clinical trials and has stimulated research by nurses on issues of concern in nursing practice. As members of research teams, nurses have incorporated nursing-care considerations into investigational protocols and overall treatment plans for research patients. Development of expanded nursing roles has served as a stimulus for the development and evaluation of teaching tools and structured educational programs for patients. The role of the clinical research nurse has enabled nurses to develop great sophistication with regard to the design, performance, and evaluation of clinical research and to begin to perform independent studies on the efficacy of nursing interventions in cancer care.

Bibliography

1. Benoliel, J. Q. The historical development of cancer nursing research in the United States. *Cancer Nursing* (August 1983). 261–268.

   Traces the development of cancer nursing research from the start of the 20th century. Describes the growth of nursing research in general and specifically as a function of the development of oncology nursing as a specialty.

2. Dorr, R., and W. Fritz. Cancer Chemotherapy Handbook. Elsevier North-Holland, Inc., New York. 1980.

   Provides a detailed discussion of the pharmacology of antineoplastic agents by class and "drug data sheets" for each agent. Includes brief sections on organ toxicity as well as ethical and legal implications.

3. Hilkemeyer, R. A historical perspective in cancer nursing. *Oncology Nursing Forum* (Spring 1982). 47–56.

   A personal account of the tremendous changes experienced in the practice of cancer nursing.

4. Hubbard, S. M., and M. G. Donehower. The nurse in a cancer research setting. *Seminars in Oncology* (March 1980). 9–18.

   In one of several articles in this issue on "The Nurse Oncologist," the authors describe the evolution of cancer nursing research during the first decades of clinical drug trials. The role is explained according to responsibilities and the physician/nurse/patient relationship.

5. Hubbard, S. M. Chemotherapy and the cancer nurse. *In* Cancer Nursing, L. B. Marino, editor. C. V. Mosby Co., St. Louis. 1981.

   Describes the role of the nurse caring for persons receiving chemotherapy. Includes explanations of the process of clinical drug trials and the implications for nursing care.

6. Hubbard, S. M. Clinical research and cancer nursing. *Oncology Nursing Forum* (Fall 1981). 17–23.

   An extensive overview of the evolution of nursing research in the field of cancer including a review of the literature.

7. Hubbard, S. M., and C. Seipp. Administration of cancer treatments: practical guide for physicians and oncology nurses. *In* DeVita, V. T., S. Hellman, and S. A. Rosenberg, editors. Cancer: Principles and Practice of Oncology. J. B. Lippincott Co., Philadelphia. 1982.

   Within the context of a large oncology textbook, this chapter focuses on practical information related to the care of patients receiving chemotherapy, radiation therapy, or surgery for cancer.

8. Knobf, M. K. Intravenous therapy guidelines for oncology practice. *Oncology Nursing Forum* (Spring 1982). 30–34.

   A practical article that presents guidelines for care of patients requiring IV therapy. Focuses on the prevention of infection and phlebitis from IV devices.

9. Knobf, M. K., D. S. Fischer, and D. Welch-McCaffrey. Cancer Chemotherapy: Treatment and Care. G. K. Hall & Co., Boston. 1984.

   A practical handbook that includes brief descriptions of currently used chemotherapeutic agents in tabular form. Each drug is explained according to its mechanism of action, indications, metabolism, dose and route of administration, toxicity, preparation, and storage. Text also provides brief sections on management of common side effects.

10. Miller, S. A. The role of the oncology nurse. *In* Carter, S. K., E. Glatstein, and R. B. Livingston. Principles of Cancer Treatment. McGraw-Hill Book Co., New York. 1982.

    Presents the roles of the oncology nurse involved in surgery, radiation therapy, chemotherapy, and immunotherapy. Stresses necessary areas of expertise for each modality as well as general areas of patient education and rehabilitation.

CHAPTER 4

PREVENTION AND EARLY DETECTION*

Bonny Libbey Johnson

Standard: The client and family possess adequate information about cancer prevention and detection.

Outcome criteria: The client and family
1. recognize factors that place an individual at risk and may lead to cancer, such as use of tobacco, improper nutrition, and immunosuppressive agents.
2. state cancer's warning signs.
3. identify a plan for seeking health care assistance whenever any alteration in health status occurs.
4. describe applicable cancer self-detection measures.

Prevention and early detection are two distinct but related approaches to reducing the morbidity and mortality of cancer. Whether any disease can be *prevented* depends upon the degree of knowledge about and control over the cause, as well as upon adequate access to the population at risk. *Early detection* is of paramount importance when the cause is not known or cannot be controlled and when the course of disease may be altered by early treatment, during an asymptomatic state. Therefore, programs for prevention and early detection are designed for populations or individuals at risk for or with cancer who are not yet symptomatic.

---

*The standards and outcome criteria that appear at the beginning of Chapters 4 through 13 are reprinted with permission from the Oncology Nursing Society Clinical Practice Committee. *Outcome Standards for Nursing Practice.* American Nurses' Association, Kansas City, Mo. 1979.

Conceptual considerations

The principal role of the nurse as a provider of information in the prevention and early detection of cancer requires a basic understanding of the etiology and epidemiology of the disease. In addition, an understanding of the motivations for individual health-seeking behaviors and of the appropriate and available health-care services will ensure effective management.

The concept of disease prevention has been classified according to three levels, focusing on health maintenance rather than disease cure. These levels are described as follows:

Primary prevention.   Risk of cancer is reduced or eliminated by avoidance of causative agents (e.g., cigarettes) or by removal of target organ (e.g., rectal polyps).

Secondary prevention.   The natural course of disease is favorably altered by early detection and effective and prompt treatment (e.g., breast self-examination).

Tertiary prevention.   The morbidity of cancer is reduced by prompt and effective antitumor treatment, symptom control, and rehabilitation.

The focus of this chapter is on primary and secondary prevention. The remaining chapters aim to describe the nursing component of tertiary prevention.

Epidemiologic considerations

Current American Cancer Society (ACS) statistics for the incidence of cancer by site are shown in Table 4–1. Such statistics are important for determining the prevailing tumor types to target for public education and screening programs and also show changes in incidence, which may reflect alterations in life-styles or changes in environmental factors related to cancer causation.

On the basis of what is currently known or suspected to cause cancer in the USA and the overall incidence of specific tumor types, it is estimated that up to 80% of cancers are associated with environmental factors. The degree to which these factors influence the incidence of cancer is reflected in Figure 4–1. It is on the basis of these estimates that the National Cancer Institute (NCI) has initiated a Cancer Prevention Awareness Program. Seven well-defined risk factors have been selected as major areas for primary prevention programs because they: (1) affect a high percentage of Americans, (2) pose a substantial threat to health, and (3) are amenable to reduction or control by individuals at risk. These factors are: diet, tobacco, viruses, occupational exposures, alcohol, radiation, and estrogens.

TABLE 4-1
Estimated New Cases and Deaths for Major Sites of Cancer—1984

Site	Number of cases	Deaths
Lung	139,000	121,000
Colon/rectum	130,000	59,400
Breast	115,900	37,600
Prostate	76,000	25,000
Urinary	57,100	19,400
Uterus	55,000	9,700
Oral	27,500	9,350
Pancreas	25,100	23,000
Leukemia	24,400	16,700
Ovary	18,300	11,500
Skin, melanoma	17,700	7,400*

*Melanoma 5,500, other skin 1,900.
Reprinted with permission from Cancer Facts and Figures, 1984. American Cancer Society, Inc. New York. 1983.

Considerations in prevention

Certain of these factors are defined as either initiators or promotors (*see* Chapter 1). An **initiator**, such as cigarette smoke or radiation, causes irreversible cellular damage and potential malignant change. A **promotor** is believed to stimulate malignant transformation following the effect of an initiator. Alcohol, when combined with tobacco use, appears to be such a promoting factor in the causation of head/neck cancers. This knowledge is useful in defining appropriate preventive strategies aimed at reducing or eliminating exposure to promotors, because their effect is reversible. Table 4-2 summarizes known or suspected risk factors according to the body site most affected. The most common types of cancer appear to be strongly related to external, and therefore controllable, risk factors.

The role of **dietary deficiency or excess** in cancer causation is considered a risk factor in ~35% of all cancers. To date, preventive programs focus on the relationship between high-fat, low-fiber diet and cancers of the GI tract. Of note is an apparent positive effect of vitamins A and C in preventing cancer. The excessive use of **alcohol** in the diet is associated with an increased risk for cancers of the head and neck, liver, and GI tract. Alcohol is believed to act as a promotor in causing cancer, enhancing the carcinogenic effect of smoking, in particular.

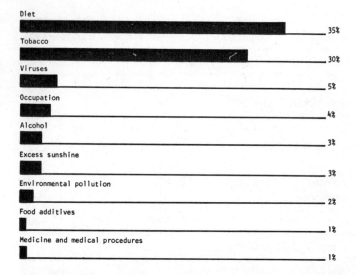

Figure 4–1. Percentage* of cancer cases attributable to various risk factors. *Average of varying estimates available from the literature. *Adapted from* Office of Cancer Communications. Cancer Prevention: A Program to Inform the Public about Cancer Risk and Risk Reduction. National Cancer Institute, Bethesda, Md. January 1984.

According to ACS statistics, the use of **tobacco** in our society is responsible for 75% of lung cancer cases and is implicated in cancers of the head and neck, esophagus, pancreas, and bladder, as well. Cigarettes account for 30% of all cancer deaths, or ~150,000 people/yr. While a slight decline in the number of adult smokers is evident, ⅓ of the US adult population smokes, and, according to the US Office on Smoking and Health, the average smoker smokes more heavily. The risk for smoking-related cancer increases with number of years smoking, number of cigarettes, and depth of inhalation. Changing to low-tar/nicotine cigarettes appears to reduce the risk for cancer only slightly. The synergistic carcinogenic effect of cigarettes and alcohol, radiation, or occupational agents (e.g., asbestos) compounds the risk.

Viruses are associated with several types of cancer: primary hepatocellular carcinoma, Burkitt's lymphoma, nasopharyngeal carcinoma, Hodgkin's disease, Kaposi's sarcoma, cancers of the cervix and genital organs, leukemias, and lymphomas. The strength of the

TABLE 4–2

Major Cancer Risk Factors Amenable to Primary Prevention*

Factor	Site of cancer
Diet: ↑fat; ↓fiber; ↓vitamins A and C	Oral cavity, pharynx, esophagus, colon/rectum
Tobacco	Lung, oral cavity, pharynx, larynx, esophagus, kidney, bladder
Viruses	
Hepatitis B	Liver
Epstein-Barr	Nose/throat, Burkitt's lymphoma
Herpes simplex II	Cervix
Occupational hazards	
Asbestos	Lung
Chromate	Lung
Nickel, uranium	Lung
Alcohol	Oral cavity, pharynx, larynx, esophagus, liver, pancreas, colon/rectum, stomach, breast (suspected), melanoma (suspected)
Radiation	
↑dose	Leukemia, thyroid, lung, breast, stomach, bone, liver
↓dose (ultraviolet light, x-rays)	Skin, site exposed to x-rays (dental, chest x-rays)
Estrogens	Uterine (especially endometrium), cervix
Premalignant conditions	
Cervical dysplasia	Cervix
Rectal polyps	Colon/rectum
Leukoplakia	Skin, oropharynx, bladder

*In order of suspected or known degree of risk.

viral association and the question of causality varies among tumor types. The presence of certain cofactors (i.e., aflatoxin, alcohol, infection) may be necessary for cancer to result. For example, the hepatitis B virus in human serum is believed to precede and lead to a high incidence of hepatocellular carcinoma; this association becomes even stronger when aflatoxin or chronic alcohol intake is a factor.

The Epstein-Barr virus (EBV), a DNA virus of the herpes group, infects B lymphocytes and, perhaps due to a genetic defect, may progress to Burkitt's lymphoma, Hodgkin's disease, or nasopharyngeal carcinoma. EBV is endemic in Africa, where the incidence of related tumors is high.

The infectious etiology for cervical cancer is believed to involve more than one viral agent. Herpes simplex virus II and cytomegalovirus are two infections that show a strong association. Both may be transmitted by sexual contact.

Estrogens have been reported to induce cancer in women when used (1) as replacement therapy after menopause (endometrial cancer); (2) for oral contraception (rare benign liver tumors); and (3) to prevent threatened abortion (clear cell adenocarcinoma of the vagina and cervix in daughters). Of particular note is the synthetic estrogen, diethylstilbesterol (DES), which is used for both (1) and (3). The benefit derived from the therapeutic use of estrogens for each individual must be weighed against her risk for developing cancer. Since the risk appears to be directly related to the dose of drug and duration of therapy, shorter courses with low doses of estrogen may be recommended.

[A detailed discussion of **chemical** and **radiation** carcinogenesis is provided in Chapter 1. Table 4–7 incorporates these risk factors into a program of prevention.]

Considerations in early detection

The concept of early detection may be applied in two ways: on an individual basis for a person at risk for specific reasons, or as the basis for mass screening of a population at risk. In either case, the underlying assumption is that the smaller the tumor is when diagnosed, the better the chance for effective treatment.

The detection of cancers early relies on two conditions: the existence of a premalignant, or detectable preclinical phase (DPCP), and the availability of appropriate tests for detection.

Cancers theoretically progress from a low to a high degree of anaplasia with metastatic potential (*see* Chapter 1). If a specific cancer demonstrates a defined, prolonged premalignant state, the chance for early detection and cure is maximized. The time during which a premalignant or malignant tumor exists prior to the onset of symptoms, or the DPCP, must be sufficient to allow purposeful diagnostic intervention. In addition, there must be available tests that can detect the tumor during the preclinical phase, as well as treatments that will alter the course of disease even before symptoms occur.

Tests for early detection of cancer are judged according to their sensitivity and specificity for a particular tumor type. Briefly stated, test **sensitivity** is reflected by the percentage of people who test positive for the disease in question. Test **specificity** refers to the percentage of people who are without the disease, who test negative. Sensitivity and specificity are closely interrelated concepts. For example, a test that has a 100% sensitivity is capable of detecting everyone who has the disease in question (no false positives). A test that is 100% specific will be negative for everyone without the disease (no false negatives). In reality, tests currently available for the early detection of cancer are neither 100% sensitive nor 100% specific, and they are affected by (1) the test itself, and (2) factors related to its application and interpretation. In addition to a high degree of sensitivity and specificity, the optimal screening test for early detection is convenient for most people, comfortable, low-cost, and without side effects. In order for any program to be well received, a system for immediate reporting of results and for follow-up must be established.

Whereas preventive programs are based upon controllable risk factors, individual programs for early detection target those at risk by virtue of both controllable and uncontrollable factors. Examples of uncontrollable risk factors and associated tumors are listed in Table 4–3.

Assessment

Prevention. An understanding of the factors that place people at risk for cancer allows the nurse to focus a preventive approach on those factors that an individual may avoid or decrease exposure to. This knowledge is combined with an assessment of the psychologic and environmental factors that guide each person's health-related behaviors. Rosenstock's Health Belief Model provides a useful framework for an assessment of a person's risk for cancer and his ability to alter that risk by behavioral change. The model briefly states that a person's health behaviors are governed by: (1) knowledge of personal susceptibility to an illness, (2) perception that the risk is severe, and (3) belief that any behavior will positively alter that risk.

These personal factors are acted upon by external, or environmental, factors such as: (1) accessibility/availability of health-care service, (2) family/peer support, (3) cost of service, and (4) logistical concerns (time, transportation, work schedule).

TABLE 4–3

Major Cancer Risk Factors Amenable to Secondary Prevention

Factor	Cancer
Endocrinopathies	
Infertility	Endometrium
Obesity	Breast, endometrium
Diabetes	Breast, endometrium
Family history of cancer	Lung, breast, thyroid
Nulliparity or late first pregnancy	Breast
Preexisting disease	
Xeroderma pigmentosum	Skin
Fibrocystic disease of the breast	Breast
Ulcerative colitis	Colon
Bloom's syndrome	Leukemia
Fanconi's syndrome	Leukemia
Mongolism	Leukemia

The NCI conducted a survey of the American public in 1983 to assess basic knowledge of risk factors and attitudes toward cancer prevention. The results show that 46% of the population surveyed believe "there is not much a person can do to prevent cancer" and 48% believe that "everything can cause cancer." It is reasonable to surmise that lack of knowledge about specific risk factors and a sense of helplessness in reducing risk will not result in an attempt to change current unhealthful behaviors (e.g., cigarette smoking, alcohol abuse, excessive sun exposure). Thus, the NCI's Cancer Prevention Awareness Program emphasizes public education about known risk factors and about methods of risk reduction.

In summary, assessment of the individual's ability to benefit from a primary prevention or risk-reduction program must include the following:

1. Knowledge base of risk factors.
2. Attitude toward cancer.
3. Knowledge of risk reduction techniques.
4. Motivation for change.

Early detection. Assessment is an integral part of any program of secondary prevention. Only when an adequate base-line assessment reveals specific risk factors can an appropriate plan be made for ongoing diagnostic examination.

On an individual basis, the standard history and physical examination provides a comprehensive format for early detection of cancer. Emphasis is placed on the following areas:

1. History:
   A. Family: family history of cancer.
   B. Social: cigarettes, alcohol use, sexual history.
   C. Occupational: exposure to chemicals, radiation, inhalants.
   D. Past medical: previous malignancy.
   E. Medications: hormone replacement(DES), cytotoxic agents.
2. Review of systems:
   A. Pulmonary: cough, pain, dyspnea, hemoptysis.
   B. GI: change in bowel habits, bleeding.
   C. Breast: nipple discharge, masses.
   D. Gynecological: vaginal discharge, dyspareunia, unusual bleeding.
   E. Skin: slow-healing sore, changing mole.
   F. Oropharynx: hoarseness >1 wk, abnormal bleeding, or pain.
3. Physical examination:
   A. Lymphadenopathy.
   B. Suspicious moles.
   C. Breast mass.
   D. Prostatic enlargement.
   E. Thyroid mass.
   F. Oral leukoplakia.

Of note is an increased risk for second tumors recognized in persons with cancer (Table 4–4). Awareness of this risk may assist the examiner in the physical examination. A summary of pertinent data derived from the history and physical examination as they relate to sites of cancer is presented in Table 4–5.

Diagnostic tests: Secondary prevention, or early detection, is facilitated by the extent to which laboratory or radiologic tests result in a correct diagnosis. Those used most commonly in the detection of cancer are presented in Table 4–6.

The term tumor markers refers to those substances (antigens, enzymes, proteins, hormones) that are secreted in response to or by tumors and can be detected in the bloodstream. For the most part tumor marker tests are extremely sensitive, because tumor marker activity occurs prior to signs and symptoms; and they are specific for the particular tumor type. The most sensitive and specific of the markers is the beta subunit of **human chorionic gonadotropin (HCG)** secreted by malignant trophoblastic disease (choriocarcinoma) and some germ-cell testicular tumors. **Carcinoembryonic antigen (CEA)** is less specific, occurring with some tumors of the colon, breast, and

TABLE 4-4
Summary of Second Cancers Following Initial Cancer

Sex	Initial cancer	Second cancer
Female	Breast	Buccal cavity Pharynx Breast Lung Ovary Corpus uteri Leukemia
	Cervix	Buccal cavity Pharynx Lung Bladder
Male	Lip and mouth	Buccal cavity Skin Lung Pharynx
	Pharynx	Esophagus Lung Prostate
	Salivary	Lung Prostate

Reprinted with permission from Newell, G. R. Cancer: etiology and prevention. *In* Nixon, D. W. Diagnosis and Management of Cancer. Addison-Wesley Publishing Co., Inc., Menlo Park, Calif. 1982. p. 37.

lung, and usually signifies a tumor burden of $>10^8$ cells. **Acid phosphatase** elevations demonstrate more advanced cancer of the prostate, and it is therefore more useful as an indicator of response to antitumor therapy than in diagnosis. Likewise, radioimmunoassay of α-fetoprotein (**AFP**) may be useful in the diagnosis of hepatoma, embryonal carcinoma, or liver metastases.

In most instances, the diagnosis of cancer is made as a result of a combination of tests and physical findings. The tests listed in Table 4-6 are specific but not limited to the diagnosis of cancer. Definitive diagnosis is made only by pathological examination of malignant cells (**cytology**) or tissue (**biopsy**) (*see* Chapter 2).

TABLE 4–5

*Major Risk Factors and Common Signs and Symptoms
for Common Cancers*

Type of cancer	Risk factors, signs, and symptoms
Colon/rectum	History of rectal polyps. Rectal polyps run in family. History of ulcerative colitis. Aged 40+. Blood in stool.
Lung	Heavy cigarette-smoker > age 50. Started cigarette-smoking at age 15 or before. Smoker working with or near asbestos.
Uterine/endometrial	Late menopause (> age 55). Diabetes, high BP, and overweight. Aged 50+. Unusual bleeding or discharge.
Uterine/cervical	Frequent sex in early teens or with many partners. Poor socioeconomic background. Poor care during or following pregnancy. Unusual bleeding or discharge.
Breast	History of breast cancer. Close relatives with history of breast cancer. Never had children; first child after age 30. Aged 35+; especially > age 50. Lump or nipple discharge.
Skin	Excessive exposure to sun. Fair complexion. Work with coal tar, pitch, or creosote.
Oral	Heavy smoker and drinker. Poor oral hygiene.
Ovarian	History of ovarian cancer among close relatives. Never had children. Aged 50+.
Prostate	Aged 60+. Difficulty in urinating.
Stomach	History of stomach cancer among close relatives. Diet heavy in smoked, pickled, or salted foods.

Reprinted with permission from Cancer Facts and Figures, 1980. American Cancer Society, Inc., New York. 1980.

TABLE 4-6
Special Diagnostic Tests

Test	Purpose	Comments
Tumor markers		
CEA	Cancers of the colon, breast, lung	High levels correlate with high tumor burden.
AFP	Hepatoma	Used to monitor treatment response. Return to normal indicates cure.
HCG/AFP	Malignant trophoblastic disease, cancer of the testes	
Acid phosphatase	Cancer of the prostate	May be used to monitor response to treatment or recurrence.
Estrogen/progesterone receptors	Cancer of the breast	Defines certain tumors that may be more responsive to hormonal therapy.
X-rays		
Mammography	Breast cancer	Average radiation exposure = 0.1–0.7 rads.
Lymphangiography	Lymph node involvement especially Hodgkin's disease lymphoma, cancer of the testes	Blue dye, injected into lymphatic channel at great toe, visualizes abdominal lymph nodes.

Radionuclide scan	Shows function and size of specific organ (brain, bone, liver, spleen, kidney)	Used for staging because ↑ sensitivity, ↓ specificity. Radioisotope injected peripherally.
Ultrasound	Visualizes structural changes, mass (stomach, pancreas, kidney, uterus, ovary)	Uses high-frequency sound waves.
Computed axial tomography CAT, CT, ACTA	Cross-section images of internal structures	X-ray ± contrast dye; ↑ specificity, especially brain tumors.
Microscopic examination Pap smear	Cancer of the cervix or uterus	Cytological examination of cells obtained by swab of vagina, endocervical canal, and exocervix.
Bone-marrow aspirate	Tumor involvement, especially by leukemia or lymphoma	Needle aspirate of marrow from iliac crest or sternum.
Sputum cytology	Bronchogenic cancer	
Stool guaiac	Cancer of the colon/rectum	Patient must eat meat-free, vitamin-C-free, high-fiber diet for 2 days, then submit 2 samples on each of 3 consecutive days.

AFP, α-fetoprotein; CEA, carcinoembryonic antigen; HCG, human chorionic gonadotropin.

Management

Prevention.   A protocol for the preventive management of persons at risk for cancer is provided in Table 4–7. The primary role of health-care providers must be to educate the public at large (e.g., the NCI Cancer Prevention Awareness Program) as well as individual consumers of health care. Coordination with existing organizations, such as the ACS, the American Lung Association, and the NCI Office of Communications, will result in maximum audience participation. Collaboration with various professionals is necessary to provide effective psychological support and counseling, nutritional guidance, surgical intervention, and/or medical follow-up.

Early detection.   Early detection programs are established with the goal of finding cancer as early as possible. Two different approaches are used to meet this goal: (1) **case-finding**, in which an individual at risk is closely assessed and monitored (e.g., person with a family history of colorectal cancer), and (2) **screening**, whereby an asymptomatic population is tested to define who may have disease and who probably does not. Both programs require: (1) knowledge of high-risk patients, and (2) available tests that are safe, effective, and affordable.

Case-finding: Early detection programs prescribed for specific individuals at risk usually occur in outpatient settings, where a one-to-one relationship between care-giver and patient allows greater communication, better patient adherence, and close follow-up. Therefore, the tests used can be more complex and the benefits/risks more carefully explained than is possible in mass screening programs.

Procedures that involve active patient participation require teaching and follow-up evaluation. Two examples are breast self-examination (BSE) and testicular self-examination (TSE).

Figure 4–2 demonstrates the 3-step process of BSE recommended by the ACS. Position changes facilitate complete assessment of the breast by displacing normal breast tissue around any possible masses. Gentle palpation while showering eliminates extra movement of the breast by friction. Patients are instructed to perform BSE monthly 1 wk after menses, or if postmenopausal, at the same time each month.

TSE is especially indicated for men aged 20 to 35, for men whose testes never descended or descended into the scrotal sac after age 6, and for men with a family history of testicular cancer. Young men should be taught to examine each testicle with both hands, gently rolling the sac between the thumb and fingers, feeling for a small lump.

Implicit in any self-examination procedure is that the individual be instructed to call the appropriate health-care-giver if an abnormality is suspected or detected.

The ACS has recommended guidelines for early detection of cancer in asymptomatic persons (Table 4–8). They emphasize that these are not appropriate as a mass-screening program, since the risk/benefit ratio is not yet established. The guidelines are based on (1) research demonstrating the effectiveness of each procedure for smaller samples of patients, and (2) the known natural history of the most common tumor types. An attempt is made to make the cost incurred commensurate with the benefit expected.

Screening: Cancers amenable to cost-effective public screening programs are those that (1) cause significant morbidity and mortality, (2) have a prolonged DPCP, and (3) may be detected by tests that are safe and low-cost. The higher the yield of positive results from any one screening test, the more effective the program is considered to be.

To date, cancers of the cervix, breast, and colon/rectum have been shown to be amenable to screening programs. Studies have been undertaken to demonstrate the role of screening for cancers of the lung, prostate, head/neck, testis, bladder, stomach, and for melanoma.

The following major tumor types are described in order to further explain specific screening programs and reasons for their success or failure.

Cervical cancer.   There is a subtle but important distinction between prevention and early detection of this disease with the use of the Pap smear. The Pap smear allows **prevention** of invasive disease by detecting cervical dysplasia or cervical intraepithelial neoplasia (CIN), a premalignant condition. The Pap smear is also critically important in the **early detection** of carcinoma in situ (CIS), which carries a 100% 5-yr survival rate when treated surgically. Progression of CIS to invasive carcinoma of the cervix (ICC) with involvement of local or regional tissues carries 79% and 45% average rates of 5-yr survival respectively. Because CIS may last for years before progressing to ICC and because spontaneous regression can occur, close monitoring with repeated Pap smears will assist the physician in understanding the natural course of each patient's disease.

Breast cancer.   One out of 11 American women will develop breast cancer during her lifetime, accounting for 115,000 new cases/yr. The principle tests available for the early detection of breast cancer are BSE, physical examination, and mammography. A survey of American women by the ACS revealed that 35% perform BSE monthly, though the impact of this statistic on early diagnosis is not known. The role of screening remains unclear, because the risk factors for developing breast cancer are not fully understood. In a large prospective study of American women carried out by the ACS to determine the significance of several suspected risk factors, ⅔ of the breast cancer cases could not be explained on the basis of these factors.

TABLE 4-7

Nursing Protocol for the Preventive Management of Persons at Risk for Cancer

Factor*	Intervention
Diet	Provide nutritional consultation for balanced diet; vitamins A and C, low fat, high fiber. Individualize diet according to general health status. Assist maintenance of ideal body weight.
Tobacco	Educate: prevent youths from starting; motivate smokers to take active role in quitting. Counsel: multicomponent plan under professional guidance; achieve intolerance by smoking to excess; low tar/nicotine cigarettes; nicotine chewing gum; cold turkey. Provide follow-up support; maintain attitude of experimentation; individualize plans as needed; enlist support of family/friends. Decrease cues to smoke: encourage nonsmoking areas in public places or workplace; run a media campaign; act as a role model by not smoking. Use outside resources: NCI Office of Cancer Communications (physician's kit; "Helping Smokers Quit"); ACS, ALA; self-help groups (Smokenders, Seventh-Day Adventists).
Viruses	Immunize against infecting agent, such as hepatitis B vaccine. Educate: avoid exposure to venereal disease: avoid promiscuity; use barrier contraceptive; improved general hygiene.
Occupational hazards	Provide public education to inform persons at risk about chemicals, dusts, radiation. Use masks or respirators when appropriate. Maintain close monitoring of persons at risk.
Alcohol	Educate: encourage moderate consumption; promote cessation if exposed to (1) upper respiratory tract carcinogens, (2) hepatitis B surface antigen. Counsel; obtain psychologic consultation for behavioral modifications; use self-help groups (AA).

Radiation	Educate: avoid unnecessary x-ray tests; avoid excess sun exposure: minimize time exposed to midday sun; use sunscreens as needed (fair-skinned need sun protection factor of 8–15); take extra caution with sun exposure while on sensitizing drugs (e.g., tetracycline).
Estrogens	Educate: avoid prolonged use of exogenous estrogens (DES). Maintain close monitoring of persons exposed to DES.
Premalignant condition	
Large-bowel polyps	Suggest surgical consultation for possible removal. Provide follow-up: annual stool guaiac; sigmoidoscopy q 2–3 yr.
Cervical dysplasia	Repeat Pap smears to confirm. Advise colposcopy with biopsy if necessary. Refer for surgical treatment depending on extent of lesion: cryosurgery; conization; hysterectomy.

*Ordered according to degree of risk.
AA, Alcoholics Anonymous; ACS, American Cancer Society; ALA, American Lung Association; DES, diethylstilbesterol; NCI, National Cancer Institute.

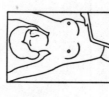

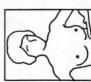

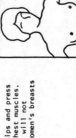

1: IN THE SHOWER

Examine breasts during bath or shower; hands glide easier over wet skin. Fingers flat, move gently over every part of each breast. Use right hand to examine left breast, left hand for right breast. Check for any lump, hard knot or thickening.

2: BEFORE A MIRROR

Inspect breasts with arms at sides. Next, raise arms high overhead. Look for any changes in contour of each breast, a swelling, dimpling of skin or changes in the nipple.

Then, rest palms on hips and press down firmly to flex chest muscles. Left and right breast will not exactly match - few women's breasts do.

3: LYING DOWN

To examine right breast, put a pillow or folded towel under right shoulder. Place right hand behind head - this distributes breast tissue more evenly on the chest. With left hand, fingers flat, press gently in small circular motions around an imaginary clock face. Begin at outermost top of right breast for 12 o'clock, then move to 1 o'clock, and so on around the circle back to 12. A ridge of firm tissue in the lower curve of each breast is normal. Then move in an inch, toward the nipple, keep circling to examine every part of breast, including nipple. This requires at least three more circles.

Now slowly repeat procedure on left breast with a pillow under left shoulder and left hand behind head. Notice how breast structure feels.

Finally, squeeze the nipple of each breast gently between thumb and index finger. Any discharge, clear or bloody, should be reported to physician immediately.

Figure 4-2.   Breast self-examination. *Reprinted with permission from American Cancer Society, Inc., New York. 1977.*

TABLE 4-8

*Protocol for the Early Detection of Cancer
in Asymptomatic Persons*

Test or procedure	Sex	Age (*yr*)	Frequency
Sigmoidoscopy	M & F	>50	every 3–5 yr after 2 negative exams 1 yr apart
Stool guaiac slide test	M & F	>50	every yr
Digital rectal examination	M & F	>40	every yr
Pap test	F	20–65; <20 if sexually active	at least every 3 yr after 2 negative exams 1 yr apart
Pelvic examination	F	20–40 >40	every 3 yr every yr
Endometrial tissue sample	F	at menopause, women at high risk*	at menopause
Breast self-examination	F	>20	every mo
Breast physical examination	F	20–40 >40	every 3 yr every yr
Mammography	F	35–40 <50 >50	base-line consult personal physician every yr
Chest x-ray			not recommended
Sputum cytology			not recommended
Health counseling and cancer checkup‡	M & F	>20 >40	every 3 yr every yr

*History of infertility, obesity, failure of ovulation, abnormal uterine bleeding, or estrogen therapy.
‡To include examination for cancers of the thyroid, testicles, prostate, ovaries, lymph nodes, oral region, and skin.
Adapted with permission from American Cancer Society. Guidelines for the cancer-related checkup: recommendations and rationale. *Ca-A Cancer Journal for Clinicians* (July/August 1980). p. 231.

Therefore, the ACS recommends that all women >35 yr of age be considered at substantial risk, with a focus on specific women at *especially* high risk. While the incidence of breast cancer is rising, the mortality remains somewhat constant, perhaps reflecting the influence of earlier diagnosis and more effective treatment.

Lung cancer. The incidence of lung cancer in the USA continues to rise (139,000 cases in 1983), and the overall 5-yr survival rate remains a low 8%. Early detection succeeds in identifying only $1/5$ of the entire group with local disease, which carries a 27% 5-yr survival rate. At present, studies have been undertaken to determine whether periodic screening of asymptomatic male smokers — using questionnaires, sputum tests for cytology, and chest x-rays — will detect lung cancer early enough to alter the natural course of disease by effective treatment. Because the DPCP appears short and available treatment inadequate, early detection programs to date appear not to affect mortality. Therefore, prevention remains the focus of large-scale programs.

Colorectal cancer. Cancer of the colon/rectum may be detected early by means of a digital examination, occult blood test of the stool (stool guaiac), or proctoscopy. The incidence of colorectal cancer is high (130,000 cases/yr) and the 5-yr survival rate for asymptomatic patients is 90% (compared with 40% overall), underscoring the importance of early detection. Screening programs using the digital examination and stool blood tests have not been cost-effective, however, for the following reasons: (1) the 1 to 2% incidence of false-positive tests necessitates a diagnostic workup, which is expensive and time-consuming; (2) digital examinations and sigmoidoscopy cannot detect tumors that originate proximal to the sigmoid colon (half of all cases); and (3) negative public attitude toward cancer of the colon/rectum makes voluntary screening difficult. Current recommendations are described in Table 4–8 for persons at risk by virtue of age; the risk factors outlined in Table 4–5 define persons at high risk.

Any discussion of public education programs for the early detection of cancer would be incomplete without inclusion of the ACS "7 Warning Signals that can Save Your Life":

1. Change in bowel or bladder habits.
2. A sore that does not heal.
3. Unusual bleeding or discharge.
4. Thickening or lumps in breast or elsewhere.
5. Indigestion or difficulty in swallowing.
6. Obvious change in wart or mole.
7. Nagging cough or hoarseness.

Although this approach to public education implies that the disease has progressed to the point of symptomatology, it remains a necessary part of the overall goal of early detection by way of increasing the public's awareness and decreasing the public's fear.

Bibliography

1. American Cancer Society. Guidelines for the cancer-related checkup: recommendations and rationale. *Ca-A Cancer Journal for Clinicians* (July/August 1980). 194–239.

    Presents rationale for recommendations made concerning both individual early detection and mass screening programs. Breaks down discussion according to specific tumor types: lung, breast, colon/rectum, and cervix.

2. Hirschman, R. S., and H. Leventhal. The behavioral science of cancer prevention. *In* Kahn, S. B., R. R. Love, C. Sherman, and R. Chakrovorty. Concepts in Cancer Medicine. Grune & Stratton, Inc., New York. 1983. 229–240.

    Provides a model for understanding and changing people's health behaviors using principles of behavioral science and biomedical science.

3. Love, R. R., and A. E. Camilli. The value of screening. *Cancer* (July 15, 1981). 489–494.

    Defines and analyzes screening tests and programs in terms of their appropriate use in cancer and cost/benefit considerations.

4. National Cancer Institute. Cancer Prevention: A Program to Inform the Public about Cancer Risk and Risk Reduction. Office of Cancer Communications, National Cancer Institute, Washington, D. C. January 1984.

    Describes the National Cancer Institute's program for prevention of cancer, which combines the efforts of the office of Cancer Communications with those of selected lay organizations to increase public awareness.

5. Newell, G. R. Cancer: etiology and prevention. *In* Nixon, D. W. Diagnosis and Management of Cancer. Addison-Wesley Publishing Co., Inc., Menlo Park, Calif. 1982. 29–41.

    Examines specific risk factors for cancer as forming the basis for the primary care physician's history-taking and preventive management approach.

6. Rosenstock, I. M. Why people use health services. *Milbank Memorial Fund Quarterly* (July 1966). 94–127.

    Describes the Health Belief Model as a means of understanding individual's health-related behaviors.

7. Sternberg, J. K. Identification and management of risk factors for cancer. *In* Kahn, S. B., R. R. Love, C. Sherman, and R. Chakravorty. Concepts in Cancer Medicine. Grune & Stratton, Inc., New York. 1983. 241–253.

    Includes are overview of known risk factors for cancer and strategies for a cancer-prevention program from the viewpont of an office practice.

8. United States Department of Health and Human Services. Cancer Prevention Research Summary. United States Department of Health and Human Services, Public Health Service, Washington, D. C. 1984. NIH Publication Nos. 84-2612 (Viruses), 84-2613 (Alcohol), 84-2614 (Tobacco), and 84-2615 (Estrogens).

    Presents literature reviews of known and avoidable cancer-causing agents and includes extensive reference lists.

9. White, L. The nurse's role in cancer prevention. *In* Newell, G. R. Cancer Prevention in Clinical Medicine. Raven Press, New York. 1983. 91-112.

    Focuses on self-care with excellent descriptions of specific self-examination techniques. Includes prescriptions for prevention/ early detection according to specific tumor type.

CHAPTER 5

INFORMATION

Deborah K. Mayer

Standard: The client and family possess knowledge about the disease and therapy in order to attain self-management, participation in therapy, optimal living, and peaceful death.

Outcome criteria: The client and family
1. describe the disease and therapy at a level consistent with their intellectual and emotional states.
2. participate in the decision-making process pertaining to the plan of care and life activities.
3. identify appropriate community and personal resources that would provide information or services.
4. describe appropriate actions in highly predictable problems, oncologic emergencies, and major side effects of disease or therapy.
5. describe the schedule when ongoing therapy is predicted.
6. describe plans for integrating valued activities into daily life.

The patient/care-giver relationship

Our society has undergone many changes that have directly and indirectly influenced the way the cancer patient is provided with information. It is no longer accepted that the physician make all the decisions for the patient or that knowledge of a diagnosis of cancer be withheld. The consumer movement of the 1960s has affected health care. As a result, the Patient's Bill of Rights was developed by the American Hospital Association. Patient-oriented standards of care have also been developed and adapted. Legislation mandating that cancer patients receive information has been enacted in a few states and others are also addressing these issues. These new approaches reflect our society's revived emphasis on individual responsibility and the right to control one's own living and dying. Today, most cancer patients prefer to receive maximum information and to participate in decision making.

The cancer patient is — like everyone else — required to make decisions all the time; however, in the course of the illness there are specific times that require specific attention to treatment options and potential life-style changes as they occur: (1) at the time of diagnosis, (2) at the first recurrence and, (3) at the terminal phase of illness.

Frequently, after receiving a diagnosis of cancer, the patient has overwhelming feelings of loss of control, which lead to feelings of helplessness and hopelessness. He has, in fact, lost control over what is happening to his body and to his life. In consequence, cancer patients are frequently depressed. A 1980 study by Cassileth found that the most hopeful patients were the ones actively involved in their own care. These patients had a better medical status. At the other end of the scale, one patient was depressed because she didn't know the "right" questions to obtain the information she needed to become involved, and she was too intimidated to ask.

In the traditional role model of the acutely ill person, the patient receives care passively in exchange for a return to health. Today, the model is not so apt for a chronic illness such as cancer, because the course of the disease is prolonged and outcome is uncertain. Models of control and power in patient-physician relationships have been studied by Schain and by Brody. These models are applicable to patient-nurse interactions as well.

In the **activity/passivity** model, the physician is active and the patient is passive. This relationship is appropriate in certain situations, such as emergencies/traumas or surgery, or, in cancer treatment, oncologic emergencies, such as hypercalcemia or spinal cord compression. The physician carries on with or without the patient's conscious contributions. This relationship is similar to a parent-child relationship, in which the child is a helpless dependent. The nurse assists the patient, implementing the care needed, as ordered by the physician. In nursing practice, such activities might include positioning and deep-breathing exercises or caring for a patient in the postoperative period.

In the **guidance/cooperation** model, the physician is the ultimate authority, but the patient is allowed to participate. An example of such a situation is the necessity for hospitalization during an evaluation of tumor status. This relationship is similar to the parent-adolescent relationship. The nurse can help clarify information needed. She may provide information that would encourage patient participation. In nursing practice, involving the patient in chemotherapy administration decisions (such as vein selection) or pain management (such as analgesic administration) are other examples.

In the **mutual participation** model, physician and patient share responsibility. Based upon mutual respect and collaborative communication, this approach is a joint endeavor, aimed at effective management of identified problems. It acknowledges the individuality, autonomy, and dignity of the patient while also acknowledging the skills, opinions, and experience of the physician. One such situation might be deciding whether to administer adjuvant chemotherapy to a woman who has breast cancer with one positive lymph node. The patient's and physician's decision is *mutually* agreed upon after discussion of the risks vs. benefits, within the perspective of the physician's knowledge of the patient and the patient's goals. This relationship is an example of an adult-adult interaction. The nurse may provide information and resources as well as listen to the patient as they explore the options. In nursing practice, this procedure might involve developing an antiemetic or pain-management regimen.

Some of these models are more appropriate in certain settings than in others, or with certain patients. The nurse can assist the patient by using the most appropriate model for the situation.

For mutual participation to be effective, the patient must have a base of accurate knowledge, at a level enabling decision making, and he must acquire and assimilate relevant information. Not all patients will be capable of this level of participation. Some are emotionally unable to use their rational or cognitive skills to make judgments. Others possess more limited capabilities, because of learning disabilities or cognitive dysfunction or lack of education. The nurse must assess the patient's educational and psychosocial abilities and then adopt the most appropriate model.

Brody suggests the following four steps to facilitate mutual participation:

1. Provide an atmosphere in which the patient feels independent. Being seated at a conference table with all participants is much less threatening to the patient than being in bed, surrounded by physicians and nurses. Appointments can be made for times when all parties can be available to meet in a comfortable setting, e.g., lounge or conference room.

2. The patient's goals and expectations should be ascertained. More realistic and feasible planning is possible when both health-care professionals and patients are working toward the same goals. For example, in one study of women with metastatic

Handbook of Oncology Nursing

breast cancer, over one third thought the intent of therapy was to cure them, when, in fact, palliation was the goal. This failure to achieve the patients' goals could lead to disillusionment.

3. Sharing of information and education is important. The patient's understanding of the seriousness of the illness should be determined. The expected benefits and costs of actions, as well as risks involved, should be reviewed. The level and amount of information should be consistent with the patient's coping strategies and needs.

4. The patient's informed suggestions and preferences should be obtained, and any disagreements negotiated. An example of such a situation might be the problem of adequate pain management with prescribed narcotics. If the patient has any reservations about taking narcotics or prefers using self-control measures, such as relaxation techniques, the prescribed management may not be as effective as planned. In this case, the patient's ideas could be explored and incorporated in the regimen, while at the same time further education on the use of analgesics and the risks associated with the medications can be provided by the nurse or physician. With relaxation incorporated into the plan for pain management and information to allay fears provided, the approach will be more acceptable and, therefore, more successful.

Mutual participation also means that health-care providers must learn to respect the independence of patients and recognize it as a therapeutic goal in itself. Health-care providers should be encouraged to adopt the view that the patient is a responsible partner in his own care, though we may lose our stereotypical "good" patient in the exchange. A shift in attitudes will be required: patients must be taught how to be more assertive and better health-care consumers and at the same time health-care providers must learn the value of shared responsibility (Table 5–1).

Patients and their families have a right to obtain information that will aid them in self-management, participation in therapy, optimal living, and peaceful death. It is the nurse's professional responsibility to make sure this information is available in a manner appropriate to each patient and situation, whether by individual teaching, group classes, or utilization of printed materials.

There are obstacles that will affect the goal. They include limited time, patients' receptivity, and the attitude and support of the institution and other health-care professionals. The nurse's obligations are not fulfilled by handing a patient a booklet, nor does this approach meet the criteria defined in this chapter or by established standards of

TABLE 5-1
Protocol for Developing Effective Nurse-Patient Relationship

Factor	Intervention
Patient need for information about illness and treatment	Encourage questioning. Establish environment conducive to questioning. Suggest patients write down questions as they occur. Provide relevant information in language and manner patient can comprehend. Supplement initial personal communication with printed or audiovisual aids.
Patient anxiety and confusion	Regard psychologic needs of patient as integral to medical treatment. Do not limit communication with patient. Match communication to knowledge, social background, interest, goals of patient.
Patient need to report medical and psychologic condition accurately	Determine patient's desire for information: information-seeker vs. information-avoider. Employ strategies that encourage patient adherence to treatment requirements, e.g., written instructions and return postcards for follow-up appointments.
Patient need to provide informed consent	Make sure patient has read and understood consent form before signing. Provide time for patient to read consent form and discuss with family. Encourage questions and discussions. Establish atmosphere conducive to questioning.

Adapted from Schain, W. Patients' rights in decision making: the case for personalism versus paternalism in health care. *Cancer* (August 15, 1980). 1035–1041.

professional nursing practice. To promote mutual participation, both the patient and health-care professional have responsibilities.

Patient education

Cancer patient education consists of structured or unstructured interventions designed to affect knowledge, attitudes, skills, or other behaviors of persons with cancer. Thus, education is an important component of total patient care. It will assist patients in their adaptation to disease and ease their rehabilitation. In a study by Jacobs conducted with patients who had Hodgkin's disease, those who received educational materials experienced a decrease in anxiety, treatment problems, depression, and life disruption, compared with a control group of patients in a peer support group. The first group also showed improvement in psychologic and social behaviors. Ensuring adequate patient education is the nurse's professional role and responsibility.

Standards for cancer patient education have been established by the Oncology Nursing Society (ONS)* based on the following assumptions:

1. Patient education can positively influence patient knowledge, skills, attitudes, and behavior, thus promoting a sense of self-control.
2. Individuals learn differently because of unique cognitive, affective, and psychomotor abilities. Information about these abilities can be obtained in the nursing history and assessment.
3. Individuals come to learning situations with certain knowledge, attitudes, expectations, and beliefs about cancer that affect their learning. Previous experience with cancer in family or friends or previous hospitalizations may influence learning.
4. Patients should be included in all phases of their educational experience. The nurse should inform the patient about needs the nurse identifies while remaining sensitive and receptive to the patient's own perceptions of his needs. Nurse/patient perceptions should be compared and negotiated.
5. Where differences in educational needs exist, learners' perceived needs must be considered and given priority in the educational plan. Unless these needs are met first, the patient will not be a receptive learner.

---

*Parts of this list are adapted with permission from the Outcome Standards for Cancer Patient Education. Oncology Nursing Society, Pittsburgh. 1982.

6. The learning environment should provide comfort, mutual trust, respect, freedom of expression, and acceptance of differences. Providing privacy and decreasing external distractions by using a conference room or lounge may establish an environment more appropriate than the patient's bedside.
7. Time must be allowed for learning to take place. Effective management may allow more teaching time for the busy staff nurse. Incorporating teaching while conducting required care procedures can be an effective technique.
8. It cannot be assumed that learning has occurred because a subject has been taught. Evaluation must take place to ascertain comprehension. What is *heard* by the patient or family is not always what is actually said. Reinforcement and clarification may be necessary.

The ONS Patient Education Standards delineate the various components of the educational process. These components apply to both structured and unstructured, formal and informal teaching situations. They include an assessment of learning needs and establishment of mutually agreed-upon goals and objectives with patients and family, the selection of appropriate educational methods, and implementation and evaluation of the educational program. The educational process is completed by thorough documentation, in nursing notes or other appropriate place.

Available resources

There are numerous resources available both for cancer patients and their families and for the nurses involved in caring for them. Unfortunately, nurses are not perceived as sources of information to the same degree that they perceive themselves as health educators. The media and physician are seen as major sources of information.

In one study, Garrison et al. found that only 37% of patients received educational information at the time of diagnosis, though 72% expressed a desire for information. These patients also were not able to identify commonly available resources such as the American Cancer Society. Of 78 patients surveyed, 68 stated they would read material if it were available to them in the physician's office or clinics. Patients and families should be aware of such material, and the nurse should help to make sure they are and that they find the pertinent publications. Patients usually want and will use any available information about cancer in general, about their specific disease, and about treatments.

A survey of 256 oncology patients as to the type of information they desired showed that in 7 of the 12 questions, >50% of the patients polled felt they absolutely needed information about the topic (Table 5–2). The questions are ones the nurse can use to assess the extent of the patient's knowledge. Patients expressed a desire for information and to participate in their own care. The importance of participation cannot be stressed often or strongly enough. It is vital in helping patients deal with feelings of helplessness and hopelessness. More information enables them to be involved in their own care and therefore to feel more in control. Teaching may take place in groups or individual sessions, structured or informal, depending on what will be most effective for the patients involved. The nurse should adapt the approach to the situation.

Many patients undergoing chemotherapy demonstrate inadequate knowledge of the drug they are taking and/or its side effects. There is no paucity of written information available on chemotherapy, on many common types of cancers, or on other treatments, all easily understandable by the layman. This is one easily accessible mechanism for providing information, and at the same time it might be a useful tool for the nurse who wishes to review pertinent information. The American Cancer Society and other resource groups are good sources for such information (*see* Appendix D).

Patients are now being taught to take a greater part in their own care, including such technical aspects as monitoring blood counts or caring for indwelling venous catheters. Generally, compliance has been high, and patients benefit by increasing their self-esteem and strengthening their relationship with their health-care provider while retaining some control. The time invested in teaching initially may well be saved later.

The I Can Cope course sponsored by the American Cancer Society is an 8-wk structured educational program, dealing with topics such as disease, diagnosis, coping with daily health problems, communicating, liking yourself, living with limits, and finding resources. This successful program was developed to help patients to adapt realistically and cope with the chronic aspects of cancer.

There are many other group and individual interventions that are well established and available. These are listed in Appendix D. These comprehensive programs have been purposefully designed, systematically applied, and are consistent. There may be others in the nurse's practice setting and community that are available.

Informed consent

One important aspect of patient participation in decision making is the matter of informed consent. According to the Department of Health and Human Services, informed consent is "the knowing consent of an individual or his legally authorized representative so

TABLE 5-2

Type of Information Desired by Patients

Question	I absolutely need this information %	I would like to have this information %	I do not want this information %
		Patient response	
What are all the possible side effects?	62.9	35.2	2.0
What will the treatment accomplish?	62.1	36.3	1.2
Is it cancer?	60.5	37.1	2.0
What is the likelihood of cure?	58.6	37.5	3.9
Are all parts of the body involved?	58.2	36.3	5.1
Exactly what will the treatment do inside my body?	57.4	37.9	4.7
What is the day-to-day (wk-to-wk) progress?	51.2	41.4	6.6
What is the specific medical name of illness?	48.4	44.5	6.3
Is it inherited, or contagious?	46.1	44.5	9.0
How effective has the treatment been for other patients?	44.5	48.4	7.0
Are there examples of cases where the treatment has been effective?	42.2	48.4	9.0
Are there examples of cases where the treatment has not been effective?	32.4	44.9	21.9

Adapted with permission from Cassileth, B., R. Zupkis, and K. Sutton-Smith. Information and participation preferences among cancer patients. Annals of Internal Medicine (June 1980). p. 834.

situated as to be able to exercise free power of choice without inducement or any element of force, fraud, deceit, distress, or any other form of constraint or coercion." Although it is the physician's legal obligation to obtain informed consent from his patients, it is the nurse's ethical obligation to make sure this consent has been obtained. There are many ethical, legal, and regulatory interactions involved, but the goal of this process is to provide a mechanism for patients to participate in treatment decisions with a full understanding of the factors relevant to their proposed care. The informed consent process is followed for any invasive procedure, but usually it is observed in greater detail and monitored more closely for higher-risk and investigational procedures or treatments.

The actual consent process consists of two parts: the oral and the written explanation. The consent form is not meant to *replace* the verbal interaction but to *supplement* and *document* it. The content of the standard consent form is required by law and enforced through institutional review boards (Table 5–3). Unfortunately, much attention has been focused on obtaining a signed consent form, rather than on the process it was meant to facilitate. In one survey conducted by Cassileth, ~80% of patients viewed consent forms as a protection of physicians' rights, although they also felt the forms were necessary and helpful in decision making.

In another study, conducted by the Psychosocial Collaborative Oncology Group, patients and their physicians were interviewed within 3 wk of signing a consent form; 50% of patients stated that they had not asked questions they had, and 75% of these patients also had lingering unspoken doubts and concerns about their treatment. The nurse, acting as patient advocate, can be helpful in avoiding this kind of situation. Patients and families should be encouraged to write down any questions they may have. The nurse can raise questions for the physician that the patient may have forgotten — or not thought of. The nurse should also ascertain the degree of the patient's and family's understanding after such a discussion. The nurse can then restate, reinforce, or expand on the information shared.

One factor influencing the usefulness of the consent form is its readability. Most consent forms are written at a level that is too technical and difficult for the average patient to comprehend. Four out of five surgical consent forms are written at the scientific journal level, whereas most newspapers are geared to the 7th- to 9th-grade level. This readability average will vary from region to region. Readability can easily be improved by keeping sentences shorter and by using fewer polysyllabic words. Giving patients their own copy of the consent form

TABLE 5–3
Standard for Consent Form Content

Section	Content
Purpose	A statement that the study involves research, an explanation of the purposes of the research, and the expected duration of the subject's participation.
Procedure	A description of the procedures to be followed and identification of any procedures that are experimental.
Benefits	A description of any benefits to the subject or to others that may reasonably be expected from the research.
Risks	A description of any reasonable forseeable risks or discomforts to the subject.
Alternatives	A disclosure of appropriate alternative procedures or courses of treatment, if any, that might be advantageous to the subject.
Guarantees of right to confidentiality; financial remuneration; questioning; withdrawal from study	A statement describing the extent, if any, to which confidentiality of records identifying the subject will be maintained; explanation of any compensation and/or medical treatments that are available if injury occurs; the name of the person to contact for answers to questions about the study, the subject's rights, or research-related injury; acknowledgment that participation is voluntary and that the participant will not be penalized for withdrawal.

Based on Food and Drug Administration regulations regarding the protection of human subjects. *Federal Register* (January 27, 1981). 8951.

ahead of time and encouraging them to read it with care will also improve their comprehension.

Nurses must remain sensitive to the patient's anxiety level and be aware of the amount of information given, because these factors may also influence comprehension. The following basic steps will facilitate understanding and retention:

1. Tell the patient what information will be covered during that session.
2. Cover the material using short words and sentences.
3. Organize the information into related clusters or categories, with the most important information first.
4. Summarize and review the material covered.

These steps can be followed with any aspect of patient education, including the consent process. Different approaches have been instituted to improve the consent process, any or all of which may be helpful:

1. Give the patient and family a copy of the consent form at least the day before signing it.
2. Encourage them to read it carefully.
3. Encourage them to write down any questions or concerns they wish to have addressed.
4. Set up an appointment for a time when the patient and a family member (or significant other) can meet with the physician and nurse to discuss treatment options.
5. Have the meeting in a private area where all participants sit around a table or in comfortable chairs. This approach makes the patient feel less intimidated and more on a par with other people involved.
6. Tape record discussions, if possible, to provide the patient with the mechanism for future references.
7. Ascertain patient's comprehension and understanding afterwards by asking the patient questions related to the discussion.
8. Document the consent process in the patient's record.

By following these guidelines, the nurse may help the patient and physician keep the *intent* of the consent process in view. The time spent at the beginning may well be saved later on because the patients and family are more involved in their care.

Bibliography

1. Brody, D. The patient's role in clinical decision-making. *Annals of Internal Medicine* (November 1980). 718–722.

This paper discusses the concept of mutual participation in clinical decision making. Potential advantages are compared to traditional concepts and approaches.

2. Cassileth, B., R. Zupkis, and K. Sutton-Smith. Information and participation preferences among cancer patients. *Annals of Internal Medicine* (June 1980). 832–836.

   This study evaluated the response of 256 oncology patients to the Information Styles Questionnaire and the Beck Hopelessness Scale. Trends were identified in the areas of age, education, and race.

3. Cassileth, B., R. Zupkis, and K. Sutton-Smith. Informed consent — why are its goals imperfectly realized. *New England Journal of Medicine* (April 1980). 896–900.

   This study evaluated the immediate recall of 200 cancer patients after signing a consent form. Education, medical status, and the care with which patients read the form were related to recall.

4. Garrison, J., J. Abner, M. Oakley, and P. Hagen. Accessibility and utilization of educational materials for cancer patients. *Oncology Nursing Forum* (Spring 1983). 60–62.

   Seventy-eight cancer patients were surveyed to determine the accessibility and utilization of education materials.

5. Jacobs, C., R. Ross, I. Walker, and F. Stockdale. Behavior of cancer patients: a randomized study of the effects of education and peer support groups. *American Journal of Clinical Oncology* (June 1983). 347–350.

   Eighty-one Hodgkin's disease patients were evaluated with the Cancer Patient Behavior Scale before and after entering either a support group, an educational group, or a control group.

6. Johnson, J., and M. Flaherty. The nurse and cancer patient education. *Seminars in Oncology* (March 1980). 63–70.

   This article provides a nice overview of patient education. It defines and outlines how programs are developed by using seven existing models as examples.

7. Johnson, J. The effects of a patient education course on persons with a chronic illness. *Cancer Nursing* (April 1982). 117–123.

   This study evaluates pretests and post-tests of 52 cancer patients in either a control group or the original I Can Cope course.

8. Oncology Nursing Society. Outcome Standards for Cancer Patient Education. Oncology Nursing Society, Pittsburgh. 1982.

   These outcome standards address a conceptual framework and assumptions related to cancer patient education.

9. Redman, B. The Process of Patient Teaching in Nursing. C. V. Mosby Co.,
   St. Louis. 1976.
       A classic text that deals with teaching in nursing; various chapters cover
   definitions, theory, techniques and tool development.

10. Schain, W. Patients' rights in decision making: the case for personalism
    versus paternalism in health care. *Cancer* (August 1980). 1035–1041.
        Analysis of the nature of the physician-patient interaction and its effects
    on decision making in women with breast cancer.

CHAPTER 6

COPING

Dianne Schilke Davis

Standard: While living with cancer, the client and family manage stress within their individual physical, psychological, and spiritual capacities and their value systems.

Outcome criteria: Within a level consistent with physical, psychosocial, and spiritual capacities and their value system, the client and family
1. use appropriate resources for support in coping.
2. communicate feelings about living with cancer.
3. participate in care and ongoing decision making.
4. identify alternative resources when present coping strategies do not provide support.
5. state accomplishable goals.

Framework

The concepts of stress, coping, and crisis aid in the psychologic assessment and management of individuals with a physical illness such as cancer.

Stress. Sources of stress are numerous on biologic, psychologic, and social levels. The individual is striving to maintain a state of homeostasis, or equilibrium, both within himself and in relation to the external physical and social environments. Anything that upsets this balance is a source of stress (a stressor) for the individual and demands responses to restore homeostasis. Stress is the state of the organism as it responds to disequilibrium. The stress manifests itself in physiologic, psychologic, and behavioral changes. This chapter concerns itself primarily with the psychologic and social spheres, considering how individuals and families cope with the threats imposed by a serious and often chronic physical illness such as cancer. It should not be forgotten, however, that the cancer patient is simultaneously dealing with physiologic stressors imposed by the illness and/or treatment. These stresses may decrease the energy that the patient can mobilize to handle psychosocial stressors.

Coping. This can be broadly defined as adaptation to stressful situations. The aims of competent coping are to contain distressing emotions and to maintain self-esteem while realistically solving problems. Thus, coping strategies have both internal and external objectives (Table 6–1). Defense mechanisms are internally oriented coping processes. These are the psychologic maneuvers that the individual uses to deal with painful thoughts and feelings, such as anxiety, fear, anger, and depression. Examples of defense mechanisms are: (1) keeping unpleasant thoughts and feelings out of conscious awareness (repression), (2) trying to minimize those that become conscious by tightly controlling the recognition or expression of associated emotions (constriction of affect), (3) avoiding the recognition of some aspect of external reality (denial), and (4) focusing concern on some less-threatening problem (displacement). Defense mechanisms operate automatically, or unconsciously, to protect the individual from emotional upset.

TABLE 6–1

Goals and Methods of Coping

	Internally oriented	Externally oriented
Goals	Manage painful effect Maintain self-esteem	Solve problems
Methods	Unconscious defense mechanisms: e.g., constriction of affect; denial; rationalization; displacement.	Cognitive: e.g., take things one step at a time; consider alternatives; draw on past experience.
	Conscious tension-reducing strategies: e.g., suppression; distraction; relaxation techniques; exercise; wish-fulfilling fantasy; alcohol or drug use.	Behavioral: e.g., seek more information; talk with care-givers or family about the problem; negotiate feasible alternatives; seek direction from authority and comply.
	Defensive reappraisal.	

Individuals also engage in activities consciously designed to reduce tension. Individuals may try to forget about their problems (suppression), do other things to distract themselves, or reduce tension by drinking, overeating, or drugs. Exercise or relaxation techniques can also be used for their tension-reducing effects.

Defensive reappraisal allows the individual to change his perception or appraisal of a situation so that threat is reduced, without there being any actual change in the situation. The cancer patient who announces that "they got it just as it was turning to cancer" is using this strategy. Attempts to maintain self-esteem are also internally oriented strategies and often depend on the individual's feeling in control of himself and the environment.

In contrast to psychologic defenses, problem solving is conscious and externally oriented coping. Problem-solving methods may be either cognitive or behavioral. Examples of cognitive strategies are: taking things one step at a time, considering alternatives, or drawing on past experience. Behavioral methods are: seeking more information, negotiating feasible plans, or seeking direction from an authority and complying.

Sometimes problem solving and maintaining emotional equilibrium are mutually exclusive goals. For instance, the woman who promptly consults her primary health-care-giver when she notices a lump in her breast is practicing intelligent problem solving, because early diagnosis facilitates cure. But she is — at least transiently — increasing her anxiety level by confronting the possibility of a diagnosis of cancer. Many people delay diagnosis because the thought of cancer arouses so much fear that they do not allow themselves to acknowledge the implications of their early symptoms. Patients also vacillate between realistic problem solving and attempts to remain calm. One minute the patient may be actively making plans for transportation to the chemotherapy clinic, and the next minute the same person may be unwilling to acknowledge that the tumor is malignant. A specific behavior, e.g., talking with others, may be used both for the resolution of a problem and for emotional relief through catharsis or avoidance.

Individuals tend to have a particular coping style, i.e., the tendency to approach problems with a given set of behaviors and defense mechanisms. This includes the tendency to vigilantly seek all information relevant to the problem, or to minimize the importance of this step in problem solving. Examples of coping styles are tackling, avoiding, or capitulating when faced with a problem. What happens in the course of a particular coping episode is described as a coping strategy. The strategy is determined by the person's coping style and by particular aspects of the problem and by the opportunities presented by this new situation.

Adaptive coping must include attention to both problems and feelings. It may be tempting to consider the more rational problem solving to be "good" coping and the strategies focused on dealing with emotional upset to be "bad." But the person who is overwhelmed with anxiety or depression is usually unable to mobilize rational problem-solving capacities. The appropriateness of any particular coping strategy is also related to the nature of the problems demanding resolution. Problem situations initiate the need for coping, shape the form of coping, and determine what coping strategies are likely to lead to adaptive problem resolution. Denial that prevents the individual from seeking diagnosis and early treatment may be maladaptive. The same strategy used by the patient who has had all the appropriate treatment and is coping with an uncertain prognosis may allow that patient to get on with living, in spite of the possibility of recurrence. The failure of coping behaviors to accomplish these dual aims of problem solving and feeling management leads to crisis.

Crisis.   Caplan has defined crisis as the state of the individual who is confronted with an important problem or an obstacle to an important life goal that cannot be immediately resolved through the use of ordinary problem-solving methods. When confronted with a problem, the individual first attempts its resolution with habitual problem-solving methods. Continued impact of the stressor and lack of success in problem solving lead to increased tension, upset, and ineffectuality. The mobilization of additional internal and external resources may lead to the solution of the problem or to a redefinition of the problem with relinquishment of certain goals. If neither of these things happens, a period of disorganization, or crisis, ensues. Eventually, usually within 6 wk, some kind of adaptation is achieved. The reorganization may be at the premorbid level of psychosocial functioning, or at a higher or lower level. If the individual has learned new methods of problem solving or discovered additional external resources, the crisis resolution may leave him psychologically healthier and more able to cope with future stressors. If, however, the crisis has depleted the individual's adaptive resources and left him bitter and defeated, he may be more crisis-prone in the future.

Three interrelated factors are necessary to produce a crisis: (1) the stressor — a hazardous event that poses a threat or challenge, (2) the individual or family definition of that event as stressful, and (3) inadequate crisis-meeting resources. Crisis-meeting resources include both individual coping strategies and interpersonal and environmental resources, such as supportive family and friends, adequate finances, health insurance, and stable employment. Though some aspect of the cancer or its treatment is likely to be defined as stressful by most cancer patients, not all patients will be in crisis. Some individuals have adequate internal and external resources to cope without major disorganization.

Several factors make cancer the kind of illness that is likely to create coping problems for afflicted individuals and their families. Cancer often strikes previously healthy people. For these individuals, illness is a novel situation, and they may not have developed the resources to deal with it, such as knowing where and how to obtain treatment. Cancer is often equated with suffering and death. It presents a threat to bodily integrity, if not life itself, with fears of pain and mutilation both from the illness and its treatment. In fact, individuals may fear surgical disfigurement or the hair loss or vomiting associated with chemotherapy more than they fear the disease. Cancer often presents a threat to self-image because of changed appearance or physical function or loss of independence. The hospitalization necessary for cancer diagnosis and treatment causes separation from social support systems and requires negotiation of relationships with many care-givers. Cancer often disrupts the patient's ability to perform in social roles at work or within the family, or to participate in pleasurable activities, all of which are important sources of self-esteem and gratification. Cancer often involves the financial burdens of a chronic illness, with expensive treatments and loss of employment. It is important to ascertain which of these factors is causing the most distress for any individual cancer patient.

Psychosocial tasks of the cancer patient/family.   The cancer patient and his family must learn to cope with certain problems imposed by chronic illness and the diagnosis of cancer. Eight *psychosocial tasks* must be accomplished. The individual must adjust to *having cancer,* which Weisman describes as the "existential plight" of cancer. Acceptance of *treatment regimens* requires adjustment to periodic clinic visits, *symptom exacerbations,* and *functional or cosmetic body changes.* The individual must establish *trusting relationships* with care-givers as resources for information and support. Maintenance of *self-esteem and family role* allows the patient to get on with living and not let cancer take on a central role. The *social stigma* of cancer may cause avoidance behaviors in friends and employers. The cancer patient must manage this and learn to express *disruptive feelings* without alienating friends and family.

Psychosocial phases of cancer.   How well patients and families cope, as well as the nature of the problems with which they must deal, may vary with the stage of the illness. The patient who is diagnosed early, cured by surgery that creates no lasting functional or cosmetic disability, and who resumes his preillness life-style free of symptoms has few ongoing problems with which to cope. Contrast this case with the patient whose disease is already metastatic at the time of diagnosis, who receives chemotherapy that does not control the progression of the illness and causes severe vomiting and weight loss, whose pain is not well managed, and who progresses rapidly to death. Weisman has suggested a model for **psychosocial phasing** that is parallel to the clinical phases of cancer. This model may highlight the times at which particular problems are likely to surface, as well as help to identify patients at high risk for psychosocial crises (Table 6–2).

Phase I, *existential plight*, begins with the impact of the diagnosis and may last for 3 or 4 mo as the patient gets his first round of treatment and attempts to resume life. Life and death concerns are prominent in this phase, which is predictably a time of high emotional distress. Phase II, *accommodation and mitigation*, is a time of comparative emotional quiescence. During this phase patients adapt to changed function and any residual disability. Patients who have only the initial treatment, e.g., surgery, are likely to have a different phase II from individuals who require follow-up treatment, such as radiation or adjuvant chemotherapy. Phase III, *recurrence and relapse*, may be the most difficult and discouraging time for patients. With the return of the disease, the original hope for cure is shattered, and both patients and care-givers become more pessimistic. There follows a limbo period before phase IV, *deterioration and decline*. In this final phase,

TABLE 6–2
Expectations at Successive Psychosocial Phases

Factor	Existential plight	Accommodation and mitigation	Recurrence and relapse	Deterioration and decline
Aims	Cure	Surveillance	Control	Care
Impairment	Transient	Variable	Increased	Nearly total
Quality of life	Same or slight change	Variable	Definite limitation	Drastic revision
Goals	No more disease	No more concerns	Respite and reprieve	Relief
Attitude	Optimistic	Optimistic	Guarded	Pessimistic or resigned
Time perspective	Ambiguous or open	Open	Cautious or restricted	Closed
Denial	Temporary	Mixed	Slight	Seldom
Coping	Active	Active	Mixed	Passive

Reprinted with permission from Weisman, A. A model for psychosocial phasing in cancer. *General Hospital Psychiatry* (September 1979). p. 191.

unfinished business needs to be completed, though some problems, such as worry about returning to work, recede in importance because the patient is no longer able to do anything about them. As death approaches, control of physical symptoms in the very sick patient becomes the prominent concern.

Family considerations. Giacquinta has suggested that there are stages in family functioning — and phases within these stages — that parallel the progression of the illness in the cancer patient and that each phase presents a particular hurdle for the family to overcome. At the time of diagnosis and early treatment, the patient is usually able to continue to carry out role obligations within the family. At this point the family is in a stage of **living with cancer**. In the impact phase they must overcome their feelings of despair at the diagnosis. Functional disruption of role responsibilities may follow and may result in family members feeling isolated from each other. Family members engage in a search for meaning as they attempt to gain intellectual mastery. As they identify with the patient, family members may themselves feel vulnerable. They must decide how and when to inform others and resist the urge to retreat from outsiders. Family must also confront their own emotions and overcome feelings of helplessness.

When the patient's illness progresses to the point where he ceases to perform accustomed roles and must be cared for either at home or in the hospital, the family enters the stage of **restructuring the living-dying interval**. There is reorganization, with a redistribution of role obligations within the family. Competition between family members must be overcome. Framing memories is the final phase of this stage. Family members need help to remember their loved one as he was prior to the illness, so that he will have an identity beyond that of the dying cancer patient.

The imminent dying and actual death of the cancer patient initiates the stage of **bereavement** for the family. Separation occurs as the patient becomes less aware of the environment. Family members must overcome the hurdle of self-absorption if they are to support each other. The mourning phase brings with it the hurdle of guilt. **Reestablishment** is the final family stage. During the period of time when they were dealing with the illness, family members may have become alienated from the larger society. Now is the time to once again expand social networks in order to reestablish the large context and meaning of their lives.

Assessment

However the psychosocial tasks of the cancer patient and family are conceptualized, coping with cancer is not a simple matter. What is amazing is that so many cancer patients and families manage as well as they do. Experience tells us that some manage better than others, both in solving their real-world problems and in containing their distress. Cancer seldom solves the psychosocial problems that the patient had before diagnosis, e.g., marital discord, alcohol abuse, psychiatric problems, difficulty in establishing relationships or holding a job, socioeconomic deprivation, or a pessimistic character. Patients who have maladaptively dealt with other aspects of their lives predictably have difficulty coping with cancer as well. Conversely, individuals with an optimistic attitude and wealth of personal and social resources, who are used to confronting and solving problems, will probably cope with cancer in an equally competent manner. In addition, as mentioned previously, a cancer diagnosis at an early stage, with few symptoms and a good chance for cure, presents fewer problems with which to cope than does advanced disease with many symptoms and only palliative treatment possible.

Adaptive and maladaptive coping strategies. Research with cancer patients conducted by Weisman and others has shown that there are some coping strategies that are more likely to be adaptive than others. Adaptive strategies include:
1. Confronting problems and taking firm action based on present understanding.
2. Accepting the situation and finding something favorable in it, e.g., that having cancer makes one realign values and realize that each day should be enjoyed.
3. Talking with others to relieve distress and share concerns.
4. Cooperative compliance: seeking competent direction and then doing what one is told.

The literature on crisis indicates further strategies likely to be helpful in resolving crises, such as:
1. A task orientation.
2. Mental work directed at correctly perceiving the situation so that one can predict and anticipate outcomes and make realistic plans for the future, e.g., asking questions and seeking information.
3. Awareness of and acceptance of feelings.
4. Accepting help from others.

Coping strategies that tend to be maladaptive in solving problems and containing distress are:
1. Suppression — trying to forget or put the problem out of one's mind.
2. Fatalism — passively submitting to the inevitable.
3. Withdrawal into isolation.
4. Projection — blaming someone or something.
5. Sacrificing or atoning — blaming oneself.

6. Acting out — impulsively doing something, no matter how reckless or impractical.
7. Reducing tension with excessive alcohol or drugs.
8. Somatizing — expressing emotion through bodily complaints.
9. Dealing with events or feelings with magical thinking or excessive fantasy.

The use of denial as a coping strategy has been given particular attention in the cancer literature. Weisman points out that denial comes in many guises and degrees:

1. Repudiation of the diagnosis of cancer or the fact of illness.
2. Dissociation of the diagnosis, which is acknowledged, from its implications or secondary manifestations.
3. Refusal to acknowledge decline, deterioration, or impending death, despite full knowledge of the diagnosis and its relationship to subsequent events.

Obviously, patients must have been given a chance to hear and absorb information before we can conclude that they are denying. Care-givers and families may collude to deprive the cancer patient of information about diagnosis or prognosis, assuming that the patient would be unable to cope with the truth. Patients may shift back and forth between awareness, acceptance, and denial. The patient's decision not to talk about something at a particular time or with a particular person should not be automatically labeled as denial. The care-giver's evaluation of the usefulness of denial must be based on a consideration of what is being denied and what needs to be done that the denial keeps the patient from doing.

In general, problems must be recognized before they can be solved. Therefore, good coping usually involves some degree of confrontation and information seeking and processing. Emotions are less likely to be a drain on adaptive energy if they are acknowledged and shared with others, because appropriate verbalization not only reduces tension but promotes mastery. Individuals who fully utilize all the resources available to them are less prone to emotional crisis, a fact that underscores the importance of the ability to seek and accept help with tasks and feelings.

Assessment techniques.   Armed with this list of coping strategies likely to be adaptive or maladaptive, how does the nurse assess how well any particular patient is coping with his situation? The nurse first discovers how the patient defines the problem(s) with which he is confronted. Knowing the stage of the cancer, the treatments and their side effects, and something about the social roles and responsibilities of the patient may help to predict what he may be struggling with. But only the patient/family can say which concerns are most prominent. The care-givers' priorities to quickly diagnose and treat the illness are not necessarily shared by the patient, who may be much more concerned about who will care for young children during the hospitalization or whether a spouse will be repelled by a disfiguring scar.

Secondly, the nurse assesses what the patient is doing about the problems he has identified. The patient's behavior and verbalization can be observed for evidence of prominent coping strategies. But the patient can also be asked the question fairly directly: "What do you usually do when faced with difficult problems like this? Is that what you have done in this case?" It is important to note whether the chosen strategies primarily confront problems or avoid them. Does the patient seem more concerned about solving problems or avoiding emotional upset? How flexible is the patient's coping? Can he think of a range of possible solutions to problems?

Finally, the nurse assesses whether the patient's coping strategy is working. Is there an objective resolution of the problem, and is the patient's subjective distress kept within manageable limits? In assessing the level of emotional upset, the nurse looks for nonverbal evidence of distress, as well as verbalization of sadness, fear, or anger. The patient who is unable to concentrate, having difficulty sleeping, quietly tearful, unwilling to see friends, uninterested in self-care, or pacing the hall may be more distressed than the person who is able to express emotion more directly by talking with others.

Assessment of family members involves the same three areas: problem definition, coping strategies, and effectiveness. The family members can be expected to share some of the patient's concerns and to have some concerns of their own.

Clinically significant emotional complications.   One expects that all or most cancer patients will be emotionally upset at some point. When is the patient's emotional response severe enough to require intervention by care-givers? Senescu has suggested some behavioral criteria for determining a clinically significant emotional complication in the patient with cancer:

1. When the emotional reaction interferes with the patient's seeking or cooperating with indicated treatments.
2. When the emotional responses cause more pain and distress than the disease itself or increases the distress that is present.
3. When the emotional responses interfere with everyday functioning in work or relationships.
4. When the emotional responses cause the patient to give up or curtail sources of gratification.
5. When the emotional responses result in a disorganization of personality or behavior, i.e., the appearance of psychiatric symptoms.

Management

Strategies for cancer professionals.   The medical and nursing staff are important resources for the cancer patient and family struggling to cope with the psychosocial tasks that confront them. Care that is emotionally supportive must begin by being **technically competent.** Staff must be knowledgable and able to explain the nature of the illness and the range of treatment options to the patient and his family. The treatment recommendations made should be consistent with the most current clinical and research data. If there are promising new treatments that are not yet available in the local hospital, patients should know about them and be offered a referral to the closest comprehensive cancer center. Treatment should be administered with a high level of technical skill, so that side effects are minimized. The importance of an IV line that is started on the first try cannot be overestimated. Finally, distressing physical symptoms such as pain, anorexia, nausea, vomiting, and constipation must be assessed and managed.

Supportive care is also care that is **individualized.** The ability to individualize care depends on a knowledge of the psychosocial factors that make this patient a unique individual: What is the family constellation? On whom does the patient depend for emotional support? Is the patient still working? Are there financial concerns? What activities are a source of pleasure for the patient? What is the patient's general level of intelligence? What are the prominent coping strategies of the patient and family members? The supportive professional gives the patient time and permission to voice concerns and express emotions. Where specific patient/family concerns are identified, specific resources can often be mobilized. But the ongoing relationship with a trusted care-giver is itself a resource. The cancer patient's sense of isolation is decreased by the feeling that the professional staff care about him as a person. This rapport between patient and care-giver is most likely to occur if there is some continuity in care-givers over time.

Supportive care is **family-centered** care. The emotional needs of family members as well as those of individual patients must be met if the family is to continue to function as the patient's primary psychosocial resource.

Supportive care springs from a value system that contends that patients have the right to be informed and active participants in their own care. Care-givers must be willing to share information as well as acknowledge uncertainty, so that patients can make informed decisions. Care-givers must also acknowledge that decisions about quality of life can be made only by the patient and that these will be based on the patient/family value system that may differ from that of the professional.

Referrals to other professionals. Besides the provision of ongoing, technically competent, individualized, and family-centered care, the physicians and nurses caring for the cancer patient also provide the patient with access to a wide range of specialized services via referral.

The professionals most commonly consulted when patients/families are having difficulty coping are psychiatric clinical nurse specialists, psychiatrists, social workers, and chaplains. Though there is some overlap in the roles of these professionals in providing supportive therapy for patients, each discipline also has a unique contribution to make. The psychiatric clinical nurse specialist who is a consultant to a cancer nursing staff is in an ideal position to assist the staff nurses with assessment and management of the psychologic needs of the cancer patient and family. This consultation helps to insure that all the nursing care is delivered in a psychologically supportive fashion. The psychiatric clinical nurse specialist also has specialized direct-patient-care skills in pain management, relaxation training, and crisis intervention. The fact that she is a nurse makes her an acceptable psychiatric resource for patients and families who do not consider themselves psychiatrically ill and who may be reluctant to see a psychiatrist.

Consultation with the psychiatrist is useful when there is a differential diagnosis between psychologic and organic causes for behavior, when the patient is manifesting overt psychiatric symptoms such as paranoia, hallucinations, or suicidal behavior, or when anxiety or depression have reached a level that requires medication. The social worker is the professional with the most knowledge of community resources and concrete services and can be a valuable resource for families who are having financial difficulties or need assistance with discharge planning. The social worker's careful attention to details of social service needs can free the energies of family members to attend to the emotional needs of the patient. Examples of such needs are: an application for social security disability, the acquisition of a hospital bed or oxygen for home use, or the choice of a nursing home. The chaplain is the logical person to address the religious or existential concerns of patients and families.

Crisis intervention. The strategy most commonly used by mental-health professionals in intervening with patients with a physical illness is crisis intervention. Though the staff nurse may use techniques based on crisis theory (Table 6–3), crisis intervention as a therapeutic modality is usually left to psychiatrically trained clinicians because of the time and skill it requires. Crisis work is time-limited and focused on the resolution of current problems. The clinician takes an active, directive stance with the patient and mobilizes all available resources to restore emotional equilibrium and enhance the patient's own

TABLE 6–3
Nursing Protocol for Interventions Based on Crisis Theory

Patient problem	Intervention
Disruption of functioning with cognitive confusion	Help patient to clearly identify concerns.
	Reduce large problems to manageable pieces.
	Maintain reality focus.
	Provide information to correct misconceptions.
Inability to recognize or express feelings	Accept presenting affect.
Presence of helpless-hopeless feelings	Give permission and opportunity for the expression of feelings.
	Validate the normality of a range of feelings.
	Offer reality-based reassurances.
	Present strategies for handling tension, e.g., relaxation techniques.
Ineffective coping	Explore alternative coping strategies.
	Assist patient in redefining situation and altering goals.
	Help patient anticipate and plan for future threatening events.
	Help patient identify additional resources.
	Refer patient to mental health professional for crisis intervention.

problem-solving ability. Crisis intervention involves assessment, planning, intervention, and resolution.

In the **assessment** of the individual and his problem, the clinician uses an active, focused interview technique to ascertain a number of factors. Is a crisis state actually present? What was the precipitating event of the current crisis? What threat does this event pose to the significant roles or relationships of the patient? What losses does he anticipate? What are the range of coping strategies being employed by the patient in attempts to resolve the crisis? Are there new factors in this situation that make habitual ways of coping ineffective?

Planning of the intervention takes into consideration: the length of time since the onset of the crisis, the amount of disruption of the patient's life and the effects on significant others, strengths the patient has, external supports, coping skills he has used in the past, and possible alternatives.

The **intervention** itself has three main aspects:

1. The patient is helped to gain an intellectual understanding of the crisis. The problem is formulated by identifying and isolating those factors that led to the disruption of functioning. The intent of this formulation is to facilitate cognitive restructuring and integration with an anticipated decrease in the cognitive confusion that commonly characterizes the crisis state. The clinician maintains a reality focus and tries to discourage the use of evasion or denial to deal with problems. Information is given to correct misconceptions or unrealistic expectations. This cognitively oriented process actually begins during the assessment phase, as the patient is helped to tell his story in coherent, organized fashion and to clearly identify his concerns. The clinician helps to redefine and reduce overwhelming problems to manageable pieces.

2. The patient is helped to identify present feelings, e.g., anger, grief, guilt. For the expression and management of feelings, the clinician explicitly accepts distorted affect, irrational attitudes, and negative responses but puts these in a rational context by understanding and clarifying the development of such reactions. The clinician offers reality-based reassurances to counteract helpless-hopeless feelings. This focus on feelings provides the patient in crisis with direct relief through a constructive sharing of concerns and the catharsis that comes from unburdening oneself to another. The clinician may suggest strategies to deal with anxiety, such as relaxation techniques or diversions that have worked for the patient in the past.

3. The patient is helped to explore alternative coping strategies. Since foreknowledge and preparation for a crucial event can mitigate the hardship, the patient is helped to anticipate the hazards to be encountered so that he can develop and practice coping strategies to deal with them. The clinician attempts to recognize distorted patterns of adaptation and to steer the patient toward a more adaptive solution, e.g., the patient is encouraged to seek specific information, rather than to base his self-assurance on vague "hopes for the best." The patient is helped to gain tolerance for an inescapable event and to begin to redefine the situation and alter his goals. The patient is helped to identify and use available sources of support such as family, significant others, and hospital staff.

During the final phase of **resolution and anticipatory planning**, the clinician reinforces adaptive coping patterns and reconfirms progress made. This phase includes making realistic plans for the future and discussion and application of present learning to the handling or avoidance of future crises.

Bibliography

1. Caplan, G. Principles of Preventive Psychiatry. Basic Books, New York. 1964.

    Classic description of crisis and crisis intervention.

2. Capone, M., D. Westie, J. Chitwood, D. Feigenbaum, and R. Good. Crisis intervention: a functional model for hospitalized cancer patients. *American Journal of Orthopsychiatry* (October 1979). 598–607.

    An excellent application of the technique of crisis intervention to work with cancer patients.

3. Giacquinta, B. Helping families face the crisis of cancer. *American Journal of Nursing* (October 1977). 1585–1588.

    Useful juxtaposition of points of transition for the individual with cancer, family stages and phases, hurdles for the family to overcome in each phase, and the goals of nursing interventions with the family in each phase.

4. Johnson, E., and D. Stark. A group program for cancer patients and their family members in an acute-care teaching hospital. *Social Work in Health Care* (Summer 1980). 335–349.

    A complete description of a program that provides information and support in the group context. Includes suggestions for the management of difficult behavior in groups.

5. National Institutes of Health. Coping with Cancer — a Resource for the Health Professional. U. S. Department of Health and Human Services (September 1980). NIH Publication No. 80–2080.

    A complete and easy-to-read guide for health professionals describing the coping of patients, families, and health professionals. Includes an extensive listing of support groups and a bibliography.

6. Rogers, B., and A. Mengel. Communicating with families of terminal cancer patients. *Topics in Clinical Nursing* (October 1979). 55–61.

    Describes the "denial-protection syndrome," guidelines for assessment of family's ability to deal with death, and nursing interventions to facilitate communication with the terminal cancer patient and his family.

7. Senescu, R. The development of emotional complications in the patient with cancer. *Journal of Chronic Disease* (July 1963). 813–832.

    Behavioral criteria for a clinically significant emotional complication in the patient with cancer. Addresses common emotional responses including: dependency, reduced self-esteem, anger, guilt, loss of gratification or pleasure, and responses to the care-giver's attitudes and behavior.

8. Strauss, A., and B. Glaser. Chronic Illness and the Quality of Life. C. V. Mosby Co., St. Louis. 1975.

Excellent description of the psychosocial problems facing any patient/ family with chronic illness.

9. Weisman, A. Coping with Cancer. McGraw-Hill Book Co., New York. 1979.

Text based on extensive research by Project Omega at Harvard. Includes a definition of coping and descriptions of coping strategies; the role of denial; descriptions of patients who are vulnerable to high distress; areas of concern for cancer patients; psychosocial staging in cancer; anticipatory grief; and techniques for psychologic intervention to support adaptive coping.

10. Weisman, A. A model for psychosocial phasing in cancer. *General Hospital Psychiatry* (September 1979). 187–195.

Detailed description of the psychosocial phases of cancer, characteristics of high-emotional-distress vs. low-emotional-distress patients, predictions of how distress levels change with psychosocial phase, and suggestions for appropriate interventions.

CHAPTER 7

COMFORT

Standard: The client and family identify and manage factors that influence comfort (the minimizing of psychobiologic distress).

Outcome criteria: The client and family
1. report alterations in comfort level.
2. identify measures to modify psychosocial, environmental, and physical factors that influence comfort and enhance the continuance of valued activities and relationships.
3. state the source of pain, the treatment, and the expected outcome of the proposed intervention.
4. describe appropriate interventions for potential or predictable problems of the pain and sleep management program.

A: PAIN

George Heidrich, III

Pain produced by an injury is an important signal to the body that damage has taken place and that attention needs to be channeled to the area. Prolonged, unrelieved pain can become a pathology itself, however, and contribute to the gradual debilitation of the sufferer. Unrelieved pain can interfere with many normal activities — ones that may be essential to the cancer patient's ability to cope with the disease. Loss of appetite is common. The ability to perform even minimal exercise may be inhibited, as well as the ability to perform normal hygiene and self-care. The patient's family relationships may be constricted and centered on vain attempts at making the patient comfortable. In some situations, families may avoid the patient because their efforts to help are consistently frustrated. Whether the

145

nurse working with such a patient is in a hospice setting, a patient's home, or an acute-care facility, the challenge remains the same: discovering methods to alleviate the pain.

First, the nurse should have an understanding of the physiology of pain perception and the prevalence and physical basis of cancer pain. Second, the nurse must be able to assess the severity and extent of the patient's pain. This information will give the nurse means of evaluating the success of current pain treatment as well as a base line with which all subsequent pain-relieving measures can be compared, thus providing objective information on their success or failure. Proper pain assessment will also provide valuable information for other health-team members on the effectiveness of their prescribed interventions and will alert them to any change in disease status, e.g., metastasis.

Once the problem has been identified and the pain assessed, intervention is chosen. Some interventions will be identified and performed by the medical specialties (e.g., nerve blocks by the anesthesiologist) but in many situations the nurse will be able to make skilled interventions with nonpharmacologic and/or pharmacologic methods of pain relief. Nonpharmacologic methods can contribute significantly to pain control, provided the patient is willing to try them and that the practitioner is knowledgable. Understanding how to maximize the effect of analgesic medications while working within their limitations is important. Strategies for nursing interventions with analgesics must be based on pharmacologic principles as well as other factors that can contribute to the variability of pain response.

Physiology of pain perception

Multiple anatomic pathways are associated with the transmission of pain, and multiple centers in the brain are responsible for its perception. The experience of pain is much more complex than sensing touch, pressure, heat, or cold. Pain provides both information about the status of the tissue involved and motivation for the alteration of behavior so that pain will stop. The neural pathway that provides information about the location and quality of pain appears to have its end point in the parietal lobes of the cerebral cortex. The pain message is also transmitted to many other areas that deal with the motivational, emotional, and behavioral expressions of pain. When this neural pathway is active, the individual is motivated to attack or retreat from the source of the pain or retreat to an inactive and energy-conserving state.

The CNS has some innate means of controlling the intensity of pain. The amount of pain transmitted to the brain from a site of injury is partially controlled in the spinal cord itself. One important model of this process, called the Gate Control Theory, was put forward by Melzack and Wall. This theory proposes that pain-conducting fibers from skin, viscera, and other structures merge at central transmission (T) cells in the substantia gelatinosa, a layer of cells extending the length of the spinal cord on both sides. The T cells provide a gate through which the pain signal must pass. As noxious stimulation builds up from peripheral fibers, the gate is generally opened. Activation of larger fibers that do not conduct pain, however, may close the gate. The passage of pain signals may also be inhibited by downward transmission from centers in the brain.

Brain and CNS peptides also inhibit pain. These naturally occurring compounds (such as enkephalins and endorphins) bind to receptors in the same fashion as morphine. When synthesized in the laboratory, these compounds are powerful analgesics. How they function is not known; they may be produced in increased amounts when major stress is present.

If cancer progresses without cure, patients have an increasing risk of experiencing pain. Although significant and sustained pain is not often a problem at time of cancer diagnosis, 1/5 to 1/3 of patients with metastatic disease will report pain of a severity that adversely affects their lives. The majority of patients with terminal cancer will have to cope with significant pain; ~1/2 of those patients who receive analgesics for pain rate their relief at a level that might be considered to be good to excellent.

There are many different ways that cancer can cause pain. Both primary tumor and metastases can infiltrate or impinge on pain-sensitive tissue. The main physical mechanisms responsible for pain include tumor involvement of bone, nerve, soft tissue, or hollow viscus. Pain may also be caused by therapies for cancer, including chemotherapy, radiotherapy, and surgery. Where tumor is a direct cause of pain, ~2/3 of patients will have involvement of bone, with the remainder having invasion of soft tissue, viscus, or impingement on nerve. Pain arising from damage caused by treatment is present in from 10 to 20% of patients with problematic pain. Pain from other causes (such as osteoarthritis) may be aggravated by cancer. Although pain may be caused by a combination of stimuli, knowledge of its mechanism will help refine treatment recommendations.

Assessment

In the assessment of a patient's pain, the patient is the expert. Though the nurse may have seen numerous patients in similar stages of disease, each patient is unique. A particular patient's perception of and reaction to pain is unknown until the patient reports on it.

At the initial pain interview and as part of an ongoing nursing assessment, the site, onset, duration, conditions of relief or aggravation, character, and intensity of pain should be ascertained.

Site. This information is vitally important in a progressive disease such as cancer. A change in the location of the patient's pain can signal a change in disease status. The metastatic process may initially reveal itself as pain. A pain site diagram can be easily constructed by drawing a human body (front and back views) on graph paper. This can then be used to track changes in the patient's pain — new pain, vanishing pain, and migratory pain — thereby helping the staff determine a plan of care.

Pain charting contributes to the continuity of the patient's care. New staff members can see just where the patient has reported pain. New pain sites will then be easily recognizable, even to staff who are unfamiliar with the patient. The pain site diagram can accompany the patient home and be used as a reference point by visiting nurse service staff.

Onset and duration. In some patients there will be a clearly identifiable time or activity that will bring on the pain. The onset and duration is important in determining the type of analgesic regimen to be followed.

Conditions of relief or aggravation. Patients will readily report that walking upstairs or sleeping on a particular side or performing a particular activity is pain producing. The nurse can then intervene and adjust the environment or instruct the patient in strategies that avoid pain-inducing activities.

Character. The character of the pain may reflect a change in the disease status. If a patient has been reporting an aching pain in the hip and leg and then begins to report a sharp, stabbing pain, the cause could be a pathologic fracture or embolus.

Intensity. Intensity can be assessed by a variety of methods. A very simple one is a categorical scale. For instance, the patient is asked if the pain is slight, moderate, or severe. This type of scale is easy to use in the hurried clinical setting, and it has proven to be a reliable measure of pain intensity.

The majority of cancer patients with pain will be taking some form of analgesic medication. In addition to the basic assessment of pain, assessment of the effectiveness of the analgesic regimen is essential.

Effectiveness of analgesic regimen. To determine the analgesic effectiveness of substances, clinical studies are undertaken with patients who are experiencing pain. The agent under investigation is compared with a standard analgesic — e.g., morphine — in a double-blind study.

Before an analgesic is administered, the patient is asked to rank pain as none, slight, moderate, or severe; ½ or 1 hr after the analgesic is administered, the patient is again asked to rank his pain and to estimate the amount of relief the analgesic is supplying, whether none, slight, moderate, a lot or complete. Pain relief is then assessed every hour until the patient reports no relief and the pain intensity has returned to the premedication level. Thus a pattern develops, indicating how the patient is responding to the prescribed analgesic. This data provides information as to the onset of analgesic action, peak effect, and duration of action. A plot or graph can be drawn, attached to the patients's chart, and used to determine efficacy of the analgesic prescription. Documented reports of severe, unrelieved pain are powerful persuaders for a change in analgesic prescription. In addition, knowing the peak time of pain relief will help in planning the timing of potentially painful procedures.

An important feature of any pain relief program is the patient's own perception of its success. The patient may have unrealistic expectations of the capabilities of the analgesic prescription. In discussions with the patient about the effectiveness of pain relief, the nurse can help clarify the objectives of the program and bring about understanding of what the patient can realistically expect.

Medical management

Systemic analgesics represent the most frequently employed treatment of cancer pain; however, other therapeutic approaches to the problem should be considered. When tumor involvement is the cause of pain, tumor mass can be attacked by palliative radiotherapy or chemotherapy or by surgical resection. Neurosurgical procedures designed to affect the patient's perception of pain may provide substantial relief, although the neurosurgeons trained in palliative procedures may not be available in all settings. Percutaneous cordotomy is the most frequently used neurosurgical procedure. A radio-frequency needle is placed in the pain-conducting tracts of the cervical cord, and these tracts are destroyed. Chemical destruction of the pituitary (hypophysectomy) has been reported to reduce pain in patients with advanced disease. Stimulation of electrodes surgically placed in the periaqueductal region of the brain may also provide relief. The mechanism by which these last two procedures relieve pain is not known.

Temporary anesthetic or the more permanent destructive nerve blocks, usually performed by anesthesiologists, are also very useful in the management of cancer pain, although here again practitioners expert in these techniques may not be available in all settings. Temporary anesthetic blocks or the destructive blocking of the celiac plexus has special application to abdominal pain syndromes caused by cancer of the pancreas, liver, gallbladder, or stomach. Destructive blocks using alcohol or phenol may be useful for pain at other sites as well, especially for disease of the head and neck.

Nursing management

Transcutaneous electrical nerve stimulators (TENS) have a place in the management of cancer pain. These units provide electric stimulation to the skin in the area of pain or the area over nerves supplying the painful site. The mechanism of pain relief is not known; possibly stimulation of this type may compete with pain signals for access to awareness. TENS is a relatively safe and noninvasive pain intervention. Some types of pain appear to respond more favorably than others. For instance, the amount of relief TENS provides for pain of deep visceral origin appears to be limited. Pain originating in peripheral body parts usually responds more favorably. Positive results have been reported in the treatment of chronic pain syndromes that occasionally result from cancer surgery, e.g., mastectomy, thoracotomy.

As with any type of pain intervention, the success of TENS intervention is dependent upon the skill of the practitioner, who must be knowledgable and possess a thorough understanding of TENS application procedures. Also essential is a careful assessment of the patient's response, as well as regular follow-up assessments.

Behavioral techniques.   The use of behavioral techniques, such as biofeedback training, hypnosis, cognitive control, imagery, and various types of relaxation training, in the control of cancer pain is based on research that suggests the brain may take an active role in inhibiting or augmenting the awareness of pain. Training in these techniques should never be a substitute for administration of appropriate analgesics, but their use may often provide additional pain reduction for the large number of patients for whom analgesics do not provide complete relief. Although these techniques are psychologic in nature, neither patients nor staff should be allowed to conclude that the relief achieved through their use means that pain is psychogenic.

It is not precisely understood why behavioral techniques produce pain relief, but the production of deep relaxation and a redirecting of attention are common features of most of them. Relaxation produces a reduction in muscle tension, which in turn can reduce strain on pain-sensitive structures. Relaxation also reduces sympathetic arousal, and this reduction may help dampen transmission of and reaction to pain. Redirection of attention may operate to reduce awareness of pain.

Biofeedback uses electronic amplification of the body's physiologic signals to help the patient learn to reduce physiologic activity. The use of biofeedback enables some patients to identify and control certain physiologic activities that may be, in part, responsible for their pain. Two types of biofeedback are useful for pain control. The first uses surface electromyography (EMG) to give patients continuous and immediate information about the level of contraction of their muscles. The patient is able to follow this activity by hearing a tone (decreasing in pitch as the patient relaxes) or by watching a visual display. The second type of biofeedback uses temperature sensors to give the patient information about extremity blood flow. With greater relaxation, peripheral circulation increases and extremity temperature rises. This technique is especially helpful for ischemic pain. Increase in peripheral circulation is also associated with reduction of sympathetic arousal.

Physiologic self-monitoring is probably of little use to patients on their own. Biofeedback must be used by an active therapist who helps the patient understand the task and continually reinforces the small initial gains that are made. Learning other relaxation techniques that can be used in conjunction with biofeedback can also be helpful.

Progressive relaxation training (PRT) is a method of teaching systematic muscular relaxation. In PRT, patients contract and then relax different muscle groups in a specific order. As patients contract muscles, they begin to get a sense of how tension feels and can develop a sense of the contrast in feeling when the muscle relaxes. Trainers can make an audio cassette of the instructions that can be used to guide the patient through practice. Patients often find practicing this technique especially useful for falling asleep. The PRT technique is taught in many schools of nursing and may also be learned through published descriptions accompanied by tape recordings.

Hypnosis has a long history in the management of pain. Hypnosis can induce deep relaxation, but its major additional advantage in pain management appears to be its ability to redirect the attention of patients. When using hypnosis for pain control, most therapists teach the patient self-hypnosis. Using self-hypnosis, patients may be able to visualize themselves in a different, more comfortable place, or even in a time before pain became problematic. Patients differ in their innate ability to use hypnosis, and some patients may experience negative as well as positive emotional responses when using it. For this reason, hypnosis should only be used by professionals with extensive training in its application and the management of the emotional states that it may produce.

The use of certain types of **imagery** and **self-talk**, without the induction of hypnosis, may help control pain. Imagery for pain relief is usually used in conjunction with a relaxation technique. The patient concentrates on an image associated with an absence of pain. Self-talk, sometimes labeled cognitive control, can be useful when the patient mislabels the source of pain or minimizes his ability to cope with it. For example, patients can be taught to have positive feelings about being active, despite their pain.

There are few controlled studies demonstrating the effectiveness of behavioral techniques in the control of cancer pain, although these techniques have been demonstrated to be effective with other types of clinical pain. Using behavioral techniques can be time-consuming for the professional. If the techniques are proven to be effective, priorities may have to be modified to make time available to use them.

Analgesics. Nurses can exert influence on the prescribing physician. A nurse who is knowledgable about the pharmacology and clinical use of analgesics can have a significant effect on the types of prescriptions that are ordered and is thus a vital member of the pain management team. Morphine is the standard to which all other analgesics are compared. Table 7A–1 is an analgesic equivalency list of different narcotics compared to morphine. The equivalency list gives the clinician a guideline for determining how many milligrams of a particular narcotic, by a particular route, would be equivalent to 10 mg of morphine IM. Whereas codeine is more commonly used than morphine for mild to moderate pain, it is more toxic in higher doses. Heroin (not available in USA), hydromorphone, oxycodone, and meperidine have a shorter duration of action than morphine. Methadone is a useful narcotic because it has a high PO:IM potency ratio and a longer duration of action (4 to 6 hr). However, careful monitoring is required due to a long plasma half-life, which may lead to excessive sedation. Pentazocine is a narcotic antagonist, producing withdrawal symptoms in persons dependent on narcotics. Table 7A–2 lists a series of analgesics used PO for less severe pain. Next to each of the analgesics is the dosage at which it is comparable to the analgesic effect of 650 mg aspirin.

An individual's response to an analgesic will be somewhat dependent on his expectations. Many patients are intimidated by the hospital environment and may submit to therapy without a clear understanding of its ramifications. Anxiety and the resultant physiologic response to stress are counterproductive to the therapeutic effects of analgesic treatment. The patient should be given as much information as needed to feel comfortable with the treatment. Any medications — and specifically analgesics — whether they are given in pill, injection, suppository, or IV form, are seen not only in their therapeutic light by the patient but also as a potential threat. By thoroughly answering the patient's questions, the medicating nurse can instill a sense of

TABLE 7A-1

Relative Potencies of Analgesics Commonly Used for Severe Pain*

Drug	IM (mg)	PO (mg)
Morphine	**10**	**60**
Codeine	130	200
Heroin	4–5	—
Hydromorphone (Dilaudid)	1.5	7.5
Levorphanol (Levo-Dromoran)	2	4
Meperidine (Demerol)	75	300
Methadone (Dalophine)	10	20
Oxycodone (Percodan [aspirin + oxycodone], Percocet-5 [acetaminophen + oxycodone])	15	30
Oxymorphone (Numorphan)	1	6
Pentazocine (Talwin)	60	180

*Expressed in IM and PO doses approximately equivalent in total effect to morphine, 10 mg IM.

Adapted with permission from Foley, K. M., and A. Rogers. The Management of Cancer Pain, Vol. II: The Rational Use of Analgesics in the Management of Cancer Pain (Hoffmann-LaRoche Monograph Series). Hoffmann-LaRoche Inc., Nutley, N. J. 1981. p. 10; and Heidrich, G., and S. Perry. Helping the patient in pain. *American Journal of Nursing* (December 1982). p. 1832.

confidence in the patient. A patient who has been instructed in this manner will approach the medicating situation with more assurance and an attitude that may allow for the enhancement of the therapeutic effects of medications.

Tranquilizers. Various phenothiazines are administered with narcotics in the belief that the tranquilizer will potentiate the effect of the narcotic. A common example of this type of prescription is the administration of 25 mg promethazine (Phenergan) with 75 mg meperidine IM. There is no convincing evidence that promethazine actually increases the analgesic effect of narcotics, and some studies indicate that promethazine may be antianalgesic. The addition of promethazine to a narcotic could well help to defeat the analgesic effect of the narcotic.

TABLE 7A-2

*Relative Potencies of Analgesics Used Orally for Less Severe Pain**

Drug	PO (mg)
Aspirin	**650**
Acetaminophen (Tylenol)	650
Codeine	32
Meperidine (Demerol)	50
Pentazocine (Talwin)	30
Propoxyphene hydrochloride (Darvon)	65
Propoxyphene napsylate (Darvon-N)	100

*Expressed in doses approximately equivalent in total effect of aspirin 650 mg.
Adapted with permission from Foley, K. M. and A. Rogers. The Management of Cancer Pain, Vol. II: the Rational Use of Analgesics in the Management of Cancer Pain (Hoffmann-LaRoche Monograph Series). Hoffmann-LaRoche, Inc., Nutley, N. J. 1981, p. 10; and Heidrich, G., and S. Perry. Helping the patient in pain. *American Journal of Nursing* (December 1982). p. 1832.

Chlorpromazine (Thorazine) is another tranquilizer that is sometimes used to potentiate the effects of narcotics. In cancer patients with pain, no difference has been found between the analgesic effect of placebo and of chlorpromazine. When chlorpromazine is combined with morphine, there is also no difference in analgesia between the combination and morphine alone, although patients receiving the morphine/chlorpromazine were more sedated.

Two tranquilizers have been shown to be analgesic. One is methotrimeprazine (Levoprome), which is at present used very infrequently, and hydroxyzine (Vistaril, Atarax). Hydroxyzine at dosages of 100 mg IM appears to be as potent as 7 to 8 mg morphine. It is commonly administered in combination with a narcotic, e.g., morphine, with the usual dosage of hydroxyzine being 25 mg IM. Whether hydroxyzine is analgesic at this reduced dosage is unclear, but anecdotal reports from clinicians suggest that it is. Hydroxyzine is also an antiemetic. Nausea and vomiting are typical postoperative problems. A hydroxyzine/narcotic combination could be beneficial in this situation, as well as in others, such as chemotherapy.

Another argument for using tranquilizer/narcotic combinations is that anxiety is a significant component of pain and reaction to pain. A tranquilizer should reduce anxiety and thus the need for larger doses of narcotics. This argument fails to consider that patients are often anxious *because* of unrelieved pain. Treating the pain and resultant anxiety by using adequate dosages of analgesics is preferable to tranquilizing the patient, who remains in pain.

Some clinicians feel that narcotic/tranquilizer combinations will allow use of a lower dosage of narcotic. The reasons given are that (1) there will be less chance of addiction and/or (2) it is desirable to slow the development of narcotic tolerance so that as disease progresses, narcotics will continue to be effective as pain increases. A clear understanding of what is meant by addiction, physical dependence, and tolerance, will suggest a different approach.

Addiction, physical dependence, and tolerance. According to the World Health Organization, addiction is a **psychologic dependence**, in which there is a behavioral pattern of drug abuse that is characterized by the craving of a drug for reasons *other than pain relief* and an overwhelming preoccupation with the procurement and use of the drug. Many cancer patients as well as staff members have an unwarranted fear of addiction. This fear can lead to patients' refusal to take narcotics or taking them only if pain becomes unbearable. Usually if patients are asked whether they would want to continue to take the pain medication if pain were to disappear, they will respond that they would have no interest in continuing the medication once the pain is gone. The nurse can explain that this feeling will not change if they receive narcotics more frequently, and hence they need not fear addiction.

Physical dependence is distinct from addiction. The degree of physical dependence that develops is related to the amount and potency of the drug taken each day and the length of time that the drug is taken. If 10 mg morphine IM were administered bid for 10 days, the patient would develop some physical dependence. This means that if the narcotic were abruptly discontinued, the patient would experience the classic withdrawal symptoms of nausea, sweating, diarrhea, and irritability. In the clinical situation, narcotics are rarely discontinued abruptly. Usually as the healing process or therapeutic pain interventions begin to work, the pain gradually subsides. The patient requests analgesics less often and thereby slowly tapers himself. In a few situations, e.g., with nerve blocks, pain may be abruptly terminated. In these cases it may be necessary for the patient to receive a gradually decreasing dosage of narcotics. Usually ¼ of the original dose is sufficient to prevent withdrawal symptoms. Over the period of 1 wk the dosage can be decreased and the patient can be slowly and comfortably withdrawn from his physical dependence on narcotics.

Tolerance means that larger doses of the analgesic are necessary to produce the original analgesic effect. One of the first signs of tolerance development is that the patient will request the analgesic more frequently. The patient may have been receiving adequate relief from his analgesic but now begins to "watch the clock" and rings for the next dose of drug at the precise moment it is due. Staff may begin to believe that the patient is craving the drug, but actually the development of tolerance has decreased the analgesic effect and the patient feels increased pain.

The appropriate response to the development of tolerance is to increase the dosage of narcotic. CNS side effects do not usually result from increasing dosage in the tolerant patient. Tolerance to respiratory and CNS effects develops at essentially the same rate as tolerance to analgesic effects.

Many cancer patients' pain can be well controlled for weeks or even months on a set dose of narcotic. Some clinicians believe that the increase in requests for drug is a result of advancing disease, not of rapidly increased tolerance. Each patient should be carefully evaluated when he reports an increased level of pain no longer adequately controlled by his current analgesic regimen.

Table 7A–3 lists some of the more commonly used narcotics for the treatment of cancer pain and their effects. An understanding of the unique nature of each of these drugs and how they fit into the clinical setting is essential.

NSAIDs and narcotic combinations. Aspirin, like other non-steroidal anti-inflammatory drugs (NSAIDs), e.g., ibuprofen (Motrin), fenoprofen (Nalfon), and naproxen (Naprosyn), can offer the patient a unique means of pain control.

Unlike narcotic analgesics, which produce pain relief primarily by their action in the CNS, NSAIDs are thought to produce their relief primarily in the peripheral nervous system. The differing sites of action for these two classes of analgesics allow the clinician to use a two-pronged pharmacologic approach to pain control, e.g., the commonly used acetaminophen/codeine combination for mild to moderate pain.

The NSAIDs do not produce the tolerance and physical dependence associated with narcotic analgesics. Repeated administration of a NSAID will not necessitate increasingly larger doses to produce the original dose's analgesic effect. Nor, if the administration of a NSAID is stopped abruptly, will the patient experience a withdrawal syndrome.

NSAIDs with narcotics are particularly effective in the management of pain secondary to bony metastasis. Bone metastasis causes the localized production of prostaglandins (PGs). These localized PGs accelerate bone destruction and, by their action on the peripheral nervous system, lower the pain threshold. The NSAIDs interfere with the production of PGs. By inhibiting PG synthesis, the NSAIDs alleviate pain and retard progressive bone deterioration.

NSAID therapy can improve analgesic relief when they are added to narcotics, especially for the patient who has developed tolerance.

For example, a patient who has been receiving 2 mg levorphanol (Levo-Dromoran) PO q 4 hr may have initially experienced adequate pain relief and now reports that the analgesia no longer lasts the full 4 hr. The addition of 2 aspirin tablets to each dose of levorphanol should increase the duration of analgesic action. In another situation, a patient who has been taking 10 mg methadone PO q 4 hr may initially have experienced good results and now reports that he continues to recieve 4 hr of relief, but the amount of relief is insufficient. The addition of 2 aspirin tablets to each dose of methadone should increase the peak analgesic relief. Another approach would be to start these patients on a scheduled regimen of ibuprofen (Motrin) or naproxen (Naprosyn) q 6 to 8 hr.

An alternative to frequent aspirin dosing is the use of one of the more potent NSAIDs on a q-6-to-8-hr fixed schedule. It should be borne in mind that if a patient does not respond to a particular NSAID, another NSAID should be tried. The variability in response to narcotics seen among various patients is also seen with NSAIDs.

To varying degrees, the NSAIDs irritate the GI mucosa. Because the possibility of GI bleeding is increased, patients with GI ulcers should not receive this type of therapy. NSAIDs should also be used cautiously in patients undergoing anticoagulant therapy, chemotherapy, patients with hepatic impairment, or bleeding disorders. The success of NSAID therapy will hinge upon whether the clinicians involved understand the rationale underlying it and are skilled in the clinical use of the drugs.

Changing routes of administration.   Many cancer patients receive IM injections for pain while they are hospitalized. Often upon discharge, the patient will receive analgesics PO. Rarely is the patient converted gradually from IM to PO analgesics *before* discharge. The abrupt change from the IM to PO route can cause significant problems, usually left to the outpatient department or the visiting nurses' service to solve.

One of the major problems for the patient is that injections offered quick and potent relief of pain, whereas pills are slower to take effect. The onset of pain relief after an IM injection is typically within ½ hr and peaks by 1 hr. Many PO analgesics may take 30 to 60 min for onset and up to 2 hr to peak. The patient should be informed of these differences in time-effect for the PO vs. IM route and that he should not wait for the pain to become severe but take the analgesic when he begins to experience mild to moderate pain. Ideally, the patient would be on a scheduled analgesic regimen of q 3 to 4 hr, with a family member available to monitor him for signs of CNS depression.

Conversion from the IM route to the appropriate PO analgesic dosage before discharge is a better approach. Gradually decreasing the

TABLE 7A-3

Nursing Implications of Narcotics Used to Relieve Pain

Drug	Dose (usual) and route	Duration of action	Adverse effects	Administration information
Codeine	30–60 mg IM 30–60 mg PO	3–4 hr	Same as morphine but weaker.	Not for IV use. Addition of 650 mg aspirin/acetaminophen with PO codeine will significantly increase analgesia. Same principle applies to other PO narcotics.
Hydromorphone (Dilaudid)	1.0–2.0 mg IM 2–4 mg PO 1–2 3-mg rectal suppositories	3–4 hr 3–4 hr 5–6 hr	Same as morphine.	Quick onset of action. Short plasma half-life, which may be an advantage in patients prone to confusion.
Levorphanol (Levo-Dromoran)	2 mg IM 2–4 mg PO	4–5 hr 4–5 hr	Same as morphine.	Similar to methadone. Some patients will respond better to levorphanol than to methadone and vice versa.
Meperidine (Demerol)	50–125 mg IM 50–100 mg PO	2–4 hr 3–4 hr	Same as morphine. Normeperidine is a toxic by-product of meperidine and a powerful CNS excitant.	Contraindicated in patients with renal compromise or who have received MAO inhibitors within 14 days.

Drug	Dose	Duration	Side effects	Comments
Methadone	10 mg IM 5–20 mg PO	4–5 hr 4–5 hr	Same as morphine.	Long plasma half-life. Monitor patient for signs of overdosage. Contraindicated in patients with CNS, renal, or hepatic impairment. IM (vs. SC) route is recommended.
Morphine	10 mg IM 60 mg PO	3–5 hr 3–5 hr	Respiratory depression, hypotension, bradycardia, urinary retention, constipation.	Contraindicated in patients with impaired ventilation, asthma, elevated intracranial pressure, liver failure.
Oxycodone (Percodan, Percocet-5)	1–2 tablets	3–4 hr	Not available in USA in IM or IV form. Same as morphine (PO) but weaker.	Rapid onset of action. Short half-life.
Oxymorphone (Numorphan)	1 mg IM 1–2 5-mg rectal suppositories	4–5 hr 6 hr	Same as morphine.	Rate of absorption for rectal suppositories can be highly variable.

MAO, monoamine oxidase.

Adapted with permission from Rogers, A. 21 problems in pain control — and ways to solve them. *Your Patient and Cancer* (September 1981). 65–69, 73–75.

IM dose and substituting an equianalgesic dose PO is one way to achieve conversion. For instance, with a patient taking 6 mg levorphanol IM q 3 hr, the first step is to decrease the IM levorphanol to 4 mg and give 4 mg levorphanol PO. The faster onset of action from the IM route will still take place but, as the IM analgesic wears off, the PO route will begin to provide relief. The patient should probably be on this initial regimen for at least 24 to 48 hr, helping him to get used to the gradual change and allowing the staff to observe his response. It may be possible to lower the PO dosage beneath the equianalgesic dose. If so, it will become apparent in ≤2 days. If the patient experiences increased sedation on the new dosage, the PO dose should be lowered. Now the patient is receiving 4 mg IM and 2 mg PO and is satisfied with the analgesia provided. The next step is to decrease the IM dose to 2 mg and increase the PO dose to 6 mg. After ≤2 days of this regimen, the patient can be switched completely to the PO route, receiving 10 mg levorphanol q 3 hr.

Patients can also be converted from the IV route of narcotic administration to the PO or IM route. Equianalgesic dosages for the PO and IM narcotic vs. the IV are, to a great extent, based on clinical experience rather than analgesic studies, however. A rough rule of thumb is that the IV dosage is ~2 times as potent as the IM dosage. Thus, 50 mg meperidine IV ≅100 mg meperidine IM or 400 mg meperidine PO. To avoid having the patient take eight 50-mg tablets of meperidine PO, he can be converted gradually from meperidine to methadone or levorphanol; the number of tablets will be greatly reduced, and the patient will receive the added benefit of the longer duration of action that is inherent in these two analgesics.

Most clinical situations do not run quite as smoothly as the ones outlined above. Therefore the nurse is the key person to judge the patient's response and inform staff of changes that are needed (Table 7A-4).

Scheduling. The scheduled, or around the clock (ATC), administration of analgesia at regular intervals for the cancer patient in pain is an effective treatment approach. This method of narcotic administration has been made popular by reports of success from British hospices. By scheduling medication at a set time, the patient will receive a steady, unfluctuating supply of analgesic, which will in turn result in a fairly steady plasma level of the narcotic. If the amount of narcotic has been titrated appropriately for the patient, the level of analgesia will be adequate and constant. This method of administration eliminates patient concern about having to ask repeatedly for medication. This concern is often well justified because prn pain prescriptions have a lower priority to medicating staff than scheduled prescriptions.

Administration of analgesics on an ATC schedule also helps to prevent the emergence of pain or to routinely halt the progression of pain beyond the mild to moderate level. For the majority of cancer patients with pain, this method of analgesic administration is the procedure of choice.

One of the potential problems with ATC administration is the possibility of overdosage. Medicating staff must be vigilant for this possibility. Constant assessment of the patient's physiologic response to the analgesic must be made. The patient with progressive disease will gradually become debilitated, and an increasing number of body systems will be compromised. Hepatic, renal, and CNS disease involvement is common and may alter response to and metabolism of narcotics. Patients taking ATC analgesic are thus at a somewhat higher risk of overdosage than patients on prn administration, simply because they usually receive narcotics more frequently. If a patient is too sedated, the regular dose should be held, and consideration should be given to decreasing the milligram dosage or increasing the intervals between doses. Fortunately, the CNS depressant effects of narcotics are easily reversible by the IV administration of naloxone (*see* discussion below).

Some patients will be best served by prn analgesic prescriptions, e.g., the patient who experiences spontaneous eruptions of moderate to severe pain at infrequent and unpredictable intervals. Since this patient is basically pain free, the administration of a potent narcotic ATC would only sedate him. Pain is a natural antagonist to the effects of narcotics. Thus, some patients in severe pain can tolerate massive doses of narcotics, though if the severe pain were to be suddenly removed the patient would experience the full CNS depressant effects.

A third group of patients will need a combination of prn and ATC analgesics. These patients will usually have a chronic moderate-to-severe base-line pain that is best controlled by an ATC routine. These patients will also have periodic episodes of acute pain for which the regular ATC dosing is inadequate. This type of periodic intense pain is often managed by a supplemental prn analgesic. An example is a patient with widespread bony metastasis. Any repositioning in bed or movement to a chair can be extremely painful. A small dose of IV narcotic can be administered 5 to 10 min before the painful episode occurs. Usually the short-duration narcotics like fentanyl (Sublimaze) or meperidine are preferred because when the painful episode is over, pain quickly subsides, and the increased analgesia is no longer needed.

Treatment for overdosage.   The possibility that severe respiratory depression may occur is always present for the patient who has been receiving progressively larger doses of narcotics for pain or is

TABLE 7A–4

Nursing Protocol for the Management of Pain Problems in Cancer Patients

Factor	Intervention
Patient reports pain	Assess nature of pain: onset, intensity, character, duration, site. Determine if a new pain that warrants medical diagnosis. Attempt to make patient comfortable through repositioning and/or removing or altering noxious stimuli, e.g., padding a wooden chair. Medicate promptly if pain is the expected result of treatment or disease process.
Decreased analgesic effectiveness	Question patient as to the analgesic's onset of action, peak effect, and duration of action. Onset: How long does pain medication take to work after you receive it? Peak: When the medication is working at its best, how much pain relief does it give you: no pain relief, slight, moderate, a lot, or complete relief of your pain? Duration: How long does each dose of the medication give pain relief? 1 hr, 3 hr, ½ hr?
Slow onset of analgesic action	Evaluate for scheduled regimen of analgesic administration, e.g., q 3 hr ATC. If patient will be remaining on a prn regimen, instruct patient to ask for medication *before* the pain becomes severe. Ensure that analgesic is delivered promptly to intercept development of severe pain.
Decreased peak effect	Obtain a medical diagnosis of increased pain secondary to disease progression or development of narcotic tolerance. Change/increase analgesic regimen or add NSAID on a fixed schedule if patient has developed tolerance.

Decreased duration of action	Obtain a medical diagnosis of increased pain secondary to disease progression or development of narcotic tolerance. Increase dose of narcotic unless a more definitive treatment is attempted.
	Unless there is reason (e.g., brain metastasis) for patient to be on short-duration analgesic (meperidine, hydromorphone, oxycodone), consider administration of a narcotic with a longer duration of action, e.g., levorphanol, methadone.
Overmedicated	Evaluate for a change in dosage and/or time of analgesic administration.
Awakened by pain	Ascertain if patient wishes to be awakened and given analgesic an hour before the pain usually awakens him.
Pain during care and other activities	Ascertain if patient would like to receive analgesic upon waking or prior to activity. Explain that this intervention should help to prevent or reduce the pain experienced during care or activity. Alter patient's environment to minimize pain-producing stimuli, e.g., have the toilet articles within easy reach to minimize stretching.
Incident-related pain	Many pain-producing incidents (e.g., changing positions, cutting food on a plate, showering, stooping) can be eliminated or modified to reduce severity of pain. Instruct patients in body mechanics to help reduce strain of position changes. Ask patient to identify painful incidents — have patient keep a diary to record incidents — that occur in a 24-hr period. Nurse and patient should examine the elements of each incident and explore ways to eliminate or modify the pain-producing factors.

receiving an initial trial of narcotics. The narcotic antagonist naloxone will quickly reverse the CNS and analgesic effects of narcotics. The nurse should be familiar with the administration and action of this narcotic antagonist. Standing physician's orders and an emergency supply of naloxone may be useful for patient-care units that administer narcotics to cancer patients on a routine and frequent basis. The usual dosage of naloxone is 0.4 mg delivered as an IV bolus over 3 to 4 min. Care must be taken, however, if the patient has had an appreciable exposure to narcotics. Many cancer patients in pain will develop some physical dependence on narcotics. The abrupt administration of a 0.4 mg naloxone bolus could well put the patient into immediate and full-blown withdrawal. Therefore, the 0.4 mg dose should be mixed with 10 ml of normal saline, administered carefully, and titrated to the patient's response. Once the patient has responded and the respirations return to normal, it may be necessary to hang an IV naloxone/normal saline drip. The duration of action of naloxone is ~30 min, but the respiratory-depressant effects of some of the analgesics with longer half-life, such as methadone and levorphanol, can last for many hours.

Some cancer patients who have been maintained on a set dosage of narcotics for an appreciable period of time will also exhibit signs of overdosage. For example, the patient may have been taking levor-phanol 4 mg PO q 4 hr for 3 wk and has tolerated this regimen well. Suddenly, the patient will begin to slur his speech, nod off during conversation, and exhibit a degree of respiratory depression. It appears that he is receiving too large a dose of drug, but it may be that his disease is progressing, with a resultant deterioration in his physical status. The disease may be advancing to the brain and/or a general metabolic encephalopathy has developed. In this situation, the patient's dosage of narcotic should be reduced and a diagnosis obtained from the medical staff.

Variables affecting narcotic analgesia.

Age: The duration of pain relief provided by a narcotic is partially dependent on the age of the patient. In general, older (>29) patients will receive more analgesia from a standard dose of morphine than younger (18–29) patients. In a retrospective study of morphine analgesia in cancer patients with pain, it was found that the 18- to 19-year-old group received the least amount of analgesia from a standard dose of morphine.

It would take 16 mg morphine IM to give the younger patient the same relief that the middle-aged (30–59) patient received from only 8 mg morphine IM. The oldest age group (60–89) received twice the analgesia from 8 mg morphine IM as the middle-aged group.

This difference may be explained by the faster metabolism and elimination of narcotics in the younger patient. In the older patient, the drug will remain active longer and stay in the body for an extended period.

Clinical staff should be aware of this difference in narcotic effect based on age. Many times the younger cancer patient who is taking narcotics for pain is labeled a potential abuser because of frequent requests for the analgesic. Likewise, care should be taken when administering narcotics to the elderly. The usual therapeutic dosage of a narcotic *may* need to be reduced in the elderly because they will tend to have a more dramatic analgesic and CNS response.

Site of injection: Methadone that is injected into the gluteal area will produce significantly less analgesia than methadone injected into the deltoid muscle. Methadone is a lipid-soluble compound and thus is probably sequestered in the gluteal fat, whereas the deltoid region has significantly less fat than it has muscle. This difference in analgesic response should be borne in mind when using IM methadone and other lipid-soluble analgesics such as pentazocine (Talwin). Males and females receive essentially the same amount of analgesia from a standard dose of morphine. Since women have more gluteal fat, their analgesic response to methadone can be significantly less than that of a man receiving a gluteal injection. Inasmuch as morphine is not a lipid-soluble analgesic, this problem is not as significant. Because there is generally less blood flow to the fatty areas, however, any analgesic may have a somewhat reduced response if it is injected into fatty tissue.

These variables underscore the great variation in patients' responses to what are considered normal therapeutic dosages of narcotics. It is thus essential that a skilled and knowledgable clinician work with the cancer patient in pain. In the clinical situation, the only way to determine accurately how much drug a particular patient will need is by the careful titration of narcotic dosage to the patient's reports of pain relief (*see* Table 7A–4).

Bibliography

1. Daut, R. L., and C. S. Cleeland. The prevalence and severity of pain in cancer. *Cancer* (November 1982). 1913–1918.

     Reports on the incidence and severity of pain caused by cancer of varying etiologies. A good reference.

2. Foley, K. M. Analgesic management of bone pain. *In* Weiss, L., and H. A. Gilbert, editors. Bone Metastases. Metastases Monograph Series, Vol. 3. G. K. Hall and Co., Boston. 1981.

     Excellent chapter on the clinical management of bone metastases. Specific strategies discussed.

3. Foley, K. M. The Management of Cancer Pain, Vol. I: Pain Syndromes in Patients with Cancer (Hoffmann-La Roche Monograph Series). Hoffmann-La Roche Inc., Nutley N. J. 1981.

   Common types of pain syndromes caused by cancer and cancer therapies. A fine outline and teaching guide.

4. Foley, K. M., and A. Rogers. The Management of Cancer Pain, Vol. II: The Rational Use of Analgesics in the Management of Cancer Pain (Hoffmann-La Roche Monograph Series). Hoffmann-La Roche Inc., Nutley, N. J. 1981.

   Informative and completely practical approach to the use of analgesic medications for the control of cancer pain.

5. Heidrich, G., and S. Perry. Helping the patient in pain. *American Journal of Nursing* (December 1982). 1828–1833.

   Information on pain assessment, use of analgesics, and strategies for helping the patient.

6. Kaiko, R. F., S. C. Wallenstein, A. G. Rogers, P. Y. Grabinski, and R. W. Houde. Narcotics in the elderly. *Medical Clinics of North America* (September 1982). 1079–1089.

   Discusses the research concerning the variations in response to analgesics that are caused by age.

7. Kaiko, R. F., K. M. Foley, P. Y. Grabinski, G. Heidrich, A. G. Rogers, C. E. Inturrisi, and M. M. Reidenberg. Central nervous system excitatory effects of meperidine in cancer patients. *Annals of Neurology* (February 1983). 180–185.

   A clinical survey of patients' subjective reports and correlations of these reports to the blood levels of normeperidine.

8. Kaiko, R. F., S. L. Wallenstein, A. G. Rogers, and R. W. Houde. Sources of variation in analgesic responses in cancer patients with chronic pain receiving morphine. *Pain* (February 1983). 191–200.

   Discusses the influence of age, sex, race, and pain character on patients' response to analgesics.

9. McCaffery, M. Nursing Management of the Patient in Pain. J. B. Lippincott Co., Philadelphia. 1979. Second edition.

   A classic book. Required reading for anyone seriously concerned with the management of pain.

10. Perry, S., and G. Heidrich. Placebo response: myth and matter. *American Journal of Nursing* (April 1981). 720–725.

    Discusses the use and misuse of placebos. Focus is on understanding and enhancing the placebo response.

B: SLEEP

Suzanne Hearne Kaempfer

Pathophysiology

Sleep is a state of decreased responsiveness to external stimuli from which an individual may be aroused. As distinct from periods of wakefulness, sleep is characterized by alterations in physiologic functioning and level of consciousness, and by a reduction of physical activity to minimal levels. The actual physiologic function and nature of sleep is poorly understood, although it appears to serve both an integrative and restorative function to the CNS and thereby to the overall well-being of the individual. The inability of the human body to function normally when an individual has been deprived of sleep demonstrates the necessity of adequate sleep.

What is known about sleep patterns has been derived in part from studies of three physiologic parameters: (1) the EEG, which measures brain electrical activity from the central scalp; (2) the electrooculogram, which measures eye movement at the outer canthus of each eye; and (3) the electromyogram, which measures muscle tension (for sleep research, from beneath the chin). Using these measurements, the cyclical nature of sleep has been characterized, and distinctive stages within the sleep cycle have been identified (Fig. 7B-1).

In general, sleep may be classified as either REM (rapid eye movement) or NREM (non-REM). REM is the active phase of sleep during which sympathetic nervous system activity predominates. REM is characterized by bursts of jerky eye movements, vivid dreams, deep muscle relaxation with occasional irregular fine motor muscle movements, irregular pulse and respirations, variations in BP, increased gastric secretion, and penile erections.

In contrast, NREM is the quiet, restful phase of sleep with parasympathetic dominance. NREM consists of four stages of progressively deepening sleep (stages 1 to 4), and it is characterized by decreased BP, respirations, and metabolic rate; relative dreamlessness; slow eye movements; and profound restfulness with diminished skeletal muscle tone.

As a periodic phenomenon, a night's sleep consists of a series of 90-min cycles that repeat four to six times during a 7- to 8-hr period (see Fig. 7B-1). Each cycle consists of most or all of the stages of NREM

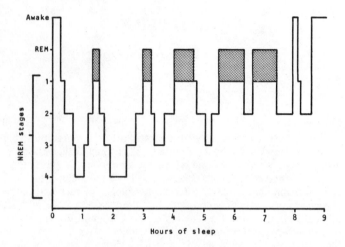

Figure 7B–1. Diagrammatic representation of a typical night's sleep. ▨ , REM; □ , NREM. *Adapted with permission from* Lee, K. Rest and comfort status. *In* Mitchell, P. H., and A. Loustau. Concepts Basic to Nursing. McGraw-Hill Book Co., New York. 1981. Third edition. p. 606.

sleep followed by REM sleep. During a typical night's sleep, the individual first progresses through the four NREM stages, then ascends through stages 3 and 2, and then enters REM, which completes the first cycle. The cycle then repeats itself beginning with stage 2 (unless the sleeper has been awakened) as follows: NREM, REM, NREM, etc. This cycle continues throughout the night, with the proportion of time spent in each stage varying.

Depending on a number of factors, the body's requirements for REM and NREM vary. The need for REM is increased by psychologic stress. In addition, the duration of REM sleep decreases throughout the life-span. For example, young adults average 7 to 8 hr of total sleep each night (20 to 25% of which is REM) and usually sleep through the night. Alternatively, elderly adults spend an average of 6 hr sleeping at night, have less REM sleep, and decreased or absent stage 4 sleep. They also tend to wake up frequently during the night, experience difficulties with sleep onset, and often have early morning awakenings.

Despite what is known about sleep, the clinical significance of both the occurrence and duration of the various sleep stages in humans is not clear. It is also difficult to determine clinically if an individual is REM or NREM deprived, whereas total sleep deprivation and insomnia are frequent and recognizable phenomena.

Insomnia, an objective and subjective experience of the inability to obtain a sufficient quantity or quality of sleep, is the most common sleep disorder, and affects one third of all adults. There are three types of insomnia: initial, intermittent, and terminal. *Initial insomnia*, or difficulty in falling asleep, is the most frequent sleep disorder in young adults. *Intermittent insomnia*, the most common form of insomnia, implies the inability to stay asleep, with frequent or prolonged awakenings during the night. *Terminal insomnia*, characterized by early morning awakening, is associated with depression, aging, daytime napping, and early retiring to bed.

The physiologic need for sleep varies for individuals, and the amount of time required in each of the different sleep stages is unknown. However, **deprivation** of total sleep needs or of different sleep stages produces observable signs. For the individual with initial sleep deprivation, signs and symptoms include a feeling of fatigue, headache, nausea, anxiety, depression, or burning eyes, and signs of somnolence, irritability, restlessness, apathy, lassitude, periods of inattention, puffy eyelids, reddened conjunctiva, and dark areas around the eyes.

As **total sleep deprivation** accumulates, more pronounced signs and symptoms include difficulty concentrating, decreased attention span, misperceptions, auditory or visual hallucinations, and muscle weakness. Objective signs of prolonged total sleep deprivation include muscle tremors, decreased coordination and reaction time, disorientation, slurred speech, and behavior changes such as aggression or withdrawal. Recovery from sleep deprivation of this type requires more hours of sleep than were previously lost, both in terms of total sleep time and of individual sleep stages.

It is also possible to have deprivation of an individual sleep stage without total sleep deprivation. REM sleep deprivation poses a particular problem to hospitalized patients. Symptoms of REM deprivation include irritability, anxiety, difficulty concentrating, hyperactivity, increased appetite, and difficulty coping with stress. Several factors inherent in the hospitalization experience contribute to the susceptibility of patients to this kind of sleep deprivation. Hospitalized patients may develop day/night sleep reversal or obtain insufficient total sleep (e.g., 3 to 4 hr of sleep in a 24-hr period). Such patients frequently sleep for only short periods (≤ 1 hr) at a time, totally eliminating periods of REM, which occurs at the end of a normal 90-min sleep cycle.

Chronic use of REM-suppressant drugs that promote sleep is another iatrogenic problem among hospital patients. Initially, the total sleep experience improves with use of these agents. As tolerance to their therapeutic effect develops, however (usually in ~2 wk), the hypnotic efficacy is lost. Furthermore, abrupt withdrawal after prolonged use of REM-suppressant drugs produces REM rebound: a marked increase in the amount of REM sleep during the days or weeks of recovery from REM deprivation. The patient experiencing REM rebound may complain of anxiety, depression, apathy, restlessness, agitation, irritability, insomnia, frequent awakenings, frequent and intense dreams, nightmares, malaise, and tiredness. But more critically, REM rebound may exacerbate medical conditions, such as angina, hypertension, cerebrovascular disease, and peptic ulcers, because REM sleep is associated with enhanced sympathetic nervous system activity.

Assessment

Of all people in industrialized countries, 12 to 15% have recurrent sleep disorders, and an additional 20 to 25% have occasional insomnia. In the general population, sleep disorders have been found to be related to such factors as situational stress, illness (or disease), effects of the aging process, and the use of drugs. In view of these findings, it is hardly surprising to find sleep disturbance to be a frequent problem among cancer patients. The cancer patient undergoing active treatment or acute care for treatment- or disease-related problems is vulnerable to sleep disorders for several reasons. Physical illness increases the individual's sleep requirements, disrupts the usual sleep/wakefulness pattern, and is often associated with anxiety and depression. In acute care settings, sleep deprivation among patients is common because of the repeated violations of sleep hygiene guidelines, which dictate awakening at the same time each day, consistency in napping patterns, use of the bed for sleep rather than for reading or working, and preservation of the natural 24-hr activity/inactivity cycle. Frequent interruptions of sleep in order to adhere to hospital routines or treatment schedules places the cancer patient at high risk for deprivation of total sleep and of various sleep stages. Sleep deprivation is an area of patient care that is likely to be overlooked, being considered less important than more acute medical problems. Table 7B–1 summarizes factors that may influence sleep.

Assessment of sleep problems in the cancer patient requires eliciting information from several sources, including the patient's subjective report of sleep difficulty, objective observations of behavioral and physiologic manifestations of sleep disruption, and reports of family members and friends on the quality of the patient's sleep. Comprehensive assessment of factors that may be affecting the patient's sleep is necessary in order to plan effective interventions. Table 7B–1 presents approaches with which to assess patients' sleep.

Medical management

Medical management of sleep disturbance in the cancer patient is an area that has received little attention in the oncology literature. The initial focus of interventions geared toward alleviating this patient-care problem is on the management of underlying conditions that may be contributing to sleep disruption. This involves treating the malignancy in order to relieve tumor-related symptoms (e.g., pain or dyspnea) that may be causing sleep loss. Medication routines should be evaluated to determine drugs or drug interactions that have potential sleep effects. It may be necessary to provide medical or psychiatric management of the anxiety and depression that accompany attempts to cope with catastrophic illness. In some cases, short-term or intermittent use of sleep medications may be prescribed for patients whose sleeplessness does not respond to other medical interventions.

Sleep medications. Hypnotics are one of the most frequently prescribed group of drugs in industrialized nations, and the second most commonly used agents among hospitalized patients. What seems to be little appreciated, however, is that the use of medications for persistent insomnia over months or years can destroy natural sleep patterns and physiologic functions. Not only do sleep medications interfere with the stages of sleep, but their prolonged use (>7 to 14 days) can produce a number of toxic effects, including tolerance, cross-tolerance, psychologic dependence, physical dependence, drug intoxication, and drug hangover. Sleep medications should not be used in the presence of uncontrolled pain because their use will exacerbate the pain.

Tolerance involves the need for increasing the doses of a medication over time in order to realize the same level of effectiveness as originally achieved. Sometimes, *cross-tolerance* between sleep medications may develop, in which case periodically changing the agent used will not prevent the development of tolerance (and the new agent may be ineffective).

Psychologic dependence is the compulsive use of and craving for a drug. Thus, the manifestations of psychologic dependence are behavioral. Physical dependence, on the other hand, is indicated by the occurrence of a physiologic withdrawal syndrome when the drug is discontinued abruptly. The severity of physical dependence depends on the specific medication, the dose, and the duration of use. Withdrawal syndrome, which may last from 24 hr to 2 wk after the last dose of the drug, can be life threatening. Initial withdrawal symptoms include insomnia, muscle tremors, irritability, weakness, anxiety, anorexia, nausea, fever, sweating, vomiting, headache, restlessness, and incoordination. As withdrawal progresses, delayed symptoms may be seen, including tinnitus, delirium, postural hypotension, incoherence, convulsions, and psychosis. These may culminate in

TABLE 7B-1

Factors That Influence Sleep and Assessment of Sleep Disturbance in Cancer Patients

Factor	Assessment
General (age and developmental level)	What are the patient's age and developmental level (infant, school age, adolescent, young adult, middle age, elderly)? How has the patient been sleeping (describe sleep habits, usual amount of sleep)?
Time retires to bed	What time does the patient usually go to bed?
Patterns of insomnia Initial	How long does it take the patient to fall asleep? Does the patient fall asleep right away? How does the patient feel before falling asleep? How often does the patient have trouble falling asleep?
Intermittent	Does the patient wake up during the night? What causes awakening? How often does the patient awaken during the night? What helps the patient get back to sleep?
Terminal	What time does the patient wake up? What wakes the patient up early? How often do early awakenings occur? Is the patient depressed? What does the patient do upon awakening early?
Patient's response to quality of sleep	Does the patient feel rested after a night's sleep? How does the patient feel after getting up? Does the patient appear to be well rested? Validate patient vs. nurse perceptions.
Naps	Does the patient nap during the day? How long? Does the patient have day/night reversal (sleeps more during the day than at night)? Does the patient have excess daytime sleepiness (e.g., due to a brain tumor)?
Recreation/exercise	Does the patient exercise? What sort of activity is involved? When does the patient exercise in relation to bedtime?

Emotional factors Anxiety	Is the patient worried about the outcome of the illness? Is there an inability to manage normal responsibilities?
Depression	What is the patient's mood? (Cheerful? Depressed?)
Stress	Has the patient received a recent diagnosis of cancer or recurrence? Are there any other obvious sources of stress in the patient's life (e.g., a new course of treatment)?
Sleep environment	What is the patient's usual sleep environment? What have been previous experiences when sleeping in an unfamiliar place?
Lighting	Does having a light on at night disturb the patient?
Ventilation	Does the patient like to sleep with a door or window open?
Bedding	How many and what type of pillows does the patient use? Is any special bedding used (blankets, mattress, or pads)?
Temperature	Does the patient need the room warm or cool to sleep well?
Noise	Do noises wake the patient or keep the patient awake? Does the patient need quiet to sleep?
Positioning	What is the patient's usual sleep position? Does the patient need to be turned q 2 hr?
Social factors	Does the patient usually sleep alone, share a room, or share the bed? Does the patient have increased social stimulation before bedtime?
Presleep routine	What does the patient do immediately before going to bed?
Beverages	Does the patient like a beverage before going to bed?
Hygiene	Does bathing at bedtime help the patient sleep?
Food	Does the patient like to eat something at bedtime?
Medication	What medications is the patient receiving? Is the patient on steroids (which can produce chronic insomnia)? Does the patient take any medications (including alcohol) to produce sleep?

Factor	Assessment
Personal beliefs about sleep	How much sleep does the patient think is necessary? What does the patient feel are the consequences of insufficient sleep?
Disease/treatment factors	What is the patient's diagnosis, disease status, and course of treatment?
Pain/discomfort	What is the source of any pain (e.g., recent surgery, mucositis)? Is pain control adequate? Is the patient febrile? Is pain preventing sleep or causing awakening?
Fatigue	Does the patient have a balance of activity and rest during the day? Has the patient undergone a late evening test or treatment?
Impaired nutritional status	Is the patient NPO? Is there nausea or vomiting?
Dyspnea/cough	Does the patient need oxygen or suctioning? Is coughing disrupting sleep?
Urinary frequency/incontinence	Is the patient receiving IV therapy or diuretics? Is the patient aware of the urge to void? If present, is the bladder catheter patent?
Diarrhea	What are the frequency and consistency of stools?
Nighttime confusion	Does the patient's mental status undergo changes from day to night? Does the patient have an electrolyte imbalance?
Altered skin integrity	Are there decubiti? Are there draining wounds or lesions that require frequent dressing changes?
Disruptive care-giver routines (tests, treatments, routine care, health team rounds)	What procedures are absolutely necessary (e.g., antibiotic administration), and which can be eliminated or postponed until the patient is awake (e.g., q 2 hr mouth care)?

*See also Table 7B–3.

status epilepticus, cardiovascular collapse, and loss of the body's temperature-regulating mechanism. Psychologic and physical dependence may occur independently or may exist simultaneously in an individual.

Drug intoxication is usually associated with the use of large doses of drugs and may occur in a patient who is unable to metabolize and excrete normal doses of the drug because of hepatic or renal dysfunction. Intoxication with sleep medications is associated with excessive CNS depression, accompanied by symptoms of ataxia, dizziness, slurred speech, and blurred vision, progressing to coma and death.

Drug hangover is frequently noted among users of sleep medications. Symptoms include residual drowsiness, heavy-headedness, impaired judgment and motor function, and decreased intellectual functioning.

Taking the potential dangers of these agents into consideration, therapeutic use of sleep medications must follow several general guidelines. Of fundamental importance is assessment of the underlying cause of the insomnia for the presence of a treatable medical condition. Furthermore, evaluation of the circumstances surrounding the development of the insomnia may uncover its responsiveness to environmental manipulation (such as adjusting the room temperature). If, on the basis of these findings, the insomnia is not attributable to a treatable cause or does not respond to nonpharmacologic measures, the use of a sleep medication may be necessary. In fact, in cases where anxiety and sleeplessness are temporary (situational), severe or intolerable to the patient, or may adversely affect the patient's medical condition, pharmacologic sleep aids are justified.

In most circumstances drugs that promote sleep should only be used for a brief or intermittent course. Brief means a maximum of 7 to 14 consecutive nights (infrequently, up to 28 consecutive nights is possible with some agents, e.g., benzodiazepines). Intermittent use permits the patient to use the sleep medication occasionally (e.g., up to 3 times/wk), but only when sleep is most needed. At all times attention must be directed to potential interactions between sleep medications and other drugs the patient is taking. Drug interactions of particular concern are enzyme induction, protein-binding displacement, and potentiation of CNS depression.

Enzyme induction involves stimulation of hepatic microsomal enzymes that metabolize drugs, thereby decreasing the pharmacologic activity of drugs disposed of in this way. For example, oral anticoagulants, systemic steroids, and phenothiazines are less effective when used in combination with barbiturates because barbiturates are known to induce enzymes in the liver.

Protein-bound hypnotics and their metabolites can displace other drugs from protein-binding sites, causing a transient increase in the unbound drug, with consequent increase in drug action. This occurs when chloral hydrate displaces diphenylhydantoin.

Potentiation of CNS depression, which may result in suppression of respiratory function and BP, is an especially dangerous drug interaction that is possible when drugs are used to promote sleep. In general, the use of sleep medications should be avoided in conjunction with narcotics; however, with some cancer patients, the use of a sleep medication in addition to a narcotic may be necessary at times. Safe administration of such a combination depends on careful assessment of the patient. For example, simultaneous use of a narcotic and a sleep medication could be indicated in a patient who had, on previous nights, slept poorly when the narcotic and hypnotic were administered alternately at intervals throughout the night.

In all instances, the use of sleep medications should include consideration of the time available for sleep after their administration, as well as upcoming activities (such as treatments) in which the patient will be involved. In the presence of hepatic, renal, or respiratory dysfunction, sleep medications should either be withheld, or appropriate dosage decrements used, with vigilance to signs of toxic accumulation of drug levels.

Table 7B–2 lists some of the pharmacologic agents used in the management of sleep disturbance. Several groups of drugs in this category deserve special mention.

At present, **benzodiazepines** are the drugs of choice in the management of sleep disorders because they are safe and effective for at least 1 mo of regular use and because they are able to produce more natural sleep (through less disruption of REM sleep) than other agents. **Antihistamines** have attracted attention for use in the management of sleep disorders in cancer patients because their anticholinergic properties may also be useful in relieving other troublesome symptoms, such as nausea and vomiting. There is no evidence, however, that antihistamines are either safer or more effective than other sleep medications. In addition, they tend to produce daytime sedation, and their anticholinergic effects may be a problem in elderly patients. Antihistamines are a major component of many over-the-counter sleep products.

Tricyclic antidepressants (TCAs) are not primary drugs for the management of sleep disorders; however, depression (with concomitant sleeplessness) is often a problem in cancer patients. In this situation, the sedative effects of TCAs may be useful in a once-daily bedtime dose and may eliminate the need for an additional hypnotic drug.

Barbiturates are generally not recommended for cancer patients because other agents are available that have fewer adverse effects and

TABLE 7B-2
Medications Used to Promote Sleep

Drug category*	Medication	Hypnotic dose (route)	Onset (duration of action)	Effect on sleep cycle
Benzodiazepines	Chlordiazepoxide (Librium)	50-100 mg (capsule, tablet)	30-60 min (6-8 hr)	Suppression of stage 4.
	Clorazepate (Tranxene)	15 mg (capsule, tablet)	1 hr (24 hr)	Suppression of stage 4.
	Diazepam (Valium)	5-10 mg (tablet)	30-60 min (3 hr)	Shortening of stage 4.
	Flurazepam (Dalmane)	15-30 mg (capsule)	20-30 min 7-8 hr)	Marked stage 4 reduction. Little or no suppression of REM.
	Lorazepam (Ativan)	2-4 mg (tablet)	Highly individual	Suppression of stage 4.
	Oxazepam (Serax)	10-30 mg (capsule, tablet)	Shorter than than diazepam	Fewer effects on sleep stages than chlordiazepoxide.
	Temazepam (Restoril)	15-30 mg (capsule)	30 min (6-8 hr)	Marked stage 4 reduction. Little or no suppression of REM.
Chloral derivative	Chloral hydrate (Noctec)	0.5-1.0 g (capsule, syrup, suppository)	30-60 min (4-8 hr)	Suppression of stage 4 in high doses.
Acetylinic alcohol	Ethchlorvynol (Placidyl)	0.5-1.0 g (capsule)	15-30 min (4-5 hr)	Suppression of REM.
Piperidinedione derivatives	Glutethimide (Doriden)	250-500 mg (capsule, tablet)	30 min (4-8 hr)	Suppression of REM and stage 4.
	Methyprylon (Noludar)	200-400 mg (capsule, tablet)	45 min (5-8 hr)	Suppression of REM and stage 4.

Drug category*	Medication	Hypnotic dose (route)	Onset (duration of action)	Effect on sleep cycle
Antihistamines	Diphenhydramine (Benadryl)	50–100 mg (capsule, tablet, syrup)	10–30 min (4–6 hr)	Suppression of REM.
	Hydroxyzine (Vistaril, Atarax)	25–100 mg (tablet, capsule, syrup)	15–30 min (4–6 hr)	Suppression of REM.
	Promethazine (Phenergan)	12.5–50.0 mg (capsule, tablet, syrup, suppository)	20 min (4–6 hr)	Suppression of REM.
Tricyclic antidepressants	Amitriptyline (Elavil)‡	75–200 mg (daily or in divided doses/ tablet)	Highly variable (20–40 hr half-life)	Suppression of REM.
	Doxepin (Sinequan)‡	75–150 mg (daily or in divided doses/ capsule, oral concentrate)	Highly variable	Suppression of REM.
	Imipramine (Tofranil)‡	100–200 mg (daily or in divided doses/ tablet, capsule)	Highly variable (10–25 hr half-life)	Suppression of REM. Decrease in number of awakenings from sleep.
Phenothiazine	Thioridazine (Mellaril)	20–200 mg (tablet, oral concentrate)	Highly variable	Suppression of stage 4.
Propanediol	Meprobamate (Equanil, Miltown)	800 mg (capsule, tablet)	1 hr (6–10 hr)	Suppression of REM.
Quinazoline	Methaqualone (Quaalude)	150–300 mg (capsule, tablet)	10–20 min (6–8 hr)	Suppression of REM.
Barbiturates	Butabarbital (Butisol)	50–100 mg (tablet, capsule, elixir)	40–60 min (6–8 hr)	Suppression of REM and stage 4.

Drug category*	Medication	Hypnotic dose (route)	Onset (duration of action)	Effect on sleep cycle
	Phenobarbital (Luminal)	100–200 mg (tablet, capsule, elixir, suppository)	10 min (6–10 hr)	Suppression of REM and stage 4.
	Secobarbital (Seconal)	100–200 mg (tablet, capsule, suppository, elixir)	15–30 min (3–5 hr)	Suppression of REM and stage 4.

* Drug categories are listed in order of importance/use.
‡ Hypnotic effect may be secondary to treatment of depression.
Adapted from Govoni, L. E., and J. E. Hayes. Drugs and Nursing Implications. Appleton-Century-Crofts, Norwalk, Conn. 1982. Fourth edition.

less potential for physical dependence. **Alcohol,** when used moderately, may decrease tension and enhance sleep onset in some patients. **Aspirin** has been found to initiate sleep onset, without affecting the normal sleep cycle, through enhanced serotonin action. Salicylates are thought to displace tryptophan, a serotonin precursor, from protein-binding sites. Serotonin is thought to promote sleep onset without disrupting the sleep cycle. As with all interventions, nursing knowledge and judgment are required in order to safely and effectively administer sleep medications to cancer patients experiencing a sleep disturbance.

Nursing management

Nursing management of the cancer patient experiencing a sleep disturbance can require considerable skill and creativity. Thorough communication between the nurse and the patient is essential to learn the patient's evaluation of a night's sleep. Communication between the physicians and the nurses caring for the patient during the entire 24-hr period is also necessary to promote continuity and uniformity of interventions. Table 7B–3 presents nursing interventions for the cancer patient who is experiencing a sleep disturbance.

Despite a unified approach to the management of sleep disorders, there will occasionally be cancer patients who suffer sleep disturbances that are refractory to all interventions. Skilled physical care, offering of the nurse's presence, and the nurse's willingness to listen may help counteract the discouragement experienced by patients and families when intractable insomnia is a problem.

TABLE 7B-3

Nursing Protocol for the Management of Sleep Problems in Cancer Patients*

Factor	Intervention
General (age and developmental level)	Observe the patient's own sleep routines as much as possible. Discuss changes and plan alternatives with the patient. Remind the patient that total sleep time decreases with advanced age.
Time retires to bed	Have the patient retire only if sleepy, not just when the time seems appropriate.
Patterns of insomnia	
Initial	Help the patient establish a relaxing, quiet period before sleep. Prevent excitement in the evening before bedtime.
Intermittent	If unable to sleep, have the patient get up and pursue some relaxing activity to produce drowsiness.
Terminal	With early awakening, have the patient get up and accomplish some useful activity (e.g., morning hygiene).
Patient's response to quality of sleep	Encourage discussion of the patient's subjective experience of sleep.
Naps	Establish regular times to go to sleep and to wake up. Increase stimulation and provide activities (e.g., after meals).
Recreation/exercise	Help the patient exercise during the day. Promote self-care and provide group participation as appropriate. Have the patient exercise for a brief period at least 2 hr before retiring to promote stage 4 sleep.

Emotional factors	
Anxiety	Explore potential causes of anxiety (e.g., financial problems, family situation, fear of death).
Depression	Offer presence, and counsel if appropriate.
Stress	Promote receptive atmosphere for expression of fears and questions. Provide adequate answers. Allow for more sleep time. Provide massage, back rub, and relaxation techniques if desired. Discourage focusing on sleep problems, because it will aggravate them.
Sleep environment	Obtain a base line on the patient's usual sleep environment, and then adapt it to the patient's needs as possible.
Lighting	Dim lighting.
Ventilation	Adjust ventilation. Leave door open or closed.
Bedding	Ensure clean linens. Smooth any wrinkles in bedding. Provide adequate covering.
Temperature	Adjust thermostat. Provide extra blankets for the elderly.
Noise	Restrict noise from staff, roommates, phones, radio, television, intercom, and visitors. Direct equipment noise (e.g., infusion pumps) away from the patient.
Positioning	Assist the patient to a preferred position if possible. Determine which movements or positions are not tolerated.
Social factors	Provide a compatible roommate if the room is shared. Provide a safe environment (side rails up, call bell in reach). Monitor the effect of visitors in relation to bedtime.

Factor	Intervention
Presleep routine	Learn about the patient's normal routine. Assist and adapt as needed.
Beverages	Avoid caffeinic beverages late in the day. Withhold fluids in the evening if nocturia is a problem.
Hygiene	Offer a bath and oral care.
Food	Avoid large meals in the evening. Offer a high-protein snack at bedtime. (Most protein foods contain L-tryptophan, an amino acid precursor of serotonin.)
Medication	Use nondrug measures to promote sleep as much as possible. Use sleep medications on a short-term or intermittent basis, and use agents that do not alter REM sleep (or withdraw REM-suppressant drugs gradually). Observe the sleep effects of a new or current medication routine.
Personal beliefs about sleep	Explore concerns about sleep, and correct misconceptions.
Disease/treatment factors	Be familiar with medications, other treatments, and expected side effects.
Pain/discomfort	Reposition the patient for comfort. Medicate for pain (give before sleep medication). Provide soothing irrigations, heat, cold, and mental diversion.
Fatigue	Prevent late evening overstimulation. Gradually increase exercise tolerance to overcome fatigue.
Impaired nutritional status	Provide oral hygiene and/or antiemetics if nausea/vomiting occur.

Dyspnea/cough	Provide extra pillows and elevate the head of the bed. Offer respiratory treatment and medications as needed.
Urinary frequency/incontinence	Have the patient void at bedtime. Limit fluid in the evening unless a high urine flow is necessary.
Diarrhea	Medicate to slow peristalsis and eliminate odors.
Nighttime confusion	To prevent nighttime confusion, reorient the patient frequently. Keep the staff and the patient's environment as consistent as possible.
Altered skin integrity	Perform wound care and dressing changes before bedtime. Eliminate odors and provide clean linens.
Disruptive care-giver routines (tests, treatments, routine care, health team rounds)	Observe the sleeping patient's condition in a nondisturbing way (minimal physical contact, no overhead light). Use any patient spontaneous awakening to complete tasks and make assessments when possible. Awaken the patient only when necessary, and, if possible, observe for REM sleep and awaken after the sleep cycle is completed. Organize nursing activities so they can be completed during one awakening (e.g., midnight vital signs, patient voiding, pain medication, antibiotic). Discuss with the physician the possibility of changing times of medication, treatments, etc., to allow for sleep. Plan with the patient procedures that will necessitate awakening.

See also Table 7B-1.

Bibliography

1. De Gennaro, M. D., R. Hymen, A. M. Crannell, and P. A. Mansky. Antidepressant drug therapy. *American Journal of Nursing* (July 1981). 1304–1310.

   Treatment of depression, major groups of antidepressants, side effects, dosages, and nursing interventions are overviewed.

2. Fordice, J. J., and D. Walder. Insomnia. *In* Weiner, M. B., G. A. Pepper, G. Kuhn-Weissman, and J. A. Romano. Clinical Pharmacology and Therapeutics in Nursing. McGraw-Hill Book Co., New York. 1979.

   Normal sleep and assessment of various sleep disorders are presented with a recognition of both pharmacologic and nonpharmacologic therapeutic measures to alleviate sleep problems. Efficacy, adverse effects, pharmacokinetics, and dosages of the major groups of hypnotic agents are briefly discussed.

3. Greenblatt, D. J., R. I. Shoder, and D. R. Abernethy. Current status of benzodiazepines (Parts I and II). *New England Journal of Medicine* (August 11 and 18, 1983). 354–358 and 410–416.

   Presents neuropharmacology, pharmacokinetics, single dose vs. multiple dose effects, clinical uses, adverse reactions, side effects, and hazards of benzodiazepines.

4. Harris, E. Sedative-hypnotic drugs. *American Journal of Nursing* (July 1981). 1329–1334.

   An overview of the major classes of sedative-hypnotic drugs is presented with attention to guidelines for use: side effects, contraindications, dosages, and half-life periods.

5. Kozier, B., and G. Erb. Fundamentals of Nursing. Addison-Wesley Publishing Co., Menlo Park, Calif. 1983. Second edition.

   Rest and sleep are examined within a nursing diagnosis framework. The nature of sleep is presented using a developmental perspective. Factors that influence sleep, assessment of the patient experiencing a sleep problem, and basic nursing interventions to promote sleep are discussed.

6. Malasanos, L., V. Barkauskas, M. Moss, and K. Stoltenberg-Allen. Health Assessment. C. V. Mosby Co., St. Louis. 1981. Second edition.

   The normal sleep cycle, various sleep disorders, and evaluation of sleep patterns are described within a unified framework of physical assessment of the total individual.

7. Walsleben, J. Sleep disorders. *American Journal of Nursing* (June 1982). 936–940.

   The various forms of sleep disorders are examined from the perspective of what has been learned about them through sleep laboratory research.

CHAPTER 8

NUTRITION

Mary E. Ropka

Standard: The client and family manage nutrition and hydration that facilitate optimal health and comfort in the presence of disease and treatment.

Outcome criteria: The client and family
1. identify foods that are tolerated and those that cause discomfort or aversion.
2. state measures that enhance food intake and retention.
3. select appropriate dietary alternative to provide sufficient nutrients when usual foods are not tolerated.
4. state methods of modifying consistency, flavor, or amounts of nutrients to ensure adequate nutrient intake.
5. state dietary modifications compatible with cultural, social, and ethnic practices.
6. state foods and fluids that provide optimal comfort during the terminal stages of illness.

Diet, nutrition, and cancer are related in at least three ways. Nutrition, specifically the diet we consume, is being investigated as a factor in causing some cancers. In addition, cancer affects the nutritional status of the patient. Nutritional status may be related to morbidity and mortality and response to treatment, thus influencing the quality and quantity of life. Finally, nutrition is used as an adjunct modality for treating cancer.

The following chapter will review the framework of normal physiology related to nutrition, the pathophysiology of the nutritional deficiencies and the consequences of cancer, both disease-related and treatment-related, nutritional assessment, and management of nutritional problems in cancer patients.

Framework

The ultimate goal of the nutritional processes is to supply the body with fluids, electrolytes, and nutrients. Various parts of the GI tract (Fig. 8-1) are structured and adapted for specific functions, including: (1) the transportation of food between areas; (2) the storage of food in different stages of digestion; (3) the digestion of food, including the secretion of digestive juices; (4) and the absorption of fluids and nutrients during the various stages of the digestive processes. The GI system (stomach and intestines, especially the small intestine) breaks down complex carbohydrates, protein, and fats into materials that are absorbable. Minerals, fluids, vitamins, and nonessential nutrients are also digested. Following digestion, absorption occurs mainly in the

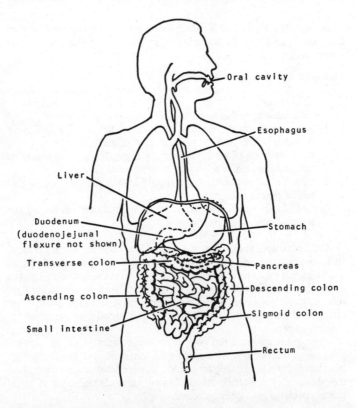

Figure 8-1. The anatomy of the GI tract.

small intestine. The absorbed nutrients then enter the circulation in a variety of ways. These physiologic processes will be discussed in more detail in terms of ingestion, digestion (including secretion) and absorption, excretion, and metabolism.

Ingestion.   Ingestion of food and fluids involves appetite, hunger, mastication, and deglutition, or swallowing. The intake of food is regulated by the body's stores of nutrients, as well as by the effects of eating on the digestive tract. The process is complicated, made up of many interrelated psychologic and physiologic factors.

The desire for specific types of food, rather than for food in general (hunger), is determined by appetite. Although appetite is controlled in areas of the brain higher than the hypothalamus, it is still closely connected to hypothalamic functioning. Ideally, the intake of food should match caloric expenditure and nutritional needs.

Defined as the intrinsic desire for food, hunger is the primary mechanism for control of food intake. The hypothalamus contains "the feeding center," which is concerned with nutritional status and is involved in the awareness of hunger and desire for food. The "satiety center," also located in the hypothalamus, inhibits the "feeding center," which normally is continually activated, and causes a decreased desire for food. The brainstem centers control the actual mechanisms of eating, such as chewing and swallowing. The cortical regions of the limbic system are also involved in feeding and preference for food.

Digestion and absorption.   Digestion involves mechanical and chemical processes that break food down into particles of the size and chemical composition that the body can absorb. Secretions from specialized cells and the motility of the GI tract are involved in the processes of digestion. Absorption by special cells transfers the digested nutrients into the body fluids. The nutrients are then transported to tissues for storage, further processing, or utilization. Most absorption occurs in the small intestine. Once they are in the body cells, nutrients are stored or further metabolized for energy or excretion (catabolism) or for synthesis of new materials for cellular growth, maintenance, or repair (anabolism). Each nutrient, including the three major ones (protein, fat, carbohydrates), requires different metabolic processes.

Mouth: Food is chewed and swallowed in the mouth, assisted by the saliva, which is secreted in amounts of 1,000 to 1,500 ml daily. Saliva contains ptyalin, which aids in starch digestion; mucin, which lubricates; and large amounts of potassium (K^+) and bicarbonate (HCO_3^-) ions. Excessive losses of saliva result in hypokalemia, dental caries, and mouth sores. Lack of saliva (xerostomia) makes it difficult to swallow or chew because saliva provides moisture in the mouth, washes away bacteria and food particles, and destroys bacteria (*see* Chapter 9 B).

Esophagus: Food moves from the oropharynx to the stomach by two types of peristalsis — primary peristalsis and secondary peristalsis. Primary peristalsis originates from the pharyngeal stage of swallowing. If food remains in the esophagus, secondary peristalsis, under vagal control, arises from the esophagus itself. Mucus is secreted by the esophagus to provide lubrication for swallowing.

Stomach: The stomach essentially consists of two parts: the corpus, or body, and the antrum. In the stomach, food is chopped and mixed into chyme by constrictor waves, or weak peristaltic waves, which move the chyme from the antrum toward the pylorus. This partially digested food is stored in the stomach until it moves along into the duodenum. Stronger peristaltic waves move the chyme into the duodenum when the pyloric valve relaxes.

Gastric secretion is under nervous control by the parasympathetic nervous system and local plexuses and under hormonal control by gastrin. These secretion mechanisms are stimulated by the vagus nerve and by food in the stomach. They are inhibited by the enterogastric reflex, which is initiated by the presence of food in the small intestine, and by hormones released by the small intestine — cholecystokinin, gastric inhibitory polypeptide, and vasoactive intestinal peptide. Two major types of secretory cells are found in the mucosa in different regions of the stomach. The **gastric, or fundic, glands**, located in the fundus and greater curvature of the body of the stomach, are lined by several types of cells that secrete mucus, pepsinogen, hydrochloric acid, and intrinsic factors. The **pyloric, or antral, glands** merge with the gastric glands in the antrum. Cells that synthesize and release gastrin are contained in these glands, as well as ones secreting mucus and pepsinogen II. Lipase and amylase are also secreted in small amounts. Little absorption occurs in the stomach (only lipid-soluble substances) because of the absence of an absorptive membrane.

Small intestine: Motility of the small intestine consists of mixing contractions and propulsive contractions. Mixing contractions, or segmentation, are local contractions of small segments of the wall of the gut that chop chyme and help move food forward slightly. Propulsive contractions, or peristalsis, move chyme toward the ileocecal valve and spread chyme along the intestinal mucosa. Distension is the usual stimulus that produces this contractile ring of peristalsis. Effective peristalsis requires a functional myenteric nerve plexus; intensity and velocity of the peristaltic contraction are altered by parasympathetic stimulation. The villi also contract to increase absorption. The ileocecal valve, located between the small intestine and the proximal large intestine, prevents the reflux of fecal contents of the colon and controls emptying of the small intestine.

The small intestine secretes about 2,000 ml/day of almost pure extracellular fluid from Lieberkühn's crypts, which are located on the entire surface of the small intestine except where Brunner's glands occur. Mucus is secreted from Brunner's glands and from goblet cells on the surface of the intestinal mucosa and in Lieberkühn's crypts. Enzymes that are secreted from the brush border of the epithelium are sucrase, maltase, isomaltase, and lactase.

The specialized anatomy of the small intestine permits most GI absorption to occur here, with absorptive capacity to spare. Absorptive mechanisms include pinocytosis, diffusion, and active transport.

Large intestine: The large intestine absorbs water and sodium; stores fecal material; forms vitamins K, B_{12}, thiamin, and riboflavin; and carries out some secretion. Digestive enzymes are not secreted by the large intestine. Water and electrolytes are secreted when the large intestine is irritated, such as by infection or laxatives. Goblet cells secrete mucus to protect the mucosa and cause the feces to be self-adherent.

Motility of the large intestine consists of mixing movements (haustrations) and propulsive movements (mass movements). Haustrations are a result of large circular constrictions and contraction of the muscle of the colon so that greater exposure of the mucosa for absorption and more mixing occurs.

The large intestine absorbs large quantities of water and electrolytes proximally. All ions are absorbed. Sodium (Na^+) moves by active transport, taking chloride (Cl^-) along with it. Water is absorbed passively as a consequence of the osmotic gradient from absorption of the Na^+ and Cl^-.

Pancreas: When acid chyme from the stomach enters the duodenum, secretin is released, along with cholecystokinin-pancreozymin (CCK-PZ). Secretin stimulates the pancreas to release water and bicarbonate from the ductal epithelium, while CCK-PZ causes the release of pancreatic enzymes from the acini. These include the proteolytic endopeptidases, trypsin and chymotrypsin; the proteolytic exopeptidases, carboxypolypeptidase and aminopeptidase; the ribonucleases, deoxyribonuclease and ribonuclease; amylase; and the lipolytic enzymes, lipase and cholesterol esterase. The bicarbonate released neutralizes the acid chyme from the stomach once it is in the duodenum. This protects the mucosa of the duodenum from damage and provides an appropriate pH for the pancreatic enzymes to function.

Liver: The liver is a complex organ that carries out many functions including: production of bile, carbohydrate storage, control of carbohydrate metabolism, reduction and conjugation of adrenal and gonadal steroid hormones, detoxification of drugs and toxins, manufacture of plasma proteins, formation of urea and ketones, and metabolism of fat.

Bile is secreted by the liver cells into the intrahepatic bile canaliculi. Bile is then carried from the liver through the common bile duct, which drains into the duodenum at a site close to or the same as the pancreatic duct. The discharge of bile from the common bile duct into the duodenum is controlled by the sphincter of Oddi. Between meals this path is closed, and bile is stored in the gallbladder. When food is eaten, the sphincter of Oddi relaxes and when the gastric contents enter the duodenum, the hormone CCK-PZ causes the gallbladder to contract and empty concentrated bile into the duodenum.

Bile contains bilirubin, bile salts, bile pigments, cholesterol, fatty acids, and water. Bilirubin and biliverdin are bile pigments that are formed from hemoglobin and give bile its characteristic golden color. Bile acids are formed in the liver from cholesterol. Some bile acids are converted by bacterial action in the intestine to secondary bile acids. Some bile acids are conjugated in the liver and are then known as bile salts. Bile salts perform a number of functions: they (1) emulsify or break up fat globules to aid digestion; (2) in their conjugated form join with fatty acids and monoglycerides to form micelles for transport to the mucosa of the intestinal villi, to be absorbed by the lymphatics; (3) activate lipases in the intestine; and (4) stimulate the uptake by cells of fatty acids and encourage the conversion of these fatty acids to triglycerides. Most of the bile acids are absorbed in the terminal ileum, transported back to the liver in the portal vein, and reexcreted in the bile (the enterohepatic circulation).

Excretion. Excretion of contents of the colon occurs as a result of the complex act of defecation. Defecation involves reflexes that are cord-mediated and those that are intrinsic through the myenteric plexus of the sigmoid colon. The long rectal muscles contract and shorten the rectum in concert with relaxation of the anal sphincter. Involuntary mass movement of the colon moves the feces into the rectum, producing the desire to defecate. Under voluntary control, the external anal sphincter relaxes, allowing expulsion of stool (*see* Chapter 11B).

Pathophysiology

The body can be considered to have three major components: skeletal mass, fat, or adipose tissue, and lean body mass. Skeletal mass is inert and does not produce energy. Fat is a rich source of energy as an alternative to carbohydrates. Lean body mass has two subcomponents:

visceral protein mass (vital organs and blood) and somatic protein mass (skeletal muscles). Figure 8–2 illustrates the relative proportions of these components in total body composition, as well as the various techniques that can be used to evaluate the different compartments.

Different biochemical and anthropometric measurements provide information about the body's fat deposits and somatic protein mass. Serum concentrations of transport proteins (serum albumin and transferrin) indicate visceral protein mass, while total lymphocyte count and reactivity to common skin-test antigens indicate immune competence.

Nutritional deficiencies develop as a progressive phenomenon. They may be categorized etiologically as a primary deficiency or a secondary deficiency. Primary deficiencies are a result of intake inadequate to meet metabolic needs. Secondary deficiencies are a result of a number of factors, acting alone or in combination. Secondary deficiencies result from poor absorption, decreased utilization, impaired transport, decreased excretion, increased destruction, or increased requirements. All of these sources of secondary deficiencies may be found in people with cancer.

As a result of the primary or secondary deficiency, (1) the nutrient tissue levels gradually decrease, leading to (2) biochemical lesions and

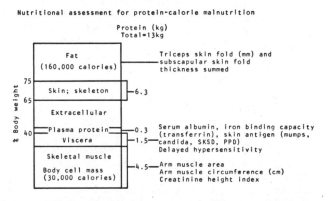

Figure 8–2. Body components and nutritional assessment. PPD, purified protein derivative of tuberculin; SKSD, streptokinase-streptodornase. *Adapted with permission from* Blackburn, G. L., B. R. Bistrian, B. S. Maini, H. T. Schlamm, and M. F. Smith. Nutritional metabolic assessment of the hospitalized patient. *Journal of Parenteral and Enteral Nutrition* (January 1977). p. 12.

tissue enzyme deficiency, eventually leading to (3) anatomical lesions, changed tissue structure, and changed organ function. An awareness of this course of progression helps determine the type of assessment technique that is appropriate at different stages in the development of the deficiency. In the first two steps of the progression, the blood, urine, and tissue can be analyzed for nutrients and enzymes/metabolites, respectively. By the third stage (anatomical lesions, etc.), clinical assessment will reveal the deficiency. Clearly, by the time the patient develops nutritional problems that are clinically detectable, the problems have probably existed for quite a while.

Malnutrition. Three major types of malnutrition are recognized. *Marasmus* results from chronic depletion of muscle or fat. The protein:calorie ratio in the intake may be acceptable, but the total dietary intake is inadequate. Fat and muscle stores are used as energy reserves. Marasmus may occur in the person with anorexia, partial intestinal obstruction, chronic illness, or old age. Usually the individual will look wasted, but marasmus may be concealed in muscular or heavyset individuals. In addition, serum albumin and transferrin may be normal. Acute visceral attrition, or *kwashiorkor,* occurs when the intake of protein is insufficient, although carbohydrate intake may be adequate. Kwashiorkor may occur from fad diets, decreased intake, or when patients are maintained on dextrose-and-water infusions without protein supplements. Kwashiorkor (in which serum albumin and transferrin are decreased) is easily overlooked in the obese person or in the person who appears well-nourished, or when laboratory data are not evaluated carefully. The combination of kwashiorkor and marasmus — or *protein-calorie malnutrition* (PCM) — is what occurs most commonly in hospitalized patients or those with a prolonged illness, such as cancer. In PCM, the serum albumin and transferrin are decreased. In all three of these types of malnutrition, the patient's immune response is decreased.

Disease-related effects of cancer. Weight loss and other nutritional problems are a frequent, but not inevitable, consequence of cancer. The incidence of malnutrition varies widely in cancer patients; when it does occur, it indicates a poor prognosis both for children and for adults. Malnutrition may become the most disabling aspect of the disease, resulting in decreased quality of life and increased morbidity and mortality. Cancer cachexia occurs as a late effect in one-half to one-third of all cancer patients and is manifested by anorexia, malaise, weight loss, and wasting. The development of malnutrition involves many factors, both physiologic and psychologic, and results in weakness and fatigue, dehydration, fluid and electrolyte imbalance, impaired wound healing and decreased skin integrity, immunocompromise, and increased risk of infection (*see* Chapter 9). The major nutritional consequences of cancer can be divided into three main areas: systemic metabolic consequences, inadequate ingestion, and impaired digestion and absorption.

Systemic metabolic consequences: These are believed to include at least three aspects: (1) alterations in the metabolism of carbohydrates, proteins, and fats, resulting in increased energy expenditure; (2) tumor-host competition for nutrients; and (3) ectopic hormone secretion. It is most important to remember that current knowledge is based on evidence that is preliminary and at times conflicting. It must also be remembered that there are many different types of cancers, whose behavior depends on the tissue of origin and the specialized cells within that tissue. There are varying degrees of malignancy, as well. The following discussion is intended to review the current information, not to give definitive answers.

One of the major systemic consequences of cancer is its effects on **metabolism of nutrients** and **increased energy expenditure** on the part of the host's cells. Tumors are believed to rely heavily on carbohydrates for energy, but the metabolic processes used are inefficient. Cancer cells are thought to have an imbalance in *carbohydrate metabolism*, using glycolysis more than respiration. Glycolysis is a anaerobic biochemical process (the Embden-Meyerhof pathway) that converts sugars, primarily glucose, to pyruvic and lactic acids to obtain energy. Glycolysis yields 4 molecules of adenosine 5'-triphosphate (ATP) for energy from every 1 molecule of glucose after lactic and pyruvic acids enter the systemic circulation. It is an inefficient process for energy production. Respiration is an aerobic biochemical process for carbohydrate metabolism. Glucose molecules are oxidized to create acetic acid, which is activated by an enzyme and further metabolized into carbon dioxide (CO_2) and hydrogen (H^+). The hydrogen is then oxidized to release energy. In contrast to glycolysis, this efficient process produces 34 molecules of ATP from 1 molecule of glucose. Not only is glycolysis less energy-efficient in carbohydrate metabolism, it also requires that more glucose molecules be available.

The body of the person with cancer responds to the increased demand for glucose required by the cancer cells and by the normal body cells with a high rate of gluconeogenesis. Gluconeogenesis is the synthesis of glucose by the liver and renal cortex from noncarbohydrate sources, such as lactate, glycerol, and amino acids. Increased Cori cycle activity, in which muscle glycogen is converted to lactic acid and then glucose, drains normal tissues for energy and stimulates significant gluconeogenesis. When protein, in the form of lean body mass, is broken down to provide amino acids for this process, the muscle wasting of PCM is thought to result.

It is suggested that the usual control, or feedback mechanisms, that function in the noncancer patient during periods of starvation do not work in cancer patients. Normally, during starvation, the body increases mobilization of fatty acids from adipose tissue, decreases gluconeogenesis from amino acids, decreases oxygen consumption, and decreases energy requirements of ATP. Thus total body protein and lean tissue mass are conserved during starvation. One possible explanation for the failure of this mechanism may be that malignant cell growth is continuous, rather than in the usual diurnal pattern of metabolic activity of normal cells. Cancer patients seem less able to utilize tissue-conserving mechanisms and to decrease gluconeogenesis from protein stores. Instead, they are thought to have inappropriately elevated energy expenditure, increased basal energy consumption, increased CO_2 production, and accelerated gluconeogenesis.

Another abnormality related to carbohydrate metabolism that has been postulated is an abnormal glucose tolerance curve in patients with malignant tumors. Cancer patients who are losing weight have been shown to be glucose intolerant. This glucose-intolerance may be caused by decreased sensitivity to insulin and/or a decreased insulin response. These individuals are unable to utilize the glucose that they have available for energy.

Protein metabolism is also thought to be altered, so that muscle tissue is used to obtain protein to meet the energy needs. Progressive muscle wasting, one of the hallmarks of cancer cachexia, is the result. Normally, protein is spared and carbohydrates are utilized as an energy source. In the tumor, protein synthesis continues at the expense of the host's nitrogen balance. The tumor becomes a "nitrogen trap," holding and using to produce protein in the tumor, nitrogen that would ordinarily be used to produce protein for normal body growth and maintenance. Furthermore, the cancer patient may have decreased albumin and protein synthesis, as well as an altered insulin regulatory mechanism. An altered insulin regulatory mechanism affects protein metabolism as well as carbohydrate metabolism. Elevated cortico-steroid and catecholamine production from fever, infection, surgery, or other physiologic stress also contributes to increased protein catabolism.

Fat metabolism is affected in cancer patients who are cachectic, resulting in increased lipolysis. Fatty acids (stored fat) are believed to be mobilized from adipose cells and released into the bloodstream for use as fuel for energy production. This process is controlled by the inhibitory effects of insulin. These inhibitory effects are compromised in cancer patients. Body stores of fat are depleted as the disease progresses.

Tumor-host competition for nutrients. It has been suggested that tumor cells may use glucose preferentially so that normal cells must use other mechanisms to obtain nutrients. It is unclear whether an increased basal metabolic rate is present in patients with cancer. It is believed that while the tumor competes effectively for nutrients when they are limited in availability, the tumor is not capable of inhibiting normal body growth. Feeding must, however, occur simultaneously with effective tumor treatment. Failure to eat, although not affecting tumor size, will be detrimental to the patient and compromise his ability to fight cancer.

Ectopic hormone secretion. Some tumors abnormally synthesize biochemical substances that have undesired systemic effects. The substances produced are hormones or are hormonelike, may be metabolically active, and are often produced normally in other body organs. Such paraneoplastic syndromes can cause severe metabolic imbalances when physiologic feedback systems are not operating. Table 8–1 lists some paraneoplastic syndromes that have nutritional consequences and includes information about the hormone secreted and the tumor.

Inadequate ingestion: Nutritional consequences of cancer result from patients' inability to eat, as well as from the body's inability to utilize nutrients once they are ingested, or from a change in the body's utilization. Many physical and physiologic factors can affect people's ability to eat, including fatigue, depression, and pain. Economic factors, such as poverty, must also be considered. Three such problems will be discussed below: (1) anatomical and mechanical alterations; (2) anorexia; and (3) altered taste perception.

Anatomical and mechanical alterations can result in anatomical and mechanical barriers to eating. Patients with cancer of the head and neck are most likely to experience such problems, and patients with brain tumors are likely candidates also. Tumors involving the oral cavity and supporting structures may cause difficulties in chewing. Painful oral lesions of the mucosa may inhibit ingestion. Facial or jaw pain also interferes with eating. Brain tumors, depending on the location, may affect chewing ability. Esophageal tumors may cause alterations in motility that manifest as odynophagia (painful swallowing). Obstruction of the esophagus can prevent the passage of food or liquids. Some gastric tumors cause pain and gastric distension, resulting in feelings of early satiety, which can decrease the patient's

TABLE 8–1

Endocrine Paraneoplastic Syndromes

Syndrome (hormone)	Tumor	Clinical manifestations with nutritional consequences
Cushing's syndrome (ACTH)	Lung cancer — all types Small cell lung cancer	Hypokalemia, hyperglycemia, edema, muscle weakness and atrophy, hypertension, and weight loss.
Diarrhea (catecholamines)	Neuroblastomas Pheochromocytomas	Secretory diarrhea (*see* Table 8–2).
Nonmetastatic hypercalcemia (PTH)	Lung cancer — all types Small cell lung cancer Other tumors	Fatigue, weakness, lethargy, renal insufficiency, anorexia, nausea, vomiting, constipation, abdominal pain.
Diarrhea (gastrin, VIP)	Zollinger–Ellison syndrome Pancreas, villous adenoma	Secretory diarrhea
Inappropriate secretion of antidiuretic hormone (ADH)	Lung cancer — all types Small cell lung cancer	Hyponatremia, hyperglycemia, urine inappropriately higher in osmolality than plasma, high urinary sodium concentrations in face of serum hyponatremia

ACTH, adrenocorticotropic hormone; ADH, antidiuretic hormone; PTH, parathyroid hormone; VIP, vasoactive intestinal peptide.

Adapted with permission from DeVita, V. T., S. Hellman, and S. A. Rosenberg, editors. Cancer: Principles and Practice of Oncology. J. B. Lippincott Co., Philadelphia. 1982. p. 1478.

intake of nutrients. When changes in the quantity or quality of foods and liquids occur, malnutrition can develop progressively, as can fluid and electrolyte disturbances.

Anorexia, or decreased appetite, is a condition resulting from a complicated process involving numerous physiologic and psychologic factors. Anorexia is frequently one of the earliest manifestations of cancer. The degree of anorexia is not necessarily related to size or type of tumor, although it increases in frequency and severity in the more advanced stages of disease. It has been shown to decrease with successful anticancer treatment, which supports the idea that it is a paraneoplastic process. Possible psychologic components include the distress of the diagnosis of cancer, discouragement or depression, anxiety, interruption of normal life-style patterns, or isolation from support people and family. Taste changes, fatigue, respiratory problems, and other disease complications also contribute to anorexia.

The specific physiologic mechanisms that cause anorexia in cancer patients are not known. Many suggestions have been made as to the mechanisms of appetite control. Most of the theories about anorexia involve decreased hunger or increased satiety, which are primarily regulated by the hypothalamus. Delayed digestion and prolonged stimulation of the volume receptors of the GI tract may decrease feelings of hunger or cause prolonged stimulation of the satiety center. Another theory suggests that anorexigenic metabolites are released from the tumor into the bloodstream. These anorexigenic metabolites are substances, such as peptides and oligonucleotides, that cause decreased appetite or hunger and alterations of metabolic processes as a result of signals to the peripheral receptors and brain centers.

Altered taste perception may profoundly affect the patient's appetite. Taste is a complex sensation and is highly dependent on smell. Normally, the four primary taste-sensation receptors are located on four different areas of the tongue and combine to give hundreds of taste sensations. Sweet receptors are located on the anterior surface and tip of the tongue. Salty and sour receptors are located on the lateral sides of the tongue. Bitter receptors are located posteriorly, on the circumvallate palate.

In general, changes in taste have been found to be associated with the extent but not the type of tumor. Decreased taste acuity is referred to as hypogeusia. Dysgeusia refers to a perverted sense of taste; for instance, a lowered urea recognition threshold is thought to result in an increased response of the taste buds to amino acid, which is manifested as an aversion to meat. A decreased response of the taste buds to sweets is believed to result in an elevated sucrose recognition threshold. In other words, food and drink must be sweeter to taste sweet to the consumer. Taste changes are thought to result from a chemical alteration rather than a physiologic alteration because taste sensations frequently return to normal as the tumor responds to treatment. Furthermore, treatments themselves (radiation and antitumor chemotherapy) may cause permanent or temporary taste alterations.

Impaired digestion and absorption: Obstruction of the lower GI tract, diarrhea, and external nutrient losses are three major nutritional problems occurring in patients with cancer, and they result from abnormal processes of digestion and absorption.

Intestinal obstruction of the lower GI tract occurs when, as a result of mechanical or neuromuscular alterations, its contents fail to progress. Obstruction can result from intrinsic involvement by tumor, extrinsic compression by metastatic cancer, or obstruction from benign lesions accompanying a metastatic process. Obstruction of the distal GI tract can occur from lymphomatous invasion of the small bowel, primary tumor of the colon or rectum, or diffuse carcinomatosis secondary to ovarian, colonic, pancreatic, or breast tumors. Peritoneal carcinomatosis is the most frequent cause of obstruction from metastatic disease (*see* Chapter 14E).

The type and location of the obstruction influence its signs and symptoms. When extrinsic or intrinsic mechanical causes of obstruction of the distal GI tract occur, the symptoms and sequelae vary with the location of the blockage.

This common and serious problem can result in severe metabolic difficulties from fluid and electrolyte imbalances or acid-base disturbances; their extent is determined by the location of the intestinal obstruction. If the obstruction is high, e.g., in the pylorus, metabolic alkalosis may result from losing gastric hydrochloric acid because of vomiting or nasogastric intubation. Dehydration is rapid when obstruction is high in the small bowel. Dehydration is less likely in obstruction of the distal large bowel because most of the fluids will already have been absorbed. Neuromuscular obstructions, or adynamic ileus, occur after general anesthesia, abdominal surgery or trauma, electrolyte imbalance (particularly hypokalemia), metabolic imbalances, peritoneal irritation, or severe pain. When mechanical obstruction occurs, replacement of fluids and electrolytes is essential, and surgical correction is frequently required.

Diarrhea implies a change in bowel habits for the patient. There is tremendous variation among individuals in "normal" bowel function. Diarrhea can be simply defined as too little of a too liquid stool. It involves increased frequency, increased fluidity, or abnormal constituents (blood, pus, or mucus) in the stools. Clinically, major changes in fluidity, frequency, or abnormal constituents are the usual hallmarks of diarrhea, but stool weight greater than 250 g/day is the definitive criterion.

Changes in digestion and absorption in the GI tract can result from cancer. As a result, diarrhea may occur. Most commonly, diarrhea is a result of cancer itself in the following instances: (1) in association with hormone-secreting tumors (carcinoid syndrome, Zollinger-Ellison syndrome, villous adenoma of the colon); (2) deficiency of pancreatic enzymes or bile salts; (3) infiltration of the small bowel by lymphomas or carcinomas; (4) blind loop from a partial upper-small-bowel obstruction; and (5) malnutrition.

Diarrhea involves different physiologic mechanisms in the above circumstances. An understanding of the physiologic mechanism causing the diarrhea helps in its identification and management. Three major physiologic mechanisms are identified: (1) excess fluid in the stools as a result of decreased net absorption in the intestines, causing an osmotic diarrhea; (2) increased net secretion by the intestines, resulting in a secretory diarrhea; and (3) the two prior mechanisms in combination, as in hypermotility states. A summary of the differences in these three pathophysiologic processes is found in Table 8–2. Fluid status, electrolytes, acid-base balance, and the availability of nutrients for energy and nutritional needs are all at risk of disturbance when diarrhea occurs.

Hormone-secreting tumors, as discussed above, are usually associated with a secretory diarrhea. Pancreatic-enzyme deficiencies and bile-salt deficiency or excess result primarily in impaired digestion of fats and some decrease in protein digestion, ultimately causing an osmotic diarrhea. Abnormalities of the wall of the intestine from infiltration of tumors, such as lymphomas, involve atrophy or destruction of the microvilli, thus decreasing absorptive surfaces. In addition, protein-losing enteropathies occur as a result of the loss of protein-rich substances when lymph channels are obstructed and when lymphatics within the intestinal villi are dilated. Even with extra-alimentary-tract malignancies, the PCM that ultimately occurs is associated with histologic abnormalities of the mucosa, with epithelial cell loss, and with decreased lactose utilization. The ability of the intestine to digest or absorb is decreased. Bacterial overgrowth occurring in the upper small bowel when it is partially obstructed can cause steatorrhea and vitamin B_{12} deficiency.

External nutrient losses occur primarily through repeated vomiting or diarrhea.

Nausea is the subjective feeling of the imminent need to vomit. It is the conscious psychic recognition of subconscious physiologic excitation in an area of the medulla closely associated with or a part of the

TABLE 8-2

Pathophysiology of Diarrhea

Type of diarrhea	Mechanism	Characteristics of diarrhea and composition of diarrheal fluid	Examples
Osmotic	Unabsorbable (e.g., oligo-saccharide) or poorly absorbable (e.g., Mg^{++}, $SO_4^=$) solute in the alimentary tract.	24-hr stool volume usually <1 liter Stool volume decreases with fasting Stool pH decreased <7	Lactose intolerance: cathartic abuse, excessive antacid use; postgastrectomy or partial gastrectomy.
Secretory	Increased secretory activity of the alimentary tract, with or without inhibition of absorption of intestinal contents; may also result from inhibition of electrolyte and water absorption.	24-hr stool volume usually >1 liter Stool volume does not decrease with fasting Stool pH ~7	Non-beta islet cell tumors of the pancreas; Zollinger-Ellison syndrome; villous adenoma; medullary carcinoma of the thyroid.
Mixed	Increased rate of transit as in hypermotility states; osmotic effect of ingested solutes may result from rapid intestinal transit and decreased net absorption.	Variable	Carcinoid syndrome; cholinergic drugs.

Adapted with permission from Greenberger, N. J. Gastrointestinal Disorders: A Pathophysiologic Approach. Year Book Medical Publishers, Inc., Chicago. 1981. Second edition. p. 195.

true vomiting center (TVC). Nausea is frequently a precursor to vomiting. Vomiting, or emesis, is the forceful expulsion of gastric contents. A complex act physiologically, vomiting is controlled by the lower brainstem, which is closely associated with respiration, to preserve safe respiration while preventing aspiration. The three elements of the act of vomiting — nausea, retching, expulsion — can occur separately or in combination. Anticipatory nausea and vomiting result from psychogenic or cerebral and limbic mechanisms. They can occur as a conditioned response to tactile, olfactory, or other stimuli associated with illness or therapy.

The physiologic mechanisms by which nausea and vomiting occur in cancer patients are thought to involve the TVC and the chemoreceptor trigger zone (CTZ). The TVC is located in the lateral region of the reticular formation of the brain. All neurologic inputs for vomiting occur here, making it the final common pathway mediating all vomiting. The TVC efferent pathways, which are all involved with the act of vomiting, include: the phrenic nerve, leading to the diaphragm; the spinal nerves to the abdominal muscles; and the visceral nerves to the stomach and esophagus. The afferent pathways leading to the TVC include: the CTZ (vagal and other spinal sympathetic nerves from the viscera), midbrain receptors for elevated intracranial pressure, the labyrinth apparatus in the middle ear, and the cerebral cortex and higher CNS structures.

The CTZ is believed to be in the area postrema, a medullary center located in the floor of the fourth ventricle. Toxic substances, including some drugs and possibly radiation therapy (RT), stimulate the CTZ, which in turn stimulates the TVC. The CTZ works with the TVC. The CTZ appears to be accessible by blood and CSF.

GI-tract fistulas result in the loss of gastric and small-bowel fluids. External losses of protein also can occur as a result of repeated taps for the relief of malignant effusions or from dilution of albumin in abnormally large extracellular fluid compartments of malignant and ascitic effusions.

Treatment-related effects of cancer. The primary modalities for treating cancer are surgery, chemotherapy, and RT. These approaches are used alone or in simultaneous or sequential combination, depending on the location, type, and extent of disease. When used in combination, the effects may be synergistic. Many of the effects of cancer treatment on nutrition are similar to those resulting from the disease itself. Effects may be local or systemic. Without exception, the various treatments for malignant tumors will have nutritional consequences. Frequently patients are already nutritionally compromised by the disease at the time they are diagnosed, thus complicating the consequences after the initiation of treatment. Effects of each of the three treatment modes will be described individually below.

Surgery: Surgery may be used as a curative treatment, totally removing tumor from the body, or as a palliative treatment, decreasing the bulk of the tumor or relieving obstruction or pressure. Surgery in any patient has immediate general metabolic systemic effects, including increased energy expenditure postoperatively, the utilization of visceral protein stores, and elevated catecholamines from the physiologic trauma of surgery. As a result, the body's needs for proteins and carbohydrates are increased if wound healing is to occur.

Specific surgical procedures can result in chronic effects on nutrition that are related to the organs resected and the degree of resection. Table 8–3 provides detailed information about the nutritional sequelae of surgical oncology procedures.

RT: Like chemotherapy, RT does not work selectively on cancer cells, but affects all cells — normal and tumor — located within the treatment field. Nutritional status will be affected by RT. Those patients who are most likely to develop nutritional problems from RT are those being irradiated in the oral cavity, larynx, pharynx, and any area that encompasses portions of the GI tract, such as in abdominal and pelvic RT. Development of problems depends on numerous factors: the part of the body involved in the field, the intensity of the radiation dose to the tumor, the time period over which the RT is administered, the volume of tissue irradiated, the nutritional status of the patient at the initiation of treatment, the sensitivity of the tissue to radiation, and the general physical and psychologic status of the individuals.

Fatigue and anorexia are two very common side effects experienced by people receiving RT. Immediate and long-term consequences of RT that influence nutritional status are outlined in Table 8–4. The immediate consequences usually begin 2 to 4 wk after RT begins and resolve within 6 wk of the end of RT. Late damage may be extensive and irreversible, occuring several months to years after RT was administered. Radiation enteritis is a well-known early and late side effect of RT. When it occurs early, it usually begins in the second week and can include diarrhea, tenesmus, rectal bleeding, and more severe proctitis. As a late and chronic condition, resulting from a permanent change in the bowel wall, radiation enteritis results in nausea, vomiting, colicky abdominal pain, and bloody diarrhea. Clinical manifestations of late consequences, in order of frequency, include abdominal pain, nausea, vomiting, and alternating constipation and diarrhea.

Chemotherapy: Antitumor chemotherapy is a potential cause of impaired nutritional states as a result of decreased intake of nutrients,

TABLE 8–3

Nutritional Consequences of Cancer Surgery

Surgery	Consequences with nutritional implications
Radical resection of oropharynx	Difficulty chewing or swallowing. Dependence on tube feedings when unable to eat. Inadequate intake to support healing and health. Altered taste perception.
Esophagectomy, esophago-gastrectomy, esophageal reconstruction	Gastric stasis and achlorhydria from vagotomy. Diarrhea. Steatorrhea. Fistula or stenosis.
Gastrectomy (partial or complete)	Dumping syndrome (cramps, diarrhea, fullness). Achlorhydria and megaloblastic anemia secondary to absence of intrinsic factor and vitamin B_{12}. Malabsorption of fats, iron, B_{12}, calcium. Delayed gastric emptying (with vagotomy). Early satiety secondary to decreased size of reservoir. Postgastrectomy syndrome (anemia, malnutrition, steatorrhea).
Intestinal resection Duodenum	Malabsorption of fat. Low iron.
Jejunum	Vitamin B_{12} deficiency, hyperoxaluria, bile salt losses.
Ileostomy and colostomy	Fluid and electrolyte disturbance.
Massive bowel resection	Malabsorption. Metabolic acidosis. Malnutrition.
Blind loop syndrome	Diarrhea. Steatorrhea. Weight loss and malnutrition. Anemia. Multiple vitamin deficiencies.
Pancreatectomy	Exocrine insufficiency leads to malabsorption. Endocrine insufficiency leads to diabetes mellitus.

TABLE 8–4

Nutritional Consequences of Radiation Therapy

| Site | Consequences | |
	Immediate	Late
Head and neck	Dry mouth (xerostomia) Taste change or loss Dysphagia Loss of appetite (anorexia) Sore mouth or throat (wk 2 or 3) Fatigue	Taste change Mandibular necrosis Xerostomia Dental caries
Esophagus	Dysphagia Sore throat Fistulas Obstruction Esophagitis Indigestion Nausea	Esophageal fibrosis Esophageal stenosis
Lung	Anorexia Shortness of breath Sore throat Nausea	
Upper abdomen	Nausea/vomiting Weight loss	Radiation enteritis Obstruction Fistula Stricture Ulcer perforation Malabsorption
Whole abdomen	Nausea/vomiting Cramping and gas Diarrhea	Same as upper abdomen
Pelvis	Diarrhea	
GI tract	Diarrhea Nausea/vomiting Anorexia	

GI toxicity from systemic effects of the chemotherapy, and dysfunction of specific major organ systems (Table 8–5). When major organ system functions are disturbed by chemotherapy, further nutritional deterioration may occur. Systemic effects that can have nutritional consequences include fever and chills, electrolyte imbalances, and weight loss.

TABLE 8–5

Nutritional Consequences of Chemotherapy

Problem	Comments
Anorexia and taste changes	Complex physical and psychologic causes. Most likely with methotrexate, cyclophosphamide, 5-fluorouracil, nitrogen mustard, and dactinomycin. Results in decreased intake and food aversions.
Nausea and vomiting	Thought to be caused by stimulation of the true vomiting center, the chemoreceptor trigger zone. Intensity, duration, onset vary with drugs and doses (cisplatin, cyclophosphamide, dacarbazine, dactinomycin, methotrexate, mitomycin-C, nitrogen mustard, nitrosoureas have severe emetic action). Results in decreased intake, fluid and electrolyte imbalances, general weakness, and weight loss.
Stomatitis and esophagitis	Very common; alimentary tract is one of the most vulnerable targets of chemotherapy because of rapid cell proliferation. Common with antibiotics, 5-fluorouracil, vinca alkaloids, methotrexate. Results in inflammation and ulceration of the oropharynx and esophagus, cheilosis, glossitis (7–14 days after administration).
Diarrhea	Similar causes as for stomatitis and esophagitis. Occurs most frequently with 5-fluorourcil, methyl-GBG, methotrexate, hydroxyurea, nitrosoureas. If severe, proctitis, mucosal ulceration, bleeding, and perforation may occur. Prolonged and uncontrolled, may result in dehydration, electrolyte imbalance, inanition.

Assessment

Nutritional status is the degree to which an individual's need for nutrients is met by his or her intake. Nutritional assessment can be performed for different purposes: to screen for potential or existing problems; to identify cause and work up existing problems; to provide an initial, complete data base for people at high risk; or to determine response to interventions or treatment. Examples of factors that can be used to identify those at risk for PCM are listed below:

1. Weight loss or gain of 10% over 1 to 3 mo.
2. Major surgery or trauma within 6 mo.
3. Living alone or preparing own meals.
4. Maintained on crystalline IV fluids for >10 days.
5. Recent medications including: catabolic steroids, immunosuppressants, antitumor agents, antibiotics, antacids.
6. RT within 6 mo.
7. Illness of >3 wk duration within past 6 mo.
8. Recurrent nausea, vomiting, diarrhea, dysphagia, esophagitis, odynophagia.
9. Inability to chew or swallow.
10. Chronic pain.
11. Inability to feed self.
12. Depression.

Although PCM is experienced by cancer patients frequently, vitamin, mineral, and fat intake, and electrolyte balance are also important considerations. The current use of megavitamin therapy and other nontraditional cancer-treatment approaches has made necessary the consideration of excesses of nutrients as well as deficits.

A surprisingly large proportion of hospitalized patients have been found to be malnourished. Assessment of nutritional status as an initial step in providing for a patient's nutritional and metabolic needs must include psychosocial as well as biophysiologic parameters. Family members and friends may be additional sources of information.

Assessment methods.   Clinical observation, anthropometric techniques, biochemical analysis, and dietary evaluation are the general methods of nutritional assessment. The specific methods that are used in assessing the nutritional status of cancer patients will vary according to the goals of the assessment, patient setting, the age of the patient, and other concurrent diseases or health conditions. A combination of measurements may be necessary to provide a complete survey of the various body components.

Clinical observation includes consideration of the physical condition of the patient, psychologic factors, socioeconomic status, medications, and other health problems. A complete physical examination will reflect the overall nutritional status of an individual. Careful attention to skin, hair, mouth, teeth, and general muscle tone may provide early clues to nutritional deficiencies. Psychologic factors that must be considered include the existence of depression, anxiety, or isolation. The ability to purchase and prepare food should be appraised. A survey of current medications used should include information about vitamins, prescriptions, over-the-counter medications, and "recreational" drugs. Additional health problems, such as diabetes, renal disease, hypertension, or malabsorption syndromes that may affect nutrition, should be identified. Much of this information is contained in any thorough nursing history.

Anthropometric measurements that may be obtained include midarm muscle circumference (MAMC), triceps skin-fold thickness (TSF), subscapular skin-fold thickness (SST), and weight for height. The purpose and process for these and other measurements are shown in Table 8–6. Once the measurements are obtained, they should be compared with the individual hospital's age- and sex-specific reference values of standards for weight, midarm circumference, midarm muscle circumference, TSF, and SST. (The reader is also referred to these tables of values in the Grant reference at the end of this chapter and in standard nutritional texts.) When tables are used to make clinical judgments, it is important not to interpret them too rigidly, thus losing sight of the wide range of individual variation that normally occurs.

Biochemical analysis contributes greatly to the nutritional assessment: *Serum albumin* indicates visceral protein levels; *serum transferrin* reflects the body's ability to make serum proteins and also indicates visceral protein stores; *total lymphocyte count* tests immunocompetence and also reflects visceral protein stores; *creatinine height index* reflects skeletal or lean body mass (somatic protein); *recall skin testing* tests T-cell-mediated immunity; and *urinary urea nitrogen* indicates skeletal muscle mass (somatic protein).

Dietary evaluation also contributes to nutritional assessment. Dietary history and intake may be evaluated by various approaches, alone or in combination, including: (1) 24-hr recall, (2) a food-frequency questionnaire, (3) a complete dietary history, (4) food diary or record, (5) direct observation, and (6) evaluation of nutrient composition according to standard nutritional criteria, such as the Basic Four Food Groups or Recommended Dietary Allowances. Assessment of the patient's knowledge of nutrition may be an alternative or a complement to other methods. This approach assumes, however, that there is a direct relationship between what people know about nutrition and what they eat.

The 24-hr recall requires the individual to complete a questionnaire or be interviewed to determine what he recalls eating in the last 24 hr or the prior day. Food-frequency questionnaires collect information on the number of times per day, week, or month that particular foods are eaten. The content of 24-hr recall may be selective or general. The method provides additional information that may be used to validate the accuracy of information gathered from other sources. The dietary

TABLE 8–6

Anthropometric Measurements for Nutritional Assessment

Measurement	Purpose	Process
Weight	Represents total of all body constituents; indicates changing nutritional reserves; basis for other anthropometric measures	Use same scale, clothing, time of day. Measure; do not accept report.
% Usual body weight (UBW)	Reflects weight change	$\% \text{ UBW} = \dfrac{\text{Current wt}}{\text{Usual wt}} \times 100.$
% Weight change	Identifies risk factor of weight loss and is considered for given time period	$\dfrac{\text{Usual wt} - \text{actual wt}}{\text{Usual wt}} \times 100.$
Midarm circumference (MAC)	Reflects muscle and fat	Using metal tape measure, measure circumference of arm at midpoint between acromial process of scapula and olecranon process of ulna.
Triceps skin-fold thickness (TSF)	Estimates SC fat stores and energy reserves (not degree of malnutrition)	Caliper measurement of nondominant arm at midpoint; measure and sum with subscapular skin-fold thicknesses; use usual weight percentile to determine expected TSF percentile.
Midarm muscle circumference (MAMC)	Reflects skeletal muscle protein mass	Indirectly estimated from midarm circumference: MAMC = MAC − $(0.314 \times \text{TSF mm})$; use usual weight percentile to determine expected MAMC percentile.
Subscapular skin-fold thickness (SST)	Estimates SC fat	Caliper measurement 1 cm below tip of right scapula; use usual body weight percentile to determine SST percentile.

history, collected by the nurse or nutritionist, provides the most complete account of nutritional intake; it may utilize 24-hr recall and the food-frequency questionnaire as part of data-gathering procedures. The history includes information about activity, economics, homelife (or hospital life), eating patterns, ethnic background, health history, medication, and appetite. If the individual is keeping a food record or diary, he is asked to record all intake of food or fluids for a given period of time. The period covered by the record depends on the regularity of the individual's food patterns. Accuracy is increased if the person records the intake immediately after eating. Observation of food intake is the most precise assessment method, but it is also the most demanding of time and energy; therefore the hospitalized patient is more easily observed than the person at home.

These methods are discussed in detail in many nutrition textbooks. Certain potential problems in evaluating dietary intake exist. They are (1) recording influences intake; (2) the patient may be unable to remember types and amounts; (3) nutrient composition of food varies with preparation; (4) accuracy varies with interviewing skills; (5) cooperation and honesty is necessary; and (6) the recorded intake may be atypical.

Management

Diarrhea. For the patient with cancer, diarrhea has numerous potential causes. The tumor itself can cause diarrhea as can malabsorption, fistulas, or pancreatic insufficiency. More commonly, diarrhea in these patients results from surgical or medical interventions for the tumor. Medications including antitumor chemotherapeutic agents, antibiotics, laxatives, and antacids also cause diarrhea in cancer patients. Other potential etiologies for diarrhea in this group of patients are bowel infections, fecal impaction, tube feedings, and anxiety and stress.

Various medications available for treating diarrhea include bulk-forming agents, adsorbents, narcotic agents, and antacids. Adsorbents, such as kaolin and pectate, are not very effective except when diarrhea is caused by an excess of bile salts. Bulk-forming agents such as methylcellulose and psyllium (Metamucil) are helpful, especially with RT patients. Various narcotic agents are available: opium derivatives (paregoric, tincture of opium, and belladonna), diphenoxylate hydrochloride (Lomotil), codeine, and loperamide hydrochloride (Imodium). Most antacids contain magnesium and act as osmotic agents to stimulate elimination. Those that do not contain magnesium but rather aluminum, such as aluminum carbonate gel (Basaljel) and aluminum hydroxide gel (Amphojel), can be used to alleviate loose stools in those patients who require frequent antacids.

When diarrhea is very severe, the individual may need to rest the bowel by restricting all oral intake except fluids containing electrolytes and sugars, which will facilitate absorption of water as well as providing fluid replacement. The diet is then gradually expanded, avoiding high fiber and other stimulants to the bowel.

Further suggestions for the care of the cancer patient with diarrhea are found in Table 8–7.

TABLE 8-7

Nursing Protocol for the Management of Diarrhea

Factor	Intervention
Activity-exercise	Assess patient's ability to care for self, including obtaining and preparing food.
	Determine energy levels and tolerance of activity and exercise.
Comfort	Evaluate discomfort caused by diarrhea (abdominal cramping, soreness around anus).
	Apply heat to abdomen for comfort.
Coping-stress	Assess family and support systems.
	Identify sources of stress and anxiety (finances, family, illness, fears).
	Encourage measures to decrease or cope with stress and anxiety (medication, counseling, relaxation training, biofeedback).
Elimination	Assess usual patterns of elimination for each individual.
	Evaluate for fecal impaction.
	Record frequency, amount, and appearance of stool.
	Evaluate bowel sounds.
	Clean rectal/anal area after each bowel movement and dry carefully.
	Apply substance for protection of skin and mucous membranes and to promote healing such as A & D ointment (Desitin) or dibucaine (Nupercainal).
	Apply a local anesthetic (ointment or spray) such as hamamelis water (Tucks).
	Use sitz baths.
	Avoid anal/rectal stimulation.

Nutritional-metabolic	Assess nutritional status, paying particular attention to hydration and electrolytes.
	Determine nutritional needs.
	Weigh patient daily.
	Evaluate dietary intake, including intake and output of fluids.
	Encourage avoidance of food and medication that aggravates the bowel.
	Appraise tube feedings as cause of diarrhea (see Table 8–10).
	Try frequent low-residue feedings if patient can tolerate (bananas, applesauce, rice) and high-carbohydrate and high-protein intake.
	If hypokalemia is evident, include foods high in potassium (baked potatoes, bananas, halibut). Supplementation or IV repletion may be necessary if diarrhea prolonged.
	Encourage drinking 2–3 quarts of fluids daily. Kooolaid, Jello, apple juice, bouillion, Gatorade, and weak tea are good sources when served at room temperature. Carbonated beverages should be allowed to flatten before being drunk.
	Avoid foods that are too hot or cold. Extreme temperatures may stimulate GI activity.
	Avoid milk and milk products to prevent lactose intolerance symptoms. Lactose-free products, such as cream substitutes, may be substituted. Lact-Aid can be used to break down the lactose in milk.
	Administer antidiarrheal medications ~½ hr before meals to minimize diarrhea.
Sleep-rest	Evaluate usual and current sleep/rest patterns; encourage resting and naps to conserve energy; plan medication administration and treatments to avoid interrupting sleep.

Nausea and vomiting. Nausea and vomiting are extremely unpleasant symptoms. Different people will cope with these experiences in different ways, depending on the severity and nature of the symptoms and on the coping styles of the individual.

Control of nausea and vomiting is an important concern for the nurse. The goal is to enhance psychologic and physical comfort for the patient; prevent pronounced physical debilitation from malnutrition, impaired mobility, and fatigue; and allow anticancer therapy to continue. Furthermore, nausea and vomiting cause fluid and electrolyte imbalances (dehydration, metabolic alkalosis from loss of potassium, chloride, and hydrogen ions); straining of abdominal muscles; and the danger of aspiration.

Nausea and vomiting in cancer patients can occur as a result of the presence of the tumor itself, but it more frequently follows chemotherapy or RT. Those cancer chemotherapeutic agents that have the most severe emetic potential are: cisplatin, dacarbazine, nitrogen mustard, dactinomycin, mithramicin, nitrosoureas, methotrexate, and mitomycin-C. It is believed that different classes of chemotherapeutic agents initiate vomiting by stimulating different sites — TVC vs. CTZ. The occurrence of nausea and vomiting is also influenced by psychologic factors, such as anxiety and fear, expectations from past experience of the patient or others, the environment's sights and smells, or conditioned responses. Other less common emetic stimuli include: fluid and electrolyte abnormalities, bowel obstruction or peritonitis, CNS metastases, hepatic metastases, uremia, local infections and septicemia, and narcotics. Careful determination of the etiology of the symptoms, by history and physical examination, is essential to planning appropriate interventions.

The specific interventions used in the treatment of nausea and vomiting will depend on its causes. Severe vomiting from chemotherapy is frequently difficult to control by currently available methods. A combination of antiemetics and sedation can be used at times when the patient prefers sedation. Two major approaches to relieving nausea and vomiting are the use of pharmacologic measures and of behavioral approaches.

Pharmacologic therapy is most commonly relied upon, even though clinical studies have shown drugs currently available commercially to be of marginal value. The ineffectiveness of these medications in the past may be because they have been administered in suboptimal doses or regimens. Some investigational drugs have shown promise.

Cannabinoids, the active ingredients of marijuana, have proven antiemetic properties. Delta-9-tetrahydrocannabinol has been effective for both chemotherapy- and RT-induced nausea and vomiting. Cannabinoids are not without significant toxicities including sedation, severe dysphorias, hallucinations, and syncope. Their use should be avoided with the naive and the elderly.

Metoclopramide hydrochloride (Reglan) is a procainamide derivative with peripheral and central antiemetic action. It increases GI motility and gastric emptying. The effectiveness of metoclopramide as an antiemetic is dependent on its dosage and route. When administered PO after chemotherapy, it is ineffective. In order to avoid the risk of mucosal tears in the GI tract, its use is contraindicated after resection or anastamoses. Reported side effects include extrapyramidal symptoms and anxiety or agitation, which can be alleviated by concurrently administering diphenhydramine (Benadryl).

Glucocorticoids have been suggested for use as antiemetics during anticancer therapy. Dexamethasone and methylprednisolone are used. It is postulated that they work by blocking the synthesis or release of prostaglandins.

The more traditionally used antiemetic medications include the phenothiazines, the butyrophenones, and antihistamines. The phenothiazines are potent dopamine receptor blockers that are believed to act on the CTZ. These are generally the most effective antiemetic drugs available commercially, even though experimental reports of their efficacy are conflicting. The phenothiazines are of limited use with strongly emetic agents. The phenothiazine tranquilizers are classified on the basis of their chemistry and pharmacology into three groups: the piperazine class, the aliphatic class, and the piperidine class. Chlorpromazine (Thorazine), an aliphatic compound, has limited antiemetic action during chemotherapy. Phenothiazines such as prochlorperazine (Compazine), a piperazine compound, have a more pronounced antiemetic action when the CTZ is involved. Potential side effects include sedation, orthostatic hypotension, extrapyramidal symptoms, and elevated prolactin levels.

The butyrophenones, including haloperidol (Haldol) and droperidol, are the most potent inhibitors of the CTZ. Experience with these drugs in the relief of nausea and vomiting induced by RT and chemotherapy is limited but promising. Because hypotension or other cardiorespiratory effects are not likely, these drugs are useful for patients who are elderly or debilitated.

Antihistamines, such as dimenhydrinate (Dramamine) and diphenhydramine (Benadryl), are helpful in increasing effectiveness and decreasing toxicity when given with other antiemetics. The mechanism by which these histamine (H–1) blockers work is not known. Antihistamines are also effective for vestibular disturbances.

Many nonpharmacologic **behavioral approaches** have been suggested to help alleviate posttreatment nausea and vomiting. These include: hypnosis, behavior modification, deconditioning, or desensitization, guided mental imagery, biofeedback, relaxation techniques, diversion, and meditation (*see* Chapter 7A). Suggested advantages of nonpharmacologic approaches are numerous. It is thought they may: (1) potentiate the placebo effect of medications; (2) improve patient-provider relationships; (3) transform passive patients into active patients, thus returning control to the patient; (4) improve patient compliance; and (5) promote an increased sense of well-being. For the most part, they are without side effects and are inexpensive and portable. The most significant potential problems with these nonpharmacologic approaches include difficulties in providing a conducive environment in institutional settings, the time needed to practice and perform these measures, and the requirement for patient motivation to carry them out.

Table 8–8 contains further considerations for the care of the cancer patient experiencing nausea and vomiting.

Decreased oral intake.   Oral intake can be decreased as a result of numerous symptoms and conditions in the patient with cancer. Anorexia, fatigue, pain, nausea or vomiting, anxiety, depression, and changes in environment or life-style can result in decreased intake of food and nutrients. Table 8–9 incorporates a number of approaches to encourage increased oral intake.

Enteral hyperalimentation (tube feeding) is used for cancer patients who have functioning GI tracts and yet are unable to ingest adequate nutrients orally to meet their metabolic needs. This situation may occur when the patient is unable to take food and fluids by mouth (anorexia, oral or esophageal abnormalities) or when the GI tract is not functioning normally (malabsorption, short bowel syndrome, fistulas). Hypermetabolic states, such as postsurgery, cancer, or infection, may also require that tube feedings be initiated to meet the increased demands for nutrients.

Tube feedings may be administered through various routes — orogastric, nasogastric, nasoduodenal, nasojejunal, esophagostomy, gastrostomy, or jejunostomy. Orogastric feedings are given through a tube swallowed from the mouth and offer the advantage of being able to be carried out by the patient, and of withdrawal of the tube between feedings. Needless to say, this procedure requires a capable, motivated patient. Any of the routes that utilize a tube passing through the nose are limited to ~3 wk duration to avoid the development of sores or fistulas. Gastrostomy tubes may be temporary or permanent.

Enteral hyperalimentation through a tube is a relatively safe and simple procedure that can be carried out at home. If the patient has a working gut, this method should be used in preference to parenteral (IV) routes. Complications that can occur include: fluid and electrolyte disturbances, such as dehydration and tube feeding syndrome (dehydration, hypernatremia, hyperchloremia, azotemia); aspiration; constipation; or most commonly, diarrhea. Feedings may be administered continuously or by bolus, except into the small bowel; bolus methods of administration are not appropriate in this case. Whenever bolus feedings are tolerated poorly, continuous feedings will need to be considered. The rate of administration is crucial to patient tolerance of tube feedings; usually the ideal rate is over a period of 20 to 30 min. Advantages of bolus feedings are increased patient mobility and freedom, independence, ease of maintenance, and similarity to the physiologic aspects of normal food consumption, making this method more physiologic. Continuous infusions require a volumetric pump to be safest and most accurate. Alternatively, a gravity system including an in-line solution administration set (Soluset, Buretrol) can be used. The maximum flow rate should be around 125 ml/hr. Rate of administration and concentration of the solution should be increased gradually to decrease side effects. Rate is usually increased before concentration.

A variety of types of formulas are available to use as tube feedings. Decisions about which to use will be based upon the individual's nutritional needs. The formulas vary in digestability, osmolality, viscosity, content of fat, carbohydrate, protein, and lactose, vitamins and minerals, and expense. High-osmolality formulas are poorly tolerated by some individuals, resulting in diarrhea, bloating, and flatus. Blenderized and milk-based feedings are relatively inexpensive and easy to use. Because they contain intact protein and lactose, they can only be used with a normally functioning GI tract. Their osmolality is relatively high (500 to 800 mOsm/kg). Lactose-free formulas are available, with standard calorie content (1 kilocalorie [kcal]/ml) or as high-density formulas (1.5 to 2 kcal/ml). Osmolality of these formulas is low (300 to 400 mOsm/kg). Chemically defined or elemental formulas contain nutrients in partially digested forms so that they can be used for patients with impaired GI function, such as malabsorption or short bowel syndrome, or with metabolic disorders. Elemental formulas are nutritionally incomplete, requiring supplementation of long-chain fatty acids and minerals. Modular formulas designed to supplement carbohydrate, fat, or protein specifically are also available. Nursing concerns for administering tube feedings are outlined in Table 8–10. Whether enteral hyperalimentation is accomplished through intermittent bolus administration or through continuous administration will have implications for nursing care of the individual.

Parenteral nutrition is a process by which carbohydrates, fat, and protein, along with trace elements, vitamins, and electrolytes are

TABLE 8-8

Nursing Protocol for the Management of Nausea and Vomiting

Factor	Intervention
Activity intolerance	Assess the effects of movement and activity on symptoms of N/V.
	Encourage activity to the extent that it does not aggravate N/V and provides diversion and exercise.
	Avoid sudden, rapid movements.
Anxiety	Assess nature and extent of anxiety as a contributing cause of N/V.
	Inquire about past experiences of patient and others to determine if they contribute to increased anxiety.
	Instruct patient about various relaxation techniques, if appropriate.
	Administer antianxiety medications.
Breathing	Assess risk of aspiration.
	Position and monitor patient to prevent aspiration during vomiting.
	Remove dentures or partial plates.
Comfort	Assess sources of discomfort or pain.
	Promote comfort measures, using an individualized approach based on patient needs.
	Control the environment to remove unpleasant sounds, sights, smells, and reduce stimulation of the vomiting center.
	Administer antiemetics at appropriate dosages and intervals.
	Prevent N/V from occurring initially.
	Provide mouth care after vomiting and as needed to freshen mouth.

Fluid volume deficit from active loss or decreased intake	Assess fluid and electrolyte status by history and physical examination and review of laboratory work.
	Observe and record intake and output of fluids, including the amount and character of emesis.
	Monitor weights, BP, skin turgor, urine concentration.
	Administer antiemetic medications as prescribed, paying particular attention to patterns of N/V and dosage and administration schedule of drugs.
	Provide fluids that reduce nausea and do not induce vomiting.
Inadequate nutrition	Assess nutritional status by dietary evaluation, physical examination, history, and laboratory tests.
	Evaluate food preferences and tolerance.
	Determine past measures that have been effective.
	Record the pattern of N/V and the amount and appearance of emesis.
	Evaluate ability to obtain and prepare food.
	Encourage small, frequent feedings of food that is tolerated well and of high nutritional value.
	Avoid intake of food with low nutritional value. Use foods that have been tolerated well in the past to provide positive reinforcement.
	Medicate prior to meals so that antiemetic effect is active during and immediately after meals.
	Avoid fat, spicy, or highly salted foods or foods with a strong odor.
	Remove food covers outside of the room where food will be eaten.
	Minimize stimuli that aggravate nausea (sights, smells, people).
	Provide distraction and relaxation opportunities.
Knowledge/information	Assess knowledge about the causes of N/V and measures recommended to treat them.
	Review signs and symptoms to report to the health-care provider.
Sleep/rest	Determine present and usual sleep patterns.
	Medicate with antiemetics and provide uninterrupted rest.
	Sedatives may be used if desired by patient to induce sleep during periods of N/V.

N/V, nausea and vomiting.

TABLE 8-9

Nursing Protocol for the Management of Decreased Oral Intake

Factor	Intervention
Activity	Encourage activity appropriate to abilities and energies of individual to increase appetite and utilization of nutrients.
Anorexia	Evaluate circumstances of anorexia.
	Encourage eating foods that are appealing at times when appetite is best. As much as possible, allow opportunity to choose mealtimes and food.
	Instruct about nutritional supplements, methods for adding protein and calories to diet. Assist to obtain.
	Serve foods attractively and in a pleasant environment.
	Provide companionship while eating to avoid social isolation.
	Remove all unpleasant stimuli from eating environment.
	Encourage "freshening up" before meals by washing hands, face, and providing mouth care.
	Encourage eating of small, frequent meals rather than three large ones.
	If not contraindicated, suggest a glass of wine or sherry prior to meals.
	For hospitalized patient, have friends and family bring in favorite foods.
	Keep nutritious snacks handy for nibbling.
	Teach to avoid eating or drinking foods low in calories or other nutrients.
	Limit the amount of liquids consumed with meals.
	Serve foods at appropriate temperatures.
Bowel elimination	Evaluate alterations such as constipation or diarrhea.
constipation	Relieve constipation by appropriate diet and medication (*see* Chapter 11B).
diarrhea	*See* Table 8–15 for interventions for diarrhea.

Fatigue	Assess ability to obtain and prepare food. Arrange for necessary assistance. Teach to expend minimal energies on food preparation. Encourage frequent rest periods, particularly before meals.
Knowledge/information	Assess knowledge about appropriate nutritional intake and measures to encourage it. Provide verbal and written information for patient and family regarding nutrition.
Nausea and vomiting	Assess patterns of N/V. Plan feedings to avoid predictable times. Medicate prior to eating. Avoid supine position for at least 2 hr after eating.
Oral mucositis	Evaluate condition of oral cavity. Provide measures to relieve oral discomfort prior to eating (*see* Chapter 9B). Maintain good oral hygiene.
Pain/comfort	Evaluate nature and extent of discomfort or pain for its effect on oral intake. Encourage wearing apparel that is loose and comfortable. Provide pain relief measures prior to mealtimes (*see* Chapter 7A). Plan care so that unpleasant or painful procedures do not take place before meals.
Sensory-perceptual alteration	Provide assistance with eating required as a result of weakness, paralysis, visual disturbances. Assess taste changes and alter available foods to accommodate.

N/V, nausea and vomiting.

TABLE 8-10

Nursing Protocol for the Management of Enteral Hyperalimentation (Tube Feeding)

Factor	Intervention
Skin integrity	Assess condition of skin around esophagostomy, gastrostomy, or jejunostomy. Change dressing at least daily and clean around tube with half-strength H_2O_2. Do not use alcohol. Evaluate for signs of essential fatty acid deficiency (dry, scaling skin over distal lower extremities). Give corn oil or safflower oil, 30 ml, daily or MCT oil, 15 ml, bid via the tube. Encourage activity and changing positions to avoid skin breakdown. Check nose for pressure necrosis if nasal tube is in place. Reposition tube.
Diarrhea	Evaluate past and present bowel function. Adjust formula type and rate of administration to avoid diarrhea. Administer formula at room temperature (not cold). Change administration set and tubing daily. Rinse with hot water when refilling set. Hang supply for 4 to 6 hr only.
Comfort/pain	Regulate the rate and select formula to prevent abdominal cramping, distension, vomiting, or diarrhea. Position patient comfortably during administration. Check continuous infusions for gastric residual. If >150 ml, discontinue temporarily.
Coping	Provide an opportunity for the patient and family to discuss the impact of enteral hyperalimentation feeding techniques. Provide opportunity to discuss fears regarding tube feeding and nutrition. Give information to help alleviate fears and provide support and practice opportunities. Determine the individual's usual and current concept of body image. Provide opportunity to talk about body image and self-concept.

Fluid volume	Evaluate for dehydration or fluid overload.
	Maintain accurate records of intake and output.
Oral hygiene	Encourage or provide mouth care ≥q 3–4 hr when awake.
Aspiration	Check placement of the tube in the stomach before initiating any feeding and ≥q 8 hr during continuous feeding.
	Elevate head of bed 30–45 degrees, unless the tube is in the jejunum, to prevent reflux or aspiration.
Nutrition	Assess nutritional status.
	Irrigate the tube with 5–10 ml of water prior to and following feeding.
	Select feeding type and amount based on individual needs and condition.
	Check urine q 6 hr for sugar and acetone.
	Watch for tube feeding syndrome.
	Evaluate electrolyte status.

H_2O_2, hydrogen peroxide; MCT, medium chain triglyceride.

infused into the venous system to correct nitrogen balance, allow weight gain, and help tissue repair. Parenteral nutrition can be accomplished through a large peripheral vein (peripheral hyperalimentation, PHAL) or through central venous access (central hyperalimentation, CHAL), using veins such as the cephalic, subclavian, or jugular.

PHAL is used on a short-term (5 to 7 days) basis to supplement PO intake when requirements are higher than normal or when the risk of central approaches is too great. Peripheral routes are useful only for repletion of mild to moderate malnutrition and when anabolic requirements are greater than normal but not excessive. PHAL may be used as a boost in conjunction with oral feedings.

Indications for CHAL include: (1) oral intake or enteral intake impossible, potentially hazardous, or insufficient; (2) short gut or short bowel syndrome, resulting in decreased absorption in the small intestine; (3) hypermetabolic states (sepsis); (4) inability to eat as a result of severe nausea, vomiting, anorexia, or obstruction; (5) unavailability of a suitable peripheral vein; or (6) requirement of long-term parenteral repletion.

The composition of the solutions administered by a central route are different from those administered peripherally. More hypertonic solutions can be administered centrally; thus the solutions given peripherally are 10 to 20% dextrose and those given centrally are 20 to 25% dextrose. When the very hypertonic solutions (20 to 25% dextrose) are administered, they must be given centrally through a large vein such as the subclavian in order to provide rapid dilution and to prevent irritation and thrombophlebitis. Usually, 2,000 to 3,500 ml of fluid are required daily.

Calories are usually provided by a carbohydrate source, such as dextrose. Adequate calories are required so that the amino acids infused for synthesis of protein into muscle mass can be utilized (usually 150 to 280 calories/g of nitrogen). Some calories can be provided from fat sources. The calculation of energy needs for 24 hr is made by multiplying basal energy expenditure (BEE) by a specific factor that compensates for energy expenditures incurred by activity or injury. (This calculation is described in detail in the Grant reference at the end of this chapter.)

Protein needs are supplied by amino acid compounds. Free crystalline amino acids are frequently used. The normal adult requires ~56 g of protein daily. These basic requirements may be exceeded during the physiologic stress of illness or surgery. The balance between nitrogen from protein that is used and protein that is consumed is evaluated by nitrogen balance studies. Wound healing, fistula closure, weight gain, and improved tolerance of therapy require a positive nitrogen balance (more taken in than put out).

Fat is provided by the infusion of Intralipid (10% or 20%) or Liposyn. Administration of fats is useful as an additional concentrated calorie source to provide for excessive calorie needs. It is also necessary to avoid essential fatty acid deficiencies in patients receiving CHAL for prolonged periods (>2 wk). Intralipid or Liposyn can be adminis-tered through a peripheral vein and should not pass through a filter. Administration should occur 2 to 3 times/wk at a rate of 1 ml/min for the first 15 min and then increase to 125 ml/hr. The nurse should observe for possible pyrogenic side effects, such as headache, nausea, vomiting, fever, flushing, dyspnea, or allergic responses or phlebitis.

Minerals, trace elements, vitamins, electrolytes, and insulin are frequently added to the parenteral nutrition solutions at the time of preparation by the pharmacy. Multivitamins and vitamins K and B_{12} and folic acid are needed. The electrolytes sodium, potassium, chloride, calcium, magnesium, and phosphorus are added because they are important in maintaining osmotic pressure in body fluids. Endogenous insulin supplies may be inadequate when hypertonic glucose solutions are administered. Insulin supplies are best augmented by administering insulin in the parenteral nutrition solutions, rather than administered SC on a sliding scale basis. Salt-poor albumin may be needed to restore visceral protein levels.

Complications occurring from parenteral nutrition can be catego-rized as technical, metabolic, and septic. Septic complications are serious potential dangers when administering parenteral nutrition, especially through central access. Potential technical complications are pneumothorax, subclavian artery puncture, air embolus, brachial plexus injury, hemorrhage, subclavian vein thrombus, or improper location (see Chapter 17). Metabolic complications that may occur are: hyperglycemia, hypoglycemia, hyperglycemic hyperosmolar non-ketotic coma, hypophosphatemia, fatty acid disturbances, hypomag-nesemia, or electrolyte and fluid imbalance.

Initially, central catheters for hyperalimentation were not to be used for any other purposes. Recently, multiple-lumen catheters that have up to 3 or 4 lumens have been developed. One port is designated for administering nutrition and the others may be used for central venous pressure monitoring, administering drugs, or drawing blood.

Major considerations for nurses administering CHAL are outlined in Table 8–11. Additional detailed instructions should be sought in institutional procedure manuals and nursing or nutrition textbooks.

TABLE 8-11

Nursing Protocol for Administration of Central Parenteral Nutrition

Factor	Intervention
Infection	Check the in-line fittings q hr.
	Refrigerate solutions until ½ hr prior to use.
	Additions to solutions should be done in pharmacy under laminar flow hood.
	Check clarity and expiration date on bottles before hanging.
	Use micropore 0.22-micron filter.
	Change IV tubing (except high-pressure tubing) daily using sterile technique.
	Change dressing at catheter insertion every other day, using clean technique for Hickman catheters and sterile technique for Centrasil or Intrasil catheters.
	Notify physician of signs of inflammation, purulence, thrombosis, or extravasation at insertion site.
	Maintain sterility of catheter tip.
	Apply an occlusive dressing, looping the tubing to prevent dislodgement.
	If discontinuing central catheter, send tip for culture and sensitivities.
	See also Chapter 17.
Fluid balance	Initiate and discontinue gradually.
	Infusion rate should never exceed prescribed rate by >10%.
	Infuse with a volumetric pump.
	Check rate ≥ q hr.
	Record intake and output, weight.
	Warm solution to room temperature prior to administering to decrease viscosity, allowing correct calculation of flow rate.
	Evaluate fluid balance of patient (including vital signs) q 4 hr.

Nutrition	Test urine for glucose q 6 hr. Report 3+ or 4+ readings.
	Substitute Multistix or Testape for Clinitest or Acetest tablets when receiving medications that alter readings of Clinitest and Acetest tablets. (This includes many antibiotics.)
	Evaluate serum electrolytes, glucose, intake and output, weight.
	Allow opportunity to talk about changes in eating activities.
Oral hygiene	Examine the oral areas for dryness, mucositis, or infection.
	Evaluate condition of the teeth.
	Provide mouth care on a regular basis q 4 hr while awake.
	Obtain artificial saliva if needed.
Coping	Instruct patient and family about purpose and procedure of CHAL.
	Assure that patient has knowledge and experience to care for CHAL himself if going home.
	Evaluate feelings about CHAL.
	Provide information and support during CHAL.
	Instruct regarding relaxation and diversion measures.
	Provide opportunity for discussion of feelings about appearance.
	Assess impact on usual responsibilities and role activities.
Activity	Develop exercise program to improve utilization of nutrients and improve/maintain strength.
	Offer diversional activities.

CHAL, central hyperalimentation.

Bibliography
1. Anderson, L., M. V. Dibble, R. R. Turki, H. S. Mitchell, and H. J. Rynberger. Nutrition in Health and Disease. J. B. Lippincott Co., Philadelphia. 1982. Seventeenth edition.

   Chapter 9, on nutrient utilization, provides an excellent review of the digestion and absorption processes for carbohydrates, fats and other lipids, and proteins, including helpful diagrams. Metabolism of nutrients in the human body is explained in detail.

2. Cunningham, S. G. Fluid and electrolyte disturbances associated with cancer and its treatment. Nursing Clinics of North America (December 1982). 579–593.

   Fluid and electrolyte disturbances that are problems in cancer patients are discussed. Body saline and water balance, calcium balance, potassium balance, and tumor lysis syndrome are covered.

3. DeWys, W. D. Pathophysiology of cancer cachexia: current understanding and areas for future research. Cancer Research (February 1982). 721s–726s.

   Cancer cachexia is explained by changes in energy, such as increased energy expenditure and reduced energy intake. The mechanisms by which body composition changes and carbohydrate, protein, and lipid metabolism is altered are described.

4. Donoghue, M., C. Nunnally, and J. M. Yasko. Nutritional Aspects of Cancer Care. Reston Publishing Co., Inc., Reston, Va. 1982.

   This programmed self-learning text provides a nice overview of our current knowledge about nutrition and cancer as well as a survey of interventions for clinical problems related to nutrition.

5. Grant, J. P., P. B. Custer, and J. Thurlow. Current techniques of nutritional assessment. Surgical Clinics of North America (June 1981). 437–463.

   A fresh look at nutritional assessment can be found in this article, which is particularly useful because it evaluates current methods and suggests reasonable approaches.

6. Margie, J. P., and A. S. Block. Nutrition and the Cancer Patient. Chilton Book Co., Radnor, Pa. 1983.

   Extensive information about practical aspects of nutrition and cancer are pulled together in this reference for professionals and patients. The coverage is broad: children, GI tumors, adjusting food, alternative therapies, other sources of information, and recipes.

7. National Cancer Institute. Eating hints: recipes and tips for better nutrition during cancer treatment. NIH Publication No. 81–2079. U. S. Department

of Health and Human Services, National Cancer Institute, Bethesda, Md. 1981.

The book is an excellent resource for practical approaches to common nutritional problems experienced by cancer patients and has many recipes contributed by cancer patients and their families.

8. Rivlin, R. S., M. E. Shils, and P. Sherlock. Nutrition and cancer. *American Journal of Medicine* (November 1983). 843–854.

An extensive overview of the relationships between cancer and nutrition can be found in this article. Dietary deficiencies and excesses are discussed, as are the effects of cancer and its treatment on nutritional status; nutrition as a therapeutic modality is reviewed.

9. Smith, S. A. N. Theories and intervention of nutritional deficit in neoplastic disease. *Oncology Nursing Forum* (Spring 1982). 43–46.

Cachexia from neoplastic diseases is reviewed in terms of deficit factors, assessment parameters, and the interventions of psychosocial modification, dietary modification, nutritional supplements, tube feeding, and parenteral nutrition.

10. Sokal, J. E. Measurement of delayed skin test responses. *New England Journal of Medicine* (September 4, 1975). 501–501.

Presents issues in using delayed skin tests as a clinical tool and procedures for performing and evaluating them. Practical suggestions are included.

CHAPTER 9

PROTECTIVE MECHANISMS

Standard: The client and family possess the knowledge to prevent or manage problems related to alterations in protective mechanisms (immune, hematopoietic, integumentary, and sensory-motor systems).

Outcome criteria: The client and family
1. list measures to prevent skin breakdown, mucosal trauma, infection, and bleeding.
2. identify signs and symptoms of infection, bleeding, or sensory-motor dysfunction.
3. contact an appropriate health team member when initial signs and symptoms of infection, bleeding, or sensory-motor dysfunction occur.
4. state measures to manage infection, bleeding, or sensory-motor dysfunction.

A: BONE MARROW

Judith A. Spross

Anatomy and physiology

A normally functioning bone marrow is essential to life. The cells it produces are responsible for oxygen and carbon-dioxide transport, hemostasis, and immunity. Myelopoiesis is the term used to describe the growth and development of erythrocytes (RBCs), megakaryocytes (source of platelets), and granulocytes (WBCs). It is known that in humans myelopoiesis occurs in the bone marrow. Lymphopoiesis refers to the production of lymphocytes and, based on animal evidence, it is thought that this process is also initiated in the bone marrow in humans. Both lymphopoiesis and myelopoiesis are sometimes referred to as hemopoiesis.

Stem cells are the most primitive type of cells from which granulocytes, megakaryocytes, RBCs, and lymphocytes arise. The structure of hemopoietic cell populations can be conceived of as three-layered. The committed precursor cell, though structurally unrecognizable under the microscope as a future erythrocyte or other mature cell, is already committed to a particular cell line. The growth and development of these cell lines according to the three-layered concept is pictured in Figures 9A-1 and 9A-2. These cells are released from the bone marrow as postmitotic cells and complete their maturation in blood and tissue. Proliferation, maturation, and function will be considered separately.

Granulopoiesis.   Granulocyte production is mediated by the presence of infection or inflammation in the body, as well as by the production of colony stimulating factor, stimulated by tissue macrophages. Colony stimulating factor stimulates the myelocyte progenitor pool to produce more myeloblasts, which will continue to differentiate to mature WBCs. Granulocytes are important in host defense against infection. Neutrophils, in particular, are considered the first line of defense against bacterial infection. These cells are mobile and are transported to the site of infection by a process called chemotaxis. The functions of the granulocytes and monocytes are listed in Table 9A-1. The life-span of circulating granulocytes is 12 hr, and monocytes live 4 times as long. The normal adult values for the WBC and differential are listed in Table 9A-2. In splenectomized patients, there tends to be

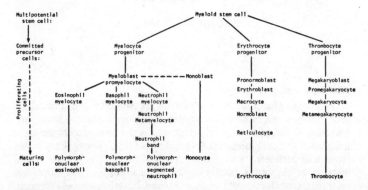

Figure 9A-1.   Myelopoiesis.

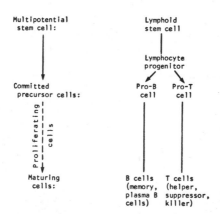

Figure 9A–2. Lymphopoiesis.

greater variation in the WBC. To determine whether a WBC is abnormal in these patients, it is important to do several counts.

Lymphopoiesis. Lymphocyte production and function are also regulated by the presence of infection or inflammation. Much of the development of lymphocytes occurs during fetal development. Transformation of stem cells to T and B cells is usually completed a few months after birth. It is thought that further lymphocyte production is initiated in the bone marrow, with maturation occurring in lymphoid tissue. Lymphocytes can be found everywhere, but they tend to concentrate in the lymphoid tissues, such as lymph nodes, thymus, spleen, and bone marrow. Lymphocytes have diverse functions. They mainly work to distinguish between self and foreign antigens, to respond to foreign antigens, and to remember the foreign antigens so that in the future a more rapid and more effective response can be mounted. To accomplish these tasks, some lymphocytes secrete substances that mediate immune reactions. Others secrete immunoglobulins. Some lymphocytes are capable of returning to a blastic stage from which they can divide again and again, giving rise to a greater number of cells that have the same properties. *See* Table 9A–1 for specific lymphocytes and their functions. Lymphocytes are mobile and tend to be long-lived, sometimes lasting years. The usual lymphocyte count is 1,000 to 4,800 cells/mm^3, or 34% of the WBC.

Immunocompetence of the host consists of humoral and cellular responses to foreign substances. Both humoral and cellular responses require adequate production of granulocytes and lymphocytes. Often, effective defense of the host against an infectious organism or other

TABLE 9A–1

Functions of Leukocytes

Leukocytes	Function
Granulocytes	
neutrophil	Moves to locus of inflammation, produces lysosomes. Phagocytosis of bacteria (first line of defense).
basophil	Release of histamine, heparin, and enzymes in acute inflammation.
eosinophil	Phagocytosis and release of enzymes to counteract effects of inflammatory mediators in allergic reactions.
Monocytes	
blood monocyte	Phagocytosis of bacteria, fungi, tumor. Synthesis of reaction-specific enzymes in response to lymphocytes.
tissue monocyte (histiocyte or tissue macrophage)	Phagocytosis, filtration of particles.
Lymphocytes	
B cells (humoral immunity)	Antibody production.
T cells (cellular immunity)	
helper and suppressor	Regulate function of other lymphocytes (e.g., mediate antibody production).
cytotoxic or "killer" cells	Specific effector function (e.g., delayed hypersensitivity reaction, graft-vs.-host disease, tumor-cell kill).

foreign protein is the result of a "cooperative" effort between the elements of humoral and cellular immunity.

Thrombopoiesis. Platelets are fragments of the megakaryocytes produced and released by the bone marrow. The production of megakaryocytes is thought to be mediated by a substance called thrombopoietin. The major functions of the platelets include: maintenance of capillary integrity, initiation of the intrinsic clotting mechanism, and clot retraction. At any one time ~⅓ of circulating platelets are sequestered in the spleen. The liver and spleen are responsible for the removal and destruction of "old" platelets. Thus, in individuals who

TABLE 9A–2

Laboratory Values for WBC Count and Differential

Cells	Quantity
WBC	4,500–11,000/mm^3
Differential	
neutrophils	54–62%
bands (immature neutrophils)	3–5%
eosinophils	1–3%
basophils	0–1%
monocytes	3–7%
lymphocytes	15–34%

have had a splenectomy, platelet counts are often higher than usual. Persons with splenomegaly may have a platelet count below normal. Platelets live for 8 to 10 days unless they are consumed during hemostasis. The average platelet count in the adult is 250,000 platelets/mm^3.

Erythropoiesis.   The production of RBCs is mediated by tissue oxygenation and renal production of erythropoietin. RBCs are released from the bone marrow as reticulocytes and mature in the blood. Maturation of RBCs is dependent on the presence of vitamin B_{12}. Other nutrients, such as amino acids and folic acid, are important to RBC development and function. The major function of RBCs is to transport hemoglobin, which in turn transports oxygen. RBCs are also important in the transportation of carbon dioxide from the tissues to the lungs. The life-span of RBCs ranges from 100 to 120 days. In the human, ~1% of RBCs turn over every day. The average number of RBCs in the adult female is 4.6 million and in the adult male, 5.4 million.

Pathophysiology of bone marrow depression (BMD)

Bone marrow dysfunction may be initiated by environmental, occupational, and hereditary factors (*see* Chapter 1). In cancer patients, BMD may occur because of a primary malignancy of the myeloproliferative tissues, metastatic cancer, or from myelosuppressive treatment. The replacement of bone marrow by primary or metastatic cancers prevents normal production and proliferation of hemopoietic elements. The hemopoietic cells that are produced may be abnormal, immature, or less functional (e.g., less able to phagocytize foreign particles). Primary malignancies of the myeloproliferative tissues, along with the specific immune defect, are listed in Table 9A–3. Myeloproliferative cancers, such as lymphoma, can metastasize to the bone marrow. Solid tumors that have a tendency to metastasize to bone marrow include lung, breast, and prostate cancer.

Though there are experimental therapies that look promising for diminishing the effects of cancer therapy on marrow, BMD can be expected with most chemotherapy and radiotherapy (RT) regimens. The effects of chemotherapy and RT on hemopoietic elements may be acute and chronic. Because hemopoietic cells are rapidly dividing, they are most susceptible to the effects of cytotoxic treatment. The effects of each modality on hemopoietic elements will be considered separately.

In the myeloid cell line **chemotherapy** affects cells in most stages, from myeloblast through myelocyte. Stem cells seem to be somewhat resistant to cycle-active drugs, such as methotrexate, but are affected by alkylators. Cells that have matured beyond the myelocyte stage are also less susceptible to chemotherapy. Thus, neutrophils in the process of differentiation are sensitive to the effects of chemotherapy. The general pattern of chemotherapy-induced neutropenia consists of a mild neutropenia for a few days after treatment, the nadir (the most pronounced decrease) for 7 to 14 days posttreatment, and recovery

TABLE 9A–3

*Primary Cancers of the Myeloproliferative Tissues
and Associated Immune Defect*

Cancer	Cell line
Acute lymphocytic leukemia	T cell or B cell
Acute myelocytic leukemia	marrow precursor cells
Chronic lymphocytic leukemia	B cell
Chronic myelogenous leukemia	granulocyte, monocyte
Multiple myeloma	B cell
Hodgkin's disease	T cell
Non-Hodgkin's lymphoma	mostly B cell
Mycosis fungoides	T cell
Sézary syndrome	T cell

within 14 to 18 days. Chemotherapy may also cause lymphopenia, suppressing both humoral- and cell-mediated immunities, a temporary effect, lasting only 2 to 3 days. BMD may be less profound when chemotherapy is intermittent, rather than continuous, because cells have a chance to recover. For the nadirs of WBCs associated with specific drugs and their duration, the reader should consult a chemotherapy handbook.

Whereas chemotherapy has a generalized effect on the bone marrow, RT tends to affect marrow activity only in the area irradiated. To understand the relative risk of bone marrow toxicity, it is useful to know which marrow sites are most active and which conventional radiation ports are most toxic to the marrow (Tables 9A–4 and 9A–5).

When RT is administered in conjunction with chemotherapy, the bone marrow toxicity is usually greater than with that of either therapy alone. In addition, prior treatment with RT may increase the bone marrow toxicity of current chemotherapy treatment. The reverse is also true.

The chronic bone marrow effects of RT and chemotherapy are similar and include atrophy or fibrosis of the bone marrow, hypocellu-

TABLE 9A–4

The Distribution of Active Bone Marrow in the Adult

Site	% of total red marrow
Head	13.1
Upper limb girdle	8.3
Sternum	2.3
Ribs (all)	7.9
Vertebrae	
cervical	3.4
thoracic	14.1
lumbar	10.9
Sacrum	13.9
Lower limb girdle (os coxae and femoral head and neck only)	26.1
Total	100.0%

Adapted from Ellis, R. E. The distribution of active bone marrow in the adult. *Physics in Medicine and Biology* (January 1961). p. 257.

TABLE 9A-5

*Proportion of Bone Marrow Irradiated by
Usual Therapeutic Techniques*

Radiation technique	Estimated % of bone marrow affected
Total body irradiation	100
Total nodal irradiation	60–70
Mantle	20–50
Para-aortic	20–25
Pelvic	15–25
Pulmonary and mediastinal	20–25
Abdominal	20–25
Cranial	25–45
Craniospinal	60–75
Chest wall and lymphatics	15–20

Reprinted with permission from Dritschilo, A., and D. Sherman. Radiation and chemical injury in the bone marrow. *Environmental Health Perspectives* (June 1981). p. 62.

larity, and sometimes the development of a second primary cancer, such as leukemia.

In addition to cancer or treatment-related causes of BMD discussed above, **gene defects** are associated with bone marrow tumors. These are listed in Table 9A-6. **Surgery** has also been reported to suppress both cellular and humoral immunity for 2 to 3 wk after surgery.

Complications of BMD. The most common and most life-threatening complication is **infection**. Infection associated with granulocytopenia (GCP) is a major cause of morbidity and mortality in cancer patients. The type of infection depends on the nature of the immune defect. Immune defects associated with cancer-related BMD are listed in Table 9A-7. The usual sites of infection in cancer patients include the respiratory tract, GU tract, alimentary tract, CNS, skin, and blood. In bone-marrow-suppressed patients, the risk for infection may be compounded by malnutrition, use of invasive procedures, obstruction of body passages, or breaks in mechanical barriers, such as skin.

Chemotherapy- and RT-induced **thrombocytopenia (TCP)** increase the cancer patient's risk of bleeding. When normal platelet

TABLE 9A–6
Gene Defects Associated with Bone Marrow Tumors

Defect	Tumor
Autosomal recessive	
Ataxia telangiectasia	leukemia
Bloom's syndrome	leukemia
Fanconi's anemia	acute myelogenous leukemia
X-linked	
Bruton's agammaglobulinemia	leukemia, lymphoreticular tumors
Wiskott-Aldrich syndrome	lymphoreticular tumors

Adapted with permission from McGuire, D. Familial cancer and the role of the nurse. *Cancer Nursing* (December 1979). p. 445.

counts drop to a level that is still >50,000 platelets/mm³ spontaneous hemorrhage is unlikely, though bleeding may occur. Minor bleeding phenomena such as petechiae and occult blood in the stool may occur at these levels but do not usually signal the onset of an acute hemorrhage. Hemorrhage at platelet levels >50,000 may occur — without these minor clinical signs — in the presence of infection, fever, chemotherapy treatment with tumor lysis, or another coagulopathy. Spontaneous hemorrhages are more likely to occur when platelets are <20,000 platelets/mm³.

Treatment-induced **anemia** tends to be overlooked because the toxic effects of chemotherapy and RT on erythropoiesis appear later than GCP or TCP and are easily treated with transfusions. Hypoproliferative normochromic, normocytic anemia tends to be the most common type of anemia in cancer patients treated with RT and chemotherapy. Other types of anemia include anemia of chronic disease and myelophthisic anemia (where marrow is replaced by tumor).

Other complications may occur secondary to hyperproliferative bone marrow disorders, e.g., hyperviscosity in multiple myeloma (*see* Chapter 15D).

Assessment

An accurate assessment of patients at risk for BMD is essential to identify risk factors, needs for patient education, and to plan and implement preventive and therapeutic nursing care. An accurate

TABLE 9A–7

Immune Defects and Associated Infections in BMD

Immune defect	Organisms

Cellular immune deficiency	Bacteria
	  gram-positive
	    Mycobacterium spp.,
	      Nocardia asteroides
	
	  gram-negative
	    Listeria monocytogenes,
	      Salmonella spp.
	
	Fungi
	  Cryptococcus neoformans,
	    Histoplasma capsulatum
	
	Protozoa
	  Pneumocystis carinii, Toxoplasma
	    gondii
	
	Viruses
	  Cytomegalovirus (CMV), herpes
	    simplex, varicella zoster

GCP	Fungi
	  Aspergillus spp., *Mucor*
	  Candida albicans (yeast)
	
	Gram-negative bacilli
	  Escherichia coli, Klebsiella
	    pneumoniae, Pseudomonas
	    aeruginosa
	
	Gram-positive cocci
	  Staphylococcus aureus,
	    Staphylococcus epidermidis

Humoral immune dysfunction	Gram-negative bacteria
	  Hemophilus influenzae
	Gram-positive bacteria
	  Streptococcus pneumoniae

BMD, bone marrow depression; GCP, granulocytopenia.

assessment may also contribute to early detection of BMD. It should be recognized that cancer is a chronic disease with remissions and relapses and that multimodal cancer therapy may have acute, chronic, and synergistic effects on the bone marrow.

When making a health assessment, it is important to be alert to the subtle changes that may indicate an impending complication in the bone-marrow-suppressed patient (Table 9A–8). For example, a headache may be the first sign of intracranial hemorrhage so that the patient would need to be examined for other signs of increasing intracranial pressure (*see* Chapter 14A). In an elderly patient, hypotension and behavioral changes may be the initial evidence of infection and sepsis. In the absence of adequate circulating neutrophils, infected lesions may not cause pain or produce pus.

After completing the health history and physical examination the nurse should be able to determine the relative risk of complications of BMD occurring. For example, the risk of acquiring a life-threatening infection increases when the absolute granulocyte count (AGC)* is <1,000 and is higher still if the AGC is <500. The risk of bleeding associated with TCP has already been discussed. Anemia is usually asymptomatic when Hb is above 8 to 10 g/100 ml. Coexisting illnesses (e.g., diabetes) usually increase the risk of complications.

Medical management

Infection.   The best way to manage complications of BMD is to prevent infection. Pizzo and Schimpff have proposed a framework for prevention that includes the following approaches: (1) bolstering host defense mechanisms; (2) avoiding damage to body barriers; (3) avoiding invasive procedures; (4) reducing acquisition of new potential pathogens; and (5) suppressing colonizing organisms. Both prophylactic and therapeutic medical approaches will be considered.

Protective environments (PE):   The total protected environment (TPE) includes isolation in a laminar flow room, GI decontamination with nonabsorbable antibiotics, and cutaneous and mucosal antisepsis. Although the TPE is effective, it is expensive, time-consuming, and cumbersome. It is best used for patients expected to have prolonged, severe GCP, such as those who receive intensive chemotherapy and/or have marrow transplantation.

Simpler methods of protective isolation include reverse isolation and isolation for BMD. Reverse isolation consists of a private room, use of mask, gown, and gloves by those entering the room, and sterile linen. Isolation for BMD usually consists of a private room, strict attention to hand-washing, protecting the patient from others with infection, and having the patient mask when outside the room. Since studies of various PEs have not shown major differences in infection

---

*The AGC is computed by multiplying the percentages of neutrophils and bands by the total WBC.

TABLE 9A–8

Health Assessment of Patient at Risk for BMD

Assessment element	Factors to consider
History	
Family history	Congenital (e.g., Fanconi's anemia); history of myeloproliferative disease.
Childhood illnesses	Look for exposure to chickenpox.
Environmental exposure	Benzene, ultraviolet rays, persons at risk for infectious disease (e.g., children who may develop chickenpox, which can cause life-threatening infection in immunocompromised person).
Immunosuppressive therapy	History of treatment with RT or chemotherapy; use of steroids; use of antibiotics (e.g., chloramphenicol has been associated with bone marrow aplasia).
Major life stressors	Stress can alter immune responses. Look for major loss or life change (e.g., divorce, death of a loved one).
Sexual history and hygiene	Homosexual men who have had hundreds to thousands of partners are known to have high titers of cytomegalovirus and also are at risk of developing AIDS with opportunistic infections. Certain sexual practices of homosexual and heterosexual individuals may increase risk of infection in immuno- compromised patients.
Sleep patterns	Lack of sleep is an added stressor on the immunocompromised patient. Patients whose marrow has been replaced by cancer may experience bone pain that alters sleep patterns.
Elimination patterns	Patients with a tendency toward constipation may use invasive procedures such as enemas, a practice contraindicated in patients with BMD. Diarrhea may cause skin excoriation, increasing risk of infection.
Nutritional patterns	Look for anorexia, unbalanced diet.
Systems review and physical examination	
General condition	Age: very old and very young patients are less immunocompetent. Weight loss.

	Fatigue: may indicate anemia. Malaise: may indicate infection.
Skin	Look for open lesions, excoriated skin, petechiae, ecchymotic areas. Skin test results (anergy or negative responses to PPD, SKSD, DCNB indicate diminished cellular immunity).
Head, eyes, ears, nose, throat	Look for tenderness, report of pain, headache, lesions, exudate, enlarged nodes, changes in vision, pupil reactions.
Respiratory	Rate, rhythm, sputum quantity, quality; pain, SOB, exercise tolerance, wheezing, consolidation, breath sounds; use of accessory muscles, results of sputum culture.
Cardiovascular	Pain, tachycardia.
GI	Pain, bleeding, diarrhea, character of stool, hemoccult results; constipation. Results of culture; perirectal pain. Ascites may prolong or worsen BMD because of slower drug metabolism and excretion. Anorectal pain in GCP may be first sign of anorectal infection (precedes objective findings by 2 to 10 days). Diffuse, abdominal cramping, fever, abdominal distension, bloody diarrhea, and decreased or absent bowel sounds may indicate neutropenic enterocolitis.
GU	Dysuria, bleeding, exudate (color, quality, quantity); loss of menses (duration, quantity); dyspareunia; urinalysis and urine culture results.
Musculoskeletal	Palpate bony areas for tenderness (especially vertebrae).
CNS	Headache, visual changes, change in level of consciousness, change in cognition, dizziness.
Laboratory values	CBC, differential, platelet count, albumin, coagulation studies.

AIDS, acquired immune deficiency syndrome; BMD, bone marrow depression; DCNB, dichloronitrobenzene; GCP, granulocytopenia; PPD, purified protein derivative; RT, radiation therapy; SKSD, streptokinase-streptodornase; SOB, shortness of breath.

rate (except for TPE), agencies tend to use the simplest precautions (private room, hand-washing, avoiding sources of infection).

Antimicrobials: Prophylactic antibiotics (systemic and oral non-absorbable) may be used in patients with BMD to prevent opportunistic infections such as those caused by the organisms listed in Table 9 A–7. Because of the dangers of superimposed infection, the emergence of resistant organisms, and other side effects of these drugs, as well as problems with efficacy, cost, and compliance, prophylactic antibiotics are generally used in the TPE. Pizzo and Schimpff recommend that oral nonabsorbable antibiotics be used only in a TPE. All prophylactic antibiotic regimens should be used with careful attention to risks and benefits, and to nursing practices that reduce the risk of contamination and colonization of the immunocompromised patient.

Fever in a cancer patient (one episode >38.5°C or 3 temperatures of >38°C in 24 hr) is considered a medical emergency, and immediate intervention is necessary. Procedures include cultures of the most logical sites for infection (blood, throat, sputum, urine, open lesions), chest x-ray, and clinical examination. The physician will prescribe antibiotics empirically.

The results of the cultures and the clinical condition of the patient are monitored closely once empiric therapy is started. Based on culture results, antimicrobial therapy may be adjusted to include agents effective against a specific organism. If the patient responds clinically, despite lack of identification of an organism, therapy is usually continued, so the patient receives a 7- to 10-day course. If fever persists despite the broad-spectrum coverage, the physician may add an antifungal agent. Some patients with persistent GCP may be on antimicrobial therapy much longer than 7 to 10 days. In this situation, the emergence of resistant organisms and superinfection are of particular concern.

Granulocyte transfusion: The effectiveness of prophylactic granulocyte transfusions has not been established. The therapeutic role of these transfusions is being studied. Granulocyte transfusions seem to improve survival in infected patients with prolonged, severe GCP. Criteria the physician may use in deciding to transfuse the granulocytopenic patient include granulocyte count <500 cells/mm^3, prolonged GCP (>10 days) anticipated, cancer diagnosis in which remission induction is likely, and fever unresponsive to antimicrobials. Donor availability may also be a factor.

Transplantation: Another promising therapy being used to overcome treatment-induced BMD is that of autologous bone marrow transplantation. Healthy marrow is harvested from the cancer patient prior to treatment and preserved to be reinfused after treatment but before the nadir of the patient's neutrophil count occurs. In the patient with marrow cancer, marrow could only be harvested autologously if the person were in remission. Allogeneic bone marrow transplantation has been used in leukemic patients when a matched donor (ideally, an identical twin) has been available. Allogeneic transplants may be complicated by the development of graft-vs.-host disease.

Immune stimulation: Therapy to stimulate more rapid granulocyte recovery has been tried and is still being studied. Agents that have been used are listed in Table 9A–9 (*see* Chapter 2).

So far, attempts at active and passive immunization in immunosuppressed cancer patients have been disappointing. Two developments that may be promising and are being studied include a varicella-zoster vaccine (active) and J-5 antiserum (passive).

TCP. The incidence of spontaneous hemorrhage in thrombocytopenic patients greatly increases when platelet counts are <20,000 platelets/mm³. TCP is not usually treated unless the platelet count is <20,000 platelets/mm³. Exceptions include a precipitous drop in platelets, spontaneous hemorrhage at counts >20,000 platelets/mm³, and for selected major surgeries when the count is between 50,000 and 100,000 platelets/mm³. The treatment of choice is platelet transfusion. Other medical approaches to TCP include the avoidance of drugs that may affect coagulation, such as aspirin, and the diagnosis and management of other coagulopathies that might increase the risk of bleeding. Patients with plasma-cell defects (e.g., multiple myeloma) often have coagulopathies in addition to TCP.

Patients should be typed for human lymphocyte antigens (HLA) for platelets to prevent alloimmunization. In a child with a body surface

TABLE 9A–9
Biological Response Modifiers

Mechanism of action	Modifier
Direct toxicity to cancer cell	Antitumor monoclonal antibodies
Initiation or augmentation of host response	Immune augmenter (BCG)
	Immunomodulator (e.g., prostaglandin)
	Immunorestorative (e.g., thymosin)
Modification of cancer cell	Interferon

BCG, Calmette-Guérin bacillus.

area (BSA) of 1 m^2, the transfusion of 1 U of platelets produces an increment of 15,000 platelets. In an adult with a BSA of 2 m^2, the increment following 1 U is 7,500 platelets. An adult will usually be transfused with 6 to 12 U. In febrile or infected patients the increment, as well as platelet survival, is reduced.

Anemia. The physician will generally try to diagnose the cause of anemia in cancer to be certain that it is a treatment-related, normochromic, normocytic anemia, because other types of anemia can be treated by vitamin and mineral supplements or reduction of chemotherapeutic dosage. The normochromic, normocytic anemia often found in patients who have had chemotherapy and RT is not usually treated unless the patient is symptomatic. In the symptomatic patient, the treatment of choice is packed red blood cells (PRBCs).

Nursing management

The nurse can be instrumental in the care of the patient with BMD. Because the complications of BMD can be life threatening to the patient, the nurse should observe carefully for any potential signs and symptoms of these complications. The assessment elements in Table 9A–8 will help the nurse focus these observations. In addition, Table 9A–10 outlines the nurse's role in the prevention and early detection of infection in BMD patients. Finally, Tables 9A–11 through 9A–13 discuss the nursing care of BMD patients with infections, TCP and bleeding, and anemia.

Bibliography

1. Fox, L. S. Granulocytopenia in the adult cancer patient. *Cancer Nursing* (June 1981). 459–466.

    Presents a review of the structure, function, and pathophysiology of the granulocyte. Discusses signs and symptoms of infection in this population and nursing care, including infection prevention and early detection.

2. Knobf, M. K. Intravenous therapy guidelines for oncology practice. *Oncology Nursing Forum* (Spring 1982). 30–34.

    Reviews risk factors associated with IV therapy and why risks of complications are increased in cancer patients. Lists principles of therapy, practices to avoid, and the rationales for these.

3. Lichtman, M., editor. Hematology and Oncology. Grune & Stratton, Inc., New York. 1980.

    Outlines normal physiology of the hemopoietic system, as well as the pathophysiology of myeloproliferative malignancies and of the bone marrow toxicities of cancer therapies.

4. Owen, H., C. Kove, and P. Cotanch. Bone marrow harvesting and high-dose BCNU therapy: nursing implications. *Cancer Nursing* (June 1981). 199–205.
   Provides an overview of the use of autologous marrow transplantation to mitigate the bone marrow toxicity of high-dose chemotherapy. Addresses the rationale, procedures, and nursing implications.

5. Patterson, P. Granulocyte transfusion: nursing considerations. *Cancer Nursing* (April 1980). 101–104.
   Discusses the role of granulocyte transfusions in the granulocytopenic cancer patient, patient response to this therapy, and detailed nursing care.

6. Pizzo, P., and S. Schimpff. Strategies for the prevention of infection in the myelosuppressed or immunosuppressed cancer patient. *Cancer Treatment Reports* (March 1983). 223–234.
   An excellent review of factors associated with infection in cancer patients and the state of the art in prophylactic therapies, as well as environmental measures to reduce acquisition of pathogens in the population at risk.

7. Schiffer, C. A., J. Aisner, and P. Daly. Platelet transfusion for thrombocytopenic cancer patients. *In* Klastersky, J., and M. Staquet, editors. Medical Complications in Cancer Patients. Raven Press, New York. 1981.
   This chapter reviews indications for platelet transfusion, preservation and storage of donated platelets, and prevention and management of alloimmunization.

8. Scogna, D. M., and C. Schoenberger. Biological response modifiers: an overview and nursing implications. *Oncology Nursing Forum* (Winter 1982). 45–49.
   Reviews the function of T and B lymphocytes and how knowledge of them has been used to develop a class of cancer therapies known as biological response modifiers. Nursing implications are presented using case studies.

9. Waterbury, L. Hematologic problems. *In* Abeloff, M., editor. Complications of Cancer. Johns Hopkins University Press, Baltimore. 1979.
   This chapter reviews the effects of cancer and its treatment on the bone marrow. Discusses indications for transfusion of various blood components.

10. Yasko, J. Guidelines for Cancer Care: Symptom Management. Reston Publishing Co., Inc., Reston, Va. 1983.
    The primary focus of this text is nursing intervention, and it is designed for self-learning. The section on BMD is comprehensive in its coverage of preventive and therapeutic nursing approaches to anemia, TCP and GCP.

TABLE 9A–10

Nursing Protocol for Prevention and Early Detection of Infection in BMD*

Problem	Intervention
General	Assess risk for infection using history, laboratory values, and clinical examination.
Need for vascular access	Practice appropriate management of peripheral IV therapy (*see* Chapter 17 for central lines):
	Aseptic technique; frequent site inspection; change IV site q 48 hr if possible.
	If patient has poor venous access and line must remain, care for site, including application of antimicrobial ointment and new dressing q 48 hr.
	Use warm, moist heat (Hydrocollator pads or towels) for 10–15 min prior to venipuncture to improve venous access.
	Ask MD to consider long-term central venous access for ongoing therapy.
	Use steel needle if patient is not seriously ill or agitated.
	Use smallest-gauge needle possible, 21 or 23 for most therapy, 18 or 19 for blood, if steel; smaller-gauge plastic catheters (21) can be used for blood.
	Use iodophor *or* alcohol to prepare site (use of both decreases antisepsis).
	Avoid shaving area; if hair needs to be removed to improve visualization or comfort, clip hair.
	Avoid irrigating a plugged IV (the thrombus may harbor microbes).
	Change IV tubing and fluids q 24 hr.
	Invasive procedures should be avoided, including rectal temperatures, rectal exams, enemas, suppositories; IM and SC injections; urinary catheterization.
	If invasive procedures must be done (e.g., bone marrow biopsy) the site should be inspected periodically for signs of infection.

| Need for protection from environmental risks | Environmental measures:
Wash hands meticulously prior to patient contact.
Restrict visitors with infections.
Have patient wear mask when appropriate.
Follow appropriate isolation technique for degree of GCP or according to investigational protocol. (In absence of laminar flow, usual procedure is private room and meticulous attention to hand-washing, patient hygiene, and housekeeping). Isolate patient from others on ward with infectious diseases.
Avoid fresh fruits and salads in severe GCP.
No *cut* flowers in room (source of *Pseudomonas* organisms).
No humidifiers.
Clean respiratory equipment q day.
Patient hygiene:
Assist patient to perform hygienic measures to decrease organisms (e.g., oral care; cleansing of high-risk sites: axillae, skin folds, perineal area; exercise if tolerated).
Immobilized patients should cough and deep-breath q 2 hr or use blow bottles. |
| Maintenance of patient's defenses | Administer vaccines as prescribed (e.g., a vaccine against pneumococcal infections).
Counsel patient regarding well-balanced diet, adequate fluid intake.
Counsel patient regarding importance of rest and sleep.
Instruct patient in stress-reduction techniques.
Lubricate dry areas (e.g., artificial tears, skin emollients).
If patient is a smoker, help patient to stop. |

BMD, bone marrow depression; GCP, granulocytopenia; MD, physician.
*These guidelines for the prevention of infection and nursing care of patients at risk or with actual infection should be adapted/modified based on the epidemiology of infections in cancer patients found in a particular institution.

TABLE 9A-11

Nursing Protocol for the Management of Infections in BMD

Problem	Intervention
General guidelines	Monitor site of infection for improvement or deterioration.
	Monitor WBC and differential.
	Implement specific isolation procedures using guidelines from Center for Disease Control and/or institutional facilities such as laminar flow room. Designate isolation procedures on door to patient's room or other types of protective isolation.
	Administer antibiotics on time. See that peak and trough drug levels are drawn if prescribed.
	Monitor and report side effects of antimicrobials.
	Observe for signs of nephrotoxicity of antimicrobials such as the aminoglycosides.
	Weigh patient 2–3 times/wk, because some drugs, such as carbenicillin, have high sodium content and may result in sodium and water retention.
	Observe for superinfection (e.g., candidiasis in patient on antibacterial drugs), signs of sepsis (*see* Chapter 15F).
	Record temperature q 4 hr. For temperature > 38.5°C follow standing orders for fever workup. Cultures usually include blood, throat, urine, sputum, lesion, and central and peripheral IV lines, as well as chest x-ray. For comfort, administer acetaminophen (Tylenol) for fever if cultures and therapy have been initiated. Implement other comfort measures as indicated or prescribed (tepid baths, cooling blanket).
	Administer analgesics as prescribed.
	Increase fluids if not contraindicated.
	Teach patient/family self-care measures: how to treat minor abrasions; preventing cross infection from one site to another; comfort measures for fever until patient can get to medical care (increasing fluids, ice bags to axillae, groin, tepid bath).
	If discharged on PO or IV antibiotics, teach regarding importance of taking each dose, side effects, signs of superinfection, safe methods of administration.

Guidelines for specific sites	Oral. *See* Chapter 9B. Lung. *See* Chapter 13. Monitor VS, breath sounds. Instruct patient on measures to loosen and expectorate secretions. Prepare patient for open lung biopsy (often performed when *Pneumocystis carinii* is suspected). Evaluate response to respiratory therapy. Tachypnea and nonproductive cough may indicate *Pneumocystis carinii*. Skin. *See* Chapter 9C. GI. Record quantity, quality of stool; culture if GI infection suspected. Auscultate bowel sounds. Record/report increased pain, tenderness, distension. For neutropenic enterocolitis administer and monitor medical therapy (including fluid and electrolyte replacement, transfusions, and antibiotics). For patients with *Candida* esophagitis, administer analgesics, antifungals, and modify diet (*see* Chapter 9B). GU. *See* Chapter 11C. Record intake and output. Observe for dimunition or exacerbation of GU signs/symptoms (e.g., flank pain). CNS. Record neurological signs q 4 hr. Report deteriorating responses.
Guidelines for specific medical therapies	Amphotericin B. Should be given only in D5W; protect infusion from light. Test dose is usually given; for patients who have a reaction, obtain premedication orders from MD. Observe for signs of hypokalemia. Aminoglycosides. See general guidelines, and observe for signs of nephrotoxicity. Granulocyte transfusion. Instruct patient about procedure, signs of reactions. Follow usual blood transfusion procedures (VS, double check, etc.) Administer first 50–75 ml slowly (about 1 hr). Transfusion can be administered over 2–4 hr. Observe for febrile reactions (transfusion may raise temperature 1 to 5 degrees). If febrile reaction occurs, administer prescribed steroid, antihistamine. (These can be used prophylactically in future transfusions.) Slower administration of transfusion may minimize febrile reactions. Chills increase intracranial pressure, which increases risk of cerebral bleeding if patient also is thrombocytopenic. Follow institutional procedures for transfusion reactions. Observe for signs of clinical response posttransfusion (reduced temperature, improvement in infected lesions).

BMD, bone marrow depression; MD, physician; VS, vital signs.

TABLE 9A–12

Nursing Protocol for the Management of Thrombocytopenia and Bleeding in BMD

Problem	Intervention
Patient teaching	Teach patient to avoid bleeding by modifying activities that may cause trauma; to ingest a diet with adequate protein and fiber; and to avoid taking medications that interfere with platelet functioning.
General guidelines	Monitor VS more frequently in patients with actual bleeding (frequency depends on site and severity). Administer platelet packs if prescribed. Usually administered IV push or via a Y-setup with NS (as with PRBCs) over 20–30 min. Volume varies with number of units (10 U = 250 ml). Observe for adverse reactions: usually chills, fever, or hives, which are usually mild. Patients may need premedication. If sensitization to platelets occurs, family donor may need to be found. Support donor as needed.
Platelets 20,000–50,000/mm^3	If invasive procedures must be done, MD may request laboratory to have several units of platelets on hold. Avoid venipuncture, parenteral injections. If these are necessary, apply pressure for 3–5 min after needle is withdrawn.
Platelets <20,000/mm^3 or >20,000/mm^3 with fever, infection, or other coagulopathy	Assess neurologic signs; report headache, change in level of consciousness or behavior or pupils. Test all output for blood daily. Observe for hemoptysis, bleeding gums, bleeding at venipuncture sites. Observe skin head-to-toe for evidence of bleeding. For females ask MD whether hormones should be used to suppress menses (often done in acute leukemia). Avoid constipation. If venipuncture is necessary, the tourniquet should not be tied tightly.
Site specific	
Skin	Prevent trauma, puncture. For large hematomas, ice bag may be helpful. Obtain prescription for use of topical thromboplastin on bleeding abrasions. Apply pressure to bleeding wounds.
Head, eyes, ears, nose, throat	For nosebleeds, use high Fowler's position and firm pressure to nostrils below the bridge of the nose. For severe nosebleeds, MD may pack nose, using gauze impregnated with phenylephrine hydrochloride (Neo-Synephrine), topical thromboplastin, topical epinephrine (1:1,000), or 10% cocaine solution. If nose is packed, provide comfort measures that will keep oral tissues moist and minimize "bad taste" (pleasant-tasting mouthwash without alcohol, ice chips, water). For oral bleeding, absorbable gelatin sponge for hemostasis (Gel-foam) or topical

thrombin (5,000 U in accompanying diluent +50 ml NS solution) may be used (prescription required). The latter preparation is swabbed onto the bleeding area with a pledget soaked in the solution. Procedure is performed q 4 hr and prn.

CNS	Platelets are not usually helpful in this situation. If prescribed, administer steroids to relieve headache. Reduce environmental stimuli to minimize exacerbation of discomfort. If there are cognitive or visual changes, employ reality and environmental orientation. Observe and report changes in VS and neurologic signs that signal further deterioration. Provide other life-support measures as indicated. Have patient avoid Valsalva maneuver. Control vomiting and cough with nursing and medical measures to minimize increasing intracranial pressure. Seizure precautions.
GI	If patient is on steroids, administer antacids. Monitor Hb and Hct. For acute bleeding, iced NS may be instilled through a nasogastric tube. Monitor platelet and PRBC transfusions. Monitor VS more frequently. Administer antiemetics if patient is vomiting blood (avoid phenothiazines). Record color of stools, emesis, quantity.
Renal	Administer analgesics for comfort. Monitor VS more frequently. Record intake and output accurately q 2–4 hr. Record color of urine.

BMD, bone marrow depression; MD, physician; NS, normal saline; PRBC, packed red blood cells; VS, vital signs.

TABLE 9A–13

Nursing Protocol for the Management of Anemia in BMD

Problem	Intervention
Fatigue	Assess current patterns of ADL and rest and sleep habits to identify factors that can be modified to promote rest. Teach patient/family: that fatigue is expected when anemia is present; to increase rest/sleep time; to rest between activities; if pattern of anemia/fatigue is cyclical with treatment regimen, have patient increase rest then and avoid planning too many activities (e.g., if fatigue and nadir occur 7 days posttreatment and last for three days, plan for more rest and fewer activities). Assist patient and family to identify sources of help for persistent, prolonged fatigue (e.g., when marrow is replaced by cancer and unresponsive to therapy). Possible resources include visiting nurse associations, church groups, family, friends, hospice.
Inadequate tissue perfusion	Transfusion of PRBCs is usually done if patient is symptomatic or Hct is <25%. To avoid hemolytic reactions, be certain type and cross-match have been checked to make sure unit is compatible with patient's blood type. Record base-line VS. Observe for transfusion reaction: fever, chills, headache, nausea, vomiting, hives; patients with history of febrile or allergic reactions with blood transfusions should have prescriptions for pretreatment medications (diphenhydramine hydrochloride and/or hydrocortisone, acetaminophen) to prevent such reactions. Monitor VS during transfusion; observe for other possible complications of blood transfusions: hyperkalemia; hypocalcemia; fluid overload. Monitor arterial blood gases as prescribed. Administer oxygen therapy as prescribed.

BMD, bone marrow depression; PRBCs, packed red blood cells; VS, vital signs.

B: MUCOUS MEMBRANES

Reidun Juvkam Daeffler

Anatomy and physiology

Mucous membranes line the alimentary canal from the lips to the anus, participating in the functions of digestion, absorption of food and fluids and elimination of residue and waste products. They also serve as a protective barrier to maintain the integrity of the organs.

The mucosal lining consists of layers of epithelial cells and various structures that correlate with the function of different organs or parts of an organ. **Mucus,** produced by glandular epithelial cells in the mucosa, facilitates movements of the contents of the canal and protects the mucosa from abrasions. The mucosa continuously renews itself; each cell has a life-span of 10 to 14 days. The mitotic index is highest in children and young individuals.

Saliva is formed by secretions of the salivary glands and the oral mucosa (Fig. 9B–1). It is usually slightly acidic, with a pH of 6.6 to 6.9, and consists of water (97 to 99%), mucin, and salts of sodium, potassium, and calcium. It also contains bacterial and fungal organisms and epithelial cells from the mucosa. Approximately 1,000 to 1,500 ml of saliva are secreted per day, depending on quantity and quality of food intake. Saliva production increases with the amount of food taken and with appetizing food. The saliva is swallowed, and much of the fluid is reclaimed by absorption.

The functions of saliva are as follows:
1. Moisten the food and lubricate the oral cavity, pharynx, and esophagus to facilitate both swallowing and contact between dry food and the taste buds in the tongue.
2. Facilitate speech by lubricating the oral structures.
3. Reduce starches to maltose with the help of the enzyme ptyalin.

Pathophysiology

The mucosal tissues in individuals with cancer may be exposed to physical, chemical, and microbial injury. The normal local reaction of tissues to such injury is **inflammation,** sometimes accompanied by constitutional symptoms, such as fever (*see* Table 9C–1). Mucosal inflammation may lead to sloughing of the cells, causing the mucosa to become thin, denuded, and ulcerated.

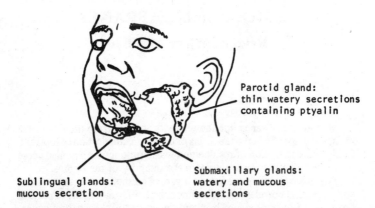

Figure 9B–1.   Salivary glands and their secretions. *Reprinted with permission from* Daeffler, R. Oral hygiene measures for patients with cancer. *Cancer Nursing* (October 1980). p. 348.

Leukocytes play a vital role in inflammation. The polymorphonuclear leukocyte (PMN) constitutes a mobile reserve for fighting infection. It destroys bacteria and liquifies cell fragments. When leukocytes are reduced in numbers or impaired in quality, susceptibility to infection occurs. Patients with leukocyte counts of <1,000 cells/mm often develop opportunistic infections — bacterial, fungal, or viral.

The factors most likely to affect mucosal integrity in the cancer patient are: (1) the disease itself, (2) antitumor therapies, and (3) nutritional compromise. The complex interrelationship of factors that contribute to mucosal alterations are illustrated in Figure 9B–2, which focuses on oral mucositis. The terms stomatitis and oral mucositis may be used interchangeably.

This section will focus on oral, pharyngeal, and esophageal mucositis, as well as rectal inflammation and abscess. Other patient problems will be discussed in subsequent chapters.

Chemotherapy.   Cytotoxic drugs affect the mucosa *directly* through toxic effects on rapidly dividing tissues and *indirectly* by myelosuppression, increasing the susceptibility to infections and bleeding.

Oral mucositis is a direct consequence of damage to the dividing cells in the basal layers of the oral mucosa, which inhibits replacement of the superficial layer of cells. Stomatitis occurs in ~40% of patients receiving chemotherapy, depending upon type of drug administered,

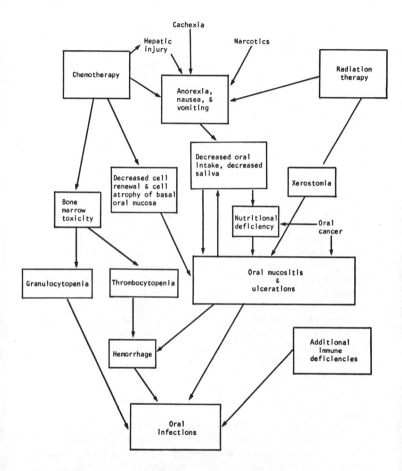

Figure 9B–2. Factors contributing to oral mucositis in cancer.

dosage, administration schedule, drug metabolism, and rescue capability.

Type of drug: Cytotoxic drugs causing mucositis are detailed in Chapter 2. In general, antibiotics and antimetabolites are likely to cause stomatitis. Methotrexate, actinomycin-D, doxorubicin, and daunomycin are especially toxic to the oral mucosa.

Dose: In some cases, stomatitis may be a dose-limiting side effect, i.e., the desired therapeutic dose may need to be reduced because of stomatitis.

Administration schedule: The incidence of stomatitis, for example, increases with *rapid* infusion of high-dose 5-fluorouracil.

Drug metabolism: The incidence of stomatitis (and other side effects, as well) is increased if an individual cannot adequately metabolize or excrete certain chemotherapeutic agents. For example, in the presence of liver dysfunction, doxorubicin cannot be metabolized; in the case of renal compromise, the body's ability to excrete methotrexate is decreased.

Rescue capability: The risk of stomatitis can be decreased by the administration of folinic acid (citrovorum factor, leucovorin) after methotrexate.

Infection is an indirect effect of chemotherapy, because cytotoxic therapy may induce neutropenia (*see* Chapter 9A). When the patient's natural barriers to infection are affected, organisms of even low virulence may have a readily accessible port of entry. The loss of an intact epithelial barrier in the mouth and in the rectum, which tend to be heavily colonized by normal flora, makes an easy entrance for systemic infection in the immunocompromised patient.

The most common oral infections are presented in Table 9B-1. Patients who are immunosuppressed and/or on antibiotic therapy are at great risk for oral candidiasis. Of the seven species of *Candida, Candida albicans* is most often the infecting organism. In some cases, preventive treatment with nystatin or clotrimazole is indicated. Frequent oral assessment will ensure prompt treatment before the infection can spread to the esophagus or become systemic. Amphotericin B, a parenteral antifungal agent, is used to treat systemic candidiasis.

Bacterial infections are less common and are successfully treated with local or systemic broad-spectrum antibiotics. The appearance of the oral mucosa, together with systemic signs of infection, signal the need for cultures of the oral cavity and prompt treatment.

Herpes simplex infection is suspected in persons with a history of cold sores; because of the immunosuppressive effects of cancer and its treatment, staff or family members with active herpes simplex infection should not have physical contact with these patients. A detailed discussion of herpes infection is included in Chapter 9C.

Thrombocytopenia occurs in association with chemotherapy-induced myelosuppression and may cause severe bleeding from mucosal surfaces. Platelet counts <50,000 platelets/mm^3 predispose

TABLE 9B-1

Common Oral Infections Secondary to Stomatitis

Infectious organism	Appearance	Management
Candida albicans (moniliasis; thrush)	Soft, whitish- or cream-colored patches covering part or all of the tongue, lips, gums, or buccal mucosa. Underneath, the mucosa is bright red and moist.	nystatin miconazole ketoconazole clotrimazole (*see* Table 9B-5)
(perlèche)	Symmetrical erosion of the labial junctions; deep cracks in the corners of the mouth, often covered with white/gray membrane.	May be associated with riboflavin deficiency
Staphylococcus aureus	Exudative, purulent, and encrusted erosions.	Broad-spectrum antibiotics
Gram-negative bacteria	Raised, creamy, moist, glistening site of infection that is nonpurulent and has smooth edges.	Broad-spectrum antibiotics
Pseudomonas aeruginosa	Raised lesions enclosed by a red halo; yellowish center turning purple to black with necrosis.	Certain broad-spectrum antibiotics (*see* Chapter 9C)
Herpes simplex virus	Vesicle that ruptures within 12 hr and becomes encrusted with dry exudate; may extend over lips. Yellowish brown membrane easily dislodges, causing severe pain.	

to bleeding as a result of invasive procedures or local trauma; spontaneous oral or GI bleeding occurs when the platelet count is <20,000 platelets/mm^3. The risk of gingival bleeding and infection increases when meticulous hygiene is not maintained and the mucosa becomes dry and friable. Whether or not the patient is thrombocytopenic, gingival bleeding may indicate an underlying infection.

Radiation therapy (RT).   Injury to surrounding mucous membranes during RT for oral cancer may result in xerostomia, dental decay, decreased oral intake, and mucositis and predispose the individual to infection and bleeding. Osteoradionecrosis and trismus are serious late effects of RT to the head and neck.

Xerostomia, or dry mouth, caused by decrease or loss of salivary secretions, occurs when the major salivary glands are irradiated (*see* Fig. 9B–1). It is related to dose and duration of treatment and usually starts during the first or second week of treatment. Although radiation-induced xerostomia may be irreversible, some patients report subjective improvement in mouth dryness in the months after therapy. Without the cleansing and lubricating functions of saliva, the risk for gingival bleeding and infection increases.

Oral mucositis is seen within the first 2 wk of RT to the head and neck and is related to the dose and the duration of treatment. Early signs include dryness, progressing to irritative hyperemia and edema, with mucosa appearing red and swollen. As treatment continues, the mucosa becomes denuded, ulcerated, and covered with a fibrinous exudate. This condition persists until 2 to 4 wk after the last treatment, when the normal healing process begins, unless it is complicated by secondary infection.

Osteoradionecrosis may occur at the site of irradiation ≥ 2 mo after therapy is completed. Necrotic ulcers develop because of fibrosis and impaired blood supply caused by the RT. These extremely painful ulcers are precipitated by trauma and are slow to heal and likely to expand.

Radiation-induced enteritis may occur any time following high-dose GI irradiation. It may present as chronic diarrhea or as a bowel obstruction and result in bowel ulceration, stricture, or fistula formation. Chronic or late radiation changes include vascular thrombosis, submucosal fibrosis, necrosis, and ulceration, and obstruction or perforation may result.

Radiation recall is a reactivation of a previous epithelial radiation effect when chemotherapeutic drugs are given soon after RT. Such radiation recall can occur in the radiation field, e.g., skin or esophagus, upon administration of methotrexate, bleomycin, cyclophosphamide, and 5-fluorouracil, but is most commonly caused by doxorubicin and actinomycin-D.

Nutritional status.   Lack of nutrients can precipitate a **nutritional-deficiency stomatitis.** Nutritional deficiencies are common in cancer patients, arising from a combination of factors, such as: (1) anorexia caused by malignancy, RT, or chemotherapy; (2) dryness or soreness of the mouth; (3) dysphagia; (4) taste alteration/loss after chemotherapy, RT; (5) surgical procedures; (6) nausea/vomiting; (7) malabsorption; (8) GI obstruction; (9) weakness; and (10) depression.

The condition of the mucosal membranes and nutritional status are interdependant. Malnutrition decreases the growth of epithelial tissue, delays healing of local ulcerations, and increases susceptibility to infection. Figure 9B–2 illustrates some of these interrelationships. Further details are discussed in Chapter 8.

Primary malignancies.   Cancerous growths may involve the mucosa directly, causing changes in functions, inflammation, tissue sloughing, necrosis, and ulceration. Examples are: (1) leukemic gingivitis and leukemic infiltrates, common in acute monocytic leukemia (leukemic infiltrates of tonsils may mimic infectious disease); (2) intestinal tumor causing partial to complete bowel obstruction; (3) colorectal cancer causing diarrhea and constipation; (4) leukoplakia, a painless, precancerous lesion easily confused with oral candidiasis, appearing as a grayish hyperkeratosis that can only be removed by tearing; (5) salivary gland tumor, most commonly found in the parotid gland.

Assessment

Oral cavity.   A base-line assessment of the oral cavity of all cancer patients is necessary to: describe presenting condition of oral cavity; identify problems that should be dealt with prior to treatment; assess oral hygiene practices, personal attitudes, and knowledge of oral health and techniques as a basis for an individualized teaching plan; and identify changes during the course of treatment.

Because of the number of stressors that affect the oral mucosa, a systematic assessment should take place on each admission to the health-care institution. Basic tools for assessing the mucosa include a tongue blade and a flashlight. Outpatients are instructed to assess themselves daily in front of a mirror with good light. They are informed that oral pain may be a late symptom of stomatitis, so visual examination is necessary for early detection.

In order to increase validity and reliability of documentation, a standardized assessment form may be helpful. Figure 9B–3 shows an example of such a form, to be used for each systematic observation. Column 1 describes the normal condition of the mouth, with each subsequent column representing degrees of deterioration. (Numerical values are included only for use in research.)

Date: _____   Time: _____   Signature: _____

Circle the term(s) in each category that best describe(s) your observations

ORGAN		1	2	3	4
LIPS Indicate site of abnormality	Texture:	Smooth, soft	Slightly wrinkled	Rough	Cracked, bleeding or ulcerated
	Color:	Pink	Red mucocutaneous junction	One or more reddened areas	Entire lip inflamed
	Moisture:	Moist	Slightly dry	Swollen, dry, blistered	Cracked and very dry
TONGUE	Texture:	Firm, smooth prominent papillae	Papillae prominent at base, Medial lingual groove deepened	Papillae all over tongue raised, Coating at the base	Ulcerated, fissured, blistered, bleeding
	Color:	Pink	Pink with reddened areas coated	Tip and papillae red, except for coated areas	Entire tongue bright red except for coating
	Moisture:	Moist	Slightly dry	Dry and swollen	Engorged, dry with indentations
MUCOUS MEMBRANES Palate Uvula Buccal Mucosa Pharynx	Texture:	Smooth	Thin and fragile	Cracked, encrusted areas	Ulcerated, sloughing Blistered Bleeding
	Color:	Pink	Pale	Red and inflamed White coating	Bright red with white, yellow, or brown spots
	Moisture:	Moist	Slightly dry	Dry and swollen	Edematous

		Smooth	Rough	Occasional lesions/blisters	Ulcerated, bleeding
GINGIVA & INTERDENTAL PAPILLAE (labial, palatal, lingual, labial)	Texture:	Smooth	Rough	Occasional lesions/blisters	Ulcerated, bleeding
	Color:	Pink	Pale with one or more reddened areas	Red	Bright red and shiny White spots
	Moisture:	Moist	Slightly dry	Swollen, dry	Edematous
SALIVA		Thin, watery Normal amount	Increase in amount	Saliva scanty, mouth dry	Saliva thick; ropy; viscid: mucid
VOICE		Normal tone and quality	Deeper, lacking resonance	Deep and raspy	Difficulty speaking
ABILITY TO SWALLOW		Swallows without difficulty Normal gag reflex	Discomfort on swallowing	Pain on swallowing Diminished gag reflex	Unable to swallow No gag reflex
TEETH	Shine:	Shiny	Slightly dull	Dull	Very dull
	Debris:	No debris	Slight debris	Debris clinging to ½ of visible enamel	Covered with debris
	Amount:	Full mouth	≥¼ of teeth lacking	≥½ of teeth lacking	No teeth remaining
	Dentures:	Well-fitting	Slightly loose	Loose and ill-fitting, with areas of irritation	Unable to wear due to irritation

Figure 9B–3. Assessment of the oral mucosa. *Adapted from Bruya, M., and N. Madeira. Stomatitis after chemotherapy. American Journal of Nursing (August 1975). p. 1350.*

Frequent assessment facilitates early detection of infections (*see* Table 9B–1). Diagnosis of infection can be made only by culture of the lesion, which should be done as early as possible so as to initiate appropriate antimicrobial treatment.

Table 9B–2 serves as a guide in planning the care of persons at risk for stomatitis after chemotherapy.

Stomatitis after local RT will usually last from 1 to 2 wk after initial treatment until 2 to 4 wk after completion of treatment.

Patients undergoing antitumor therapy may be immunosuppressed, increasing the importance of accurate and thorough assessment of the oral and rectal mucosa. These patients may develop infections without the usual signs and symptoms (*see* Chapter 9A), because the inflammatory process may be delayed or reduced. Perception of pain may be decreased, and mucosal changes may occur prior to patient complaints of discomfort.

Esophagus.   When mucositis extends from the oral mucosa to the esophagus, the patient may experience additional symptoms calling for special interventions. Early symptoms of esophagitis are: difficulty in swallowing solid foods, a "lump" in the throat, and pain on swallowing. Progression may lead to severe substernal pain.

Assessment of dysphagia includes the three phases of swallowing:

1. Oral—the patient's ability to move his tongue, keep his lips closed, and make a sucking movement with lips and cheek. These movements are necessary to chew and move food to the posterior tongue.

TABLE 9B–2

Timetable for Development of Stomatitis after Chemotherapy

Time after treatment	Effect
5–7 days	Histologic changes: drug interference with cell division and maturation.
7–14 days (less in children), or 3–5 days prior to drop in granulocyte count	Visible inflammation, oral ulceration resulting from minor trauma. Ulcerations most often <5 mm and superficial. Most severe prior to granulocyte nadir.
21 days (beginning with granulocyte recovery)	Resolution of mucositis.

2. Pharyngeal—the patient's ability to elevate his larynx.
3. Esophageal—the patient's ability to move food into the stomach.

Rectal area. Because the rectal area is less accessible for observation than the oral cavity, patient cooperation in assessment is especially important. The patient is taught to report signs and symptoms of infection and bleeding, including: rectal and perineal pain; bleeding; itching and burning; urinary burning and frequency; redness.

Visual inspection of the rectal area is part of the nursing assessment. Perianal abscess is suspected when the temperature is elevated >1 degree centigrade for more than 24 hr and when the patient experiences rectal pain. The usual signs of inflammation may be reduced or absent in the immunosuppressed patient, however, especially when being treated with corticosteroids and other anti-inflammatory agents.

Management

A healthy oral and GI mucosa is of significant value for emotional expression, verbal communication, comfort, nutrition, elimination, and fluid/electrolyte balance.

Oral hygiene is subject to special attention from oncologists, because inadequate care of the oral cavity can lead to life-threatening infections and result in dose and schedule modification of curative agents.

Although there is not yet evidence that oral hygiene measures can *prevent* mucositis from occurring after chemotherapy with cytotoxic drugs, such measures can *reduce* the incidence of life-threatening infections. Preexisting periodontal disease, as well as poor oral hygiene, predisposes to oral complications of cancer treatment, including gingival bleeding in thrombocytopenic patients. The purpose of oral care in cancer patients is to: (1) prevent infections and periodontal disease; (2) prevent gingival bleeding; (3) improve the patient's feeling of well-being; (4) maintain/improve the nutritional function of the oral cavity; (5) prevent further damage to oral structures; (6) reduce oral complications to allow for completion of the treatment plan.

The ideal approach to the management of oral complications of chemotherapy and RT is interdisciplinary, combining the expertise of dentists, nutritionists, oral surgeons, and infectious disease physicians with those of medical oncologists, radiation therapists, and nurses.

Nursing management of oral infections in the immunosuppressed patient includes:

1. Dental evaluation with attention to potentially irritating teeth surfaces; underlying gingivitis or periodontal infection; ill-fitting dentures.

2. Patient education to accomplish intensive oral hygiene before and during myelosuppressive therapy.
3. Daily oral assessment for early diagnosis of complications.
4. Management of complications: symptomatic treatment (Tables 9B–3 and 9B–4); antimicrobial treatment (see Table 9B–1 and Table 9B–5).

Oral hypothermia techniques are being evaluated as preventive measures for mucositis, but they are subject to questions as to the effect on antitumor treatment.

Nursing protocols for care of the patient with potential or actual alterations in mucous membranes are presented in Tables 9B–3, 9B–4, and 9B–6. These care plans must be individualized and adjusted for each patient, recognizing the variation in risk for mucositis, choice of regimen, and response to treatment.

Bibliography

1. Beck, S. Impact of a systematic oral care protocol in stomatitis after chemotherapy. *Cancer Nursing* (June 1979). 185–199.

    Report of a study of oral condition of 25 chemotherapy patients before and after implementation of an oral care protocol.

2. Brown, H., and M. Kiss. Standards of clinical nursing practice: the side effects of chemotherapy in the treatment of leukemia. *Cancer Nursing* (August 1982). 317–323.

    Presents a standard patient-care plan for stomatitis in the leukemia patient, developed by nurses at Memorial Sloan-Kettering Cancer Center. The care plan is organized according to nursing diagnosis.

3. Daeffler, R. Oral hygiene measures for patients with cancer. *Cancer Nursing* (October 1980). 347–356; (December 1980). 427–432; (February 1981). 29–35.

    Part I reviews nursing and medical literature on oral hygiene and summarizes a survey of oral care practices in cancer institutions; part II focuses on agents for oral care and instruments for oral hygiene; part III offers conclusions and recommendations for research, a glossary of terms, advice on diet, and process standards for oral care.

4. Oncology Nursing Society, Clinical Practice Committee. Guidelines for nursing care of patients with altered protective mechanisms. *Oncology Nursing Forum* (Winter 1982). 68–73.

    Presents guidelines for nursing management in three levels of altered mucous membrane integrity, from potential stomatitis to severe stomatitis. Presented as a standard care plan with expected outcome and nursing management for each patient problem.

5. Ostchega, Y. Preventing and treating cancer chemotherapy's oral complications. *Nursing 80* (August 1980). 47–52.

    Guidelines and rationale for oral care presented in tables and illustrations with brief narrative. Includes pictures of mucositis with infections and descriptions of clinical appearance of *Pseudomonas*, candidiasis, and herpes simplex.

6. Peterson, D. E., and S. T. Sonis. Oral complications of cancer chemotherapy: present status and future studies. *Cancer Treatment Reports* (June 1982). 1251–1256.

    Refers to the 1981 symposium on oral complication of cancer chemotherapy, recommending dental staff involvement in the oncologic team. Both infectious and noninfectious oral complications are reviewed.

7. Ross Laboratories. Mouth Care Instructions for the Chemotherapy Patient (Patient Booklet). October 1981. Ross Laboratories, Columbus, Ohio.

    A 9-page pocket-sized booklet distributed for patient education with instructions, written in easy language, for care of normal as well as sore mouth. Includes management of problems such as difficulties in eating, pain, dry mouth and lips, bleeding, and low blood count.

TABLE 9B-3

Nursing Protocol for Patients at Risk for Alteration in Oral Mucosa

Problem	Intervention

Potential mucositis caused by antitumor therapy	Assess oral mucosa for base-line condition (*see* Fig. 9B-3).
	Initiate dental referral.
	Instruct patient and evaluate outcome of instruction:
	  Oral complications of particular treatment regimen.
	  Daily oral self-examination:
	    Wash hands.
	    Use mirror and notice changes from normal oral mucosa or lips.
	    Report early signs and symptoms of mucositis: dryness, burning, redness, small white or yellow lesions, difficulty swallowing, swelling of gums or tongue, coating of mucosa, ulceration.
	  Oral hygiene program:
	    Floss daily with unwaxed dental floss (gentle).
	    Use soft toothbrush tid with sweeping motion from gingiva toward crowns of teeth, cleaning front and back surfaces. Use horizontal motion for top surfaces of teeth.
	    Remove prostheses during procedure; brush and clean and keep in water while outside of mouth.
	    Cleanse oral cavity well after meals and at bedtime using mild saline solution, plain water, or 1:5 dilution of mild mouthwash and water.
	    Avoidance of irritants to mucosa, e.g., commercial mouthwashes or dentifrice, tobacco, hot food/beverages, alcohol, spicy foods, poorly fitting dentures, lemon-glycerin swabs.

Xerostomia	Force fluids as tolerated; take frequently throughout the day. Use artificial saliva prn (commercial products contain carboxymethyl cellulose and are available in spray containers, bottles, or tubes.) Oral hygiene program after meals and bedtime (*see* above). Avoid irritants to oral mucosa (*see* above). Increase air moisture by means of humidifier or vaporizer. Include soft, moist foods with sauces (*see* Chapter 8).
	Stimulate salivary glands: sugar-free gum, sour-lemon candy (contraindicated in mucositis). oral hygiene tid and at bedtime. Provide moisture: popsicles, ice chips, artificial saliva.
Decreased or thickened saliva because of inadequate oral intake	
Indwelling endotracheal or nasogastric tube	Oral hygiene tid and at bedtime.

TABLE 9B-4

Nursing Protocol for Management of Alterations in Oral Mucosa

Problem	Intervention
Stomatitis related to antitumor therapy	Increase program to q 2 hr.
	Select mouthwash according to specific condition: NS as basic mouthwash; sterile NS if WBC < 1,000 cells/mm³; sodium bicarbonate (1 tsp in 500 ml NS or water) for thick saliva; 3% H_2O_2 and water (1:4) to remove hardened debris (mix immediately prior to use to maintain oxidizing effect); rinse with NS to remove unpleasant taste; avoid commercial mouthwashes containing alcohol, phenol, or astringents; avoid mineral oil.
Impaired ability to swish/swallow	Prevent aspiration: use side-lying or sitting position over sink or basin; use tonsil-tip suction.
	Irrigate oral cavity using cleansing device: irrigation bag with tubing; atomizer with nozzle tip; Water Pik (contraindicated if patient thrombocytopenic).
	Remove debris using foam stick (Toothette) without dentrifice moistened with mouthwash; soft toothbrush if tolerated.
Dry, cracked, or ulcerated lips	Moisten lips with lubricating jelly or artificial saliva prn.
	If lips are cracked or ulcerated, clean gently q 2 hr with 4 × 4-in. sterile pads dipped in sterile NS.
	If lips are encrusted, clean with 4 × 4-in. pads dipped in sodium bicarbonate or H_2O_2 solution, pat dry, and apply lubricating jelly.
Discomfort	
general	Consult MD regarding appropriate medication (Table 9B-5).
	Avoid hot, acidic, coarse, spicy, and fried foods, citrus juices and fruits.
	Try soft, coating foods, e.g., yogurt, sour cream, cottage cheese.
	Suggest artificial saliva prn for discomfort related to mouth dryness.
local analgesia	Administer diphenhydramine hydrochloride elixir prn alternating with dyclonine hydrochloride (Dyclone).
	Use swish and discard method if frequent local analgesia is required.
	If taste not tolerated, try making popsicle by mixing drug with desired beverage and freezing around tongue blade.
systemic analgesia	For severe discomfort, use of parenteral drugs (e.g., morphine by continuous IV drip) may be necessary.

Impaired verbal communication because of increased or thickened saliva	Provide tonsil-tip suction setup and instruct patient in suctioning technique.
	Rinse mouth with sodium bicarbonate solution to dissolve mucus (1 tsp in 500 ml NS or water).
	Respond promptly and in person to patient's call.
Potential for infection	
general (see Chapter 9A)	Maintain clean environment: hand-washing, care of cleaning devices, care of eating utensils.
	Prepare food carefully: avoid raw fruits, vegetables; foods of questionable origin.
	Use sterile NS.
oral hygiene	Use individually wrapped foam sticks and discard after use.
	Avoid damage to mucosa: Commercial mouthwashes or dentifrice, tobacco, hot food/beverages, alcohol, spicy foods, poorly fitting dentures; gently use soft toothbrush and floss.
patient teaching	Assess patient understanding of oral hygiene program and reinforce teaching as needed.
	Teach signs and symptoms of infection: pain, white patches, encrustation, ulcerations, coated areas, swelling.
early detection	Assess patient's oral cavity daily using oral assessment chart (Fig. 9B–3).
	Report signs and symptoms of infection to MD promptly.
	Culture oral mucosa when signs are present.
Infection of oral mucosa	Administer appropriate medication (Table 9B–5).
	Provide oral care prior to local administration of medication. Avoid mouthwash and oral intake for 20 min after medication to allow for effect.
	If patient intolerant of medication: try alternative method of administration (e.g., freeze in desired liquid and serve as popsicle); encourage patient and reinforce importance of treatment.
	In case of systemic antimicrobials, administer regularly to maintain blood levels.
	Maintain anti-infection protocol.
	Measure vital signs q 2 hr. Report abnormal findings promptly.
Oral bleeding	Promptly notify MD and assist: platelet transfusion; topical thrombin; e.g., 5,000 U mixed in diluent, then in 50 ml NS to swab area of bleeding repeating q 4 hr or prn for active bleeding; periodontal packs.

H_2O_2, hydrogen peroxide; MD, physician; NS, normal saline.

TABLE 9B-5

Commonly Used Drugs for Oral Application in Mucositis

Indication	Product	Administration*	Nursing implications
Pain and discomfort; local anesthetic for oral/pharyngeal/ esophageal pain	benzocaine 20%	Apply directly to painful area or swish and swallow.	Comes in a tube for spot application. Duration 20 min.
	dyclonine hydrochloride (Dyclone) 0.5%	15 min prior to meal: 5–10 ml swish for 2 min, gargle, discard.	Avoid serving hot food to patients receiving local anesthetics because sensitivity to temperature is diminished.
		Swab to painful sites prn, using an applicator.	Contraindicated in patients with compromised swallowing function.
		5–10 ml swish and swallow.	Decreases gag reflex.
		Onset: 10 min Duration: 1 hr or more	Note the longer duration of dyclonine hydrochloride as compared to lidocaine.
	lidocaine (Xylocaine) viscous 2%	10–15 ml swish and swallow/ discard q 3 hr prn Duration: 20 min	Note systemic effects of lidocaine in larger doses (cardiovascular depression, CNS depression or excitation).

Painful oral mucosa: antihistamine to soothe	Vitamin E capsule	Puncture capsule with a sterile needle and apply contents directly to painful lesions.	Recommended by oncology nurses as promoting healing as well as reducing pain. No research results available.
	diphenhydramine hydrochloride	5–10 ml swish for 2 min, gargle and discard/swallow prn	Note that drug also is used to treat motion sickness, allergic reactions (except asthma), extrapyramidal reactions. It may cause sedation, dizziness, and hypotension, especially in older patients.
	kaopectate	Mix 10 ml with pain reliever (above) to coat mucosa and keep pain reliever in place.	
	remineralizing solution	As prescribed by producer/pharmacy	
Dry mouth and throat: decreased saliva	artificial salivas (eg., Saliva Substitute, Xero-Lube, Mouth Moisturizer, Orex)	Swish 5–15 ml prn in a clean oral cavity; swallow or discard or apply on painful areas with a swab.	Commercial salivas consist of sorbitol, carboxymethyl cellulose, and a flavoring agent and have no known side effects. Dispenser bottles allow patient to squirt a small amount directly into mouth.

Indication	Product	Administration*	Nursing implications
Fungal infection: candidiasis	ketoconazole (Nizoral) tablets 200 mg	1 tablet/day for 1–2 wk.	This systemic treatment has been shown effective in oncology patients with oral thrush. Hepatic damage is a possibility.
	nystatin (Mycostatin) suspension	Swish 500,000 U q 4–6 hr, keep in mouth for 2 min, then discard/swallow (if esophageal effect desired).	NPO for 20 min after administration.
	nystatin tablet	Let dissolve slowly in mouth q 6 hr.	Use only for patients who are able to understand instructions for administration and able to keep troche/table in mouth until dissolved.
	clotrimazole (Mycelex) troche 10 mg	Dissolve lozenge slowly in mouth (5 troches/day for 2 wk).	
	miconazole or clotrimazole cream	Thin topical application on oral mucosa.	This tasteless, odorless cream has been found soothing for inflamed tissues by some oncology patients.
		May alternate q 4 hr with nystatin; swish and swallow q 4 hr.	

*All topical drugs should be applied to a clean mucosa, followed by NPO for 15–30 min.

TABLE 9B-6

Nursing Protocol for Patients at Risk for Alteration in Rectal Mucosa

Problem	Intervention
Potential for rectal abscess related to neutropenia and thrombocytopenia	Assess patient's personal hygiene practices and instruct/assist as needed: Clean perineal/perianal area after each bowel movement and prn to a minimum of bid, using a mild soap, tepid water; rinse thoroughly and carefully pat dry with soft towel. Provide clean undergarments, washed with mild detergent. Wash hands after procedure.
	Teach patient to report rectal or perineal pain, bleeding, itching, burning, redness, urinary burning or frequency.
	Prevent rectal injury by avoiding enemas and suppositories, rectal thermometers, sharp fingernails.
	Place on prophylactic bowel regimen to avoid constipation (*see* Chapter 11).
	Maintain integrity of perianal skin; give special consideration if patient receiving RT: avoid rubbing, scratching, or massaging area; avoid tight clothing; avoid medications and other chemical products; protect irritated skin with lanolin or A & D ointment.
	Use sitz baths for rectal irritation after bowel movement, observing meticulous clean technique.

Problem	Intervention
Ulceration of rectal mucosa	Maintain frequent, gentle skin and wound care with mild soap and water (sitz bath); rinse; pat dry.
	Avoid powders, lotions, perfumed soaps.
	Position patient in bed so as to keep off affected area.
	Use clothing washed in mild detergent with double rinsing.
	Avoid trauma: constipation; manipulation of area (rectal thermometers, suppositories).
	Culture wound at first sign of infection and add povidone-iodine (Betadine) to sitz-bath regimen.

RT, radiation therapy.

C: SKIN

Donna L. Couillard-Getreuer

The skin is a remarkable organ. When intact, it is capable of withstanding numerous assaults. If impaired, it is subject to a host of pathogens, including those from one's own body. In persons with cancer, skin impairment may result from treatment- or disease-related causes. The major focus of this section is the identification of patients at high risk for such impairment and related actual or potential problems. A thorough understanding of the principles behind integument function and dysfunction in cancer patients is necessary for planning, implementing, evaluating, and replanning nursing management.

Anatomy and physiology

The integument consists of the epidermis, dermis (corium), and its derivatives. The **epidermis**, or outer epithelial layer, functions as the outermost barrier to prevent loss of water. Skin pigment cells, called melanin, are contained within this level. Constant mitotic activity replaces dead cells; old cells are brought to the surface and rubbed off by normal daily activities, and new cells are constantly being made to replace them.

The **dermis** is the inner, connective tissue layer. Its variable thickness determines the total thickness of the skin. The skin is thickest on dorsal areas of the body, hands, and soles, and thinnest on the abdomen, genitalia, and ventral surfaces. The dermis is well supplied with blood, lymphatics, and afferent sensory nerve receptors.

Derivatives of the integument include the cutaneous glands, hair, nails, and teeth.

Eight major functions of the skin are commonly recognized. (1) It is a sensory organ with the ability to distinguish between varying intensities of the sensations pain, touch, and temperature. (2) Regulation of body temperature is controlled by vasoconstriction (heat) and perspiration evaporation (cooling). (3) The skin maintains a homeostatic internal environment by preventing loss of necessary fluids and electrolytes. (4) The skin also excretes—to a minor extent—excess fluids and electrolytes. (5) It possesses absorptive qualities that allow for the effectiveness of oily medications applied directly to the skin. (6) The skin remains impermeable to external gases, liquids, and pathogens as long as it is intact. (7) The skin serves as a protective barrier for the internal body. (8) Finally, the skin is partly responsible for nourishment (food, water, oxygen) of underlying structures through assistance with blood circulation.

Normal bacterial flora.　Commensal organisms living on the skin and mucosal surfaces are not static. They change with age, body site, sex, activity, habits, and the external environment. The organisms that normally inhabit the human skin are capable of causing infection if given the opportunity to enter the system through breaks in the skin and to colonize when the host's defenses are compromised.

While each person carries his own complement of microorganisms, the most common types are bacterial: (1) *Staphylococcus,* (2) *Corynebacterium,* (3) *Mycobacterium,* (4) *Streptococcus,* (5) gram-negative, and (6) aerobic spore-forming bacilli. Fungi (notably *Candida*), yeasts, and molds are frequent inhabitants as well. The concentration of pathogens is often determined by location: high concentrations are apt to occur in areas with hair, sebaceous, or sudoriferous glands, skin folds, areas in close proximity to mucosal surfaces (e.g., circumanal), and areas covered by clothing.

The most effective barrier against entry and colonization by microorganisms is the maintenance of an unbroken skin. Daily wear and tear can cause frequent minor breaks in this protective barrier, thus providing normal bacterial flora and other pathogens with the opportunity to enter the body and cause infection.

Injury and wound-healing.　Inflammation is the response of a body tissue to any injury. The inflammatory response is characterized by (1) **redness** (rubor) from increased vascularity, (2) **warmth** (calor) because of increased blood flow, (3) **pain** (dolor) from irritation of nerve endings and release of certain chemical mediators, and (4) **loss of tissue function.**

The inflammatory process begins with a vascular response, initially mediated by histamines and later by kinins. The injury stimulates increased WBC production with polymorphonuclear leukocytes (PMNs) rushing to the site of insult. These cells either ingest injured cells and bacteria or rupture and release enzymes to destroy them. Finally, monocytic macrophages arrive to phagocytize debris and dead PMNs (Table 9C–1).

When injury occurs, the hemostatic system is also activated. Coagulation, with platelet aggregation and thrombosis formation, proceeds by way of a cascading mechanism to produce fibrin and initiate the repair process (*see* Chapter 15G).

Repair of the site of injury then concludes by primary or secondary intention. **Primary intention,** with simple, clean wounds, occurs when

TABLE 9C–1

Inflammatory Process of Wound Repair

Response to injury	Process of repair
Vascular	Brief constriction of blood vessels; vasodilation of arterioles, capillaries, venules; increased permeability of vessels; transudation (extravasation of fluid into injured tissues); exudation (transport of blood cells and plasma proteins).
Cellular	Increased WBC production, PMNs primarily; chemotaxis (PMNs rush to injured site); diapedesis (RBCs pass through vessel wall); phagocytosis and lysosome release; monocytic macrophages ingest debris and dead PMNs.
Hemostasis	Coagulation; platelet aggregation; thrombosis.
Repair	Primary intention; secondary intention.

PMNs, polymorphonuclear leukocytes.

there is proliferation and migration of fibroblasts to the subcutaneous tissue. Epithelial cells then multiply to restore the surface area. Larger, ulcerated, or necrotic areas heal from within by **secondary intention.** Granulation occurs from fibroblast proliferation, capillary budding, and macrophage proliferation. Eventually, epithelial cells join to cover the surface defect.

The integument is in a state of constant mitotic activity, continually repairing injuries and insults by replacement of lost cells. The following factors contribute to a delayed healing time: (1) a large amount of tissue damage with vascular compromise; (2) coagulation disorders (e.g., thrombocytopenia); (3) medications affecting the inflammatory response (e.g., steroids, aspirin, chemotherapy); (4) impaired phagocytic function (e.g., malnutrition, sepsis, hypoxia, steroids, myelocytic leukemia, multiple myeloma); and, (5) impaired inflammatory response (e.g., from radiation, chemotherapy, hormonal manipulation, hypoxia).

The repair of any injury can be complicated by serum collections (e.g., postmastectomy), fistula or sinus formation, hemorrhage, herniation, and evisceration or dehiscence. Factors that delay or prevent wound-healing include cancer involvement, chronic trauma, poor hygiene, jaundice, pruritus, infections, neuropathies, radiation, chemotherapy, diabetes, obesity, and malnutrition.

Pathophysiology

The cancer patient is particularly vulnerable to numerous treatment- and/or disease-related impairments (*see* Tables 2–3 through 2–10).

Treatment-related causes of skin impairment. Chemotherapy causes delayed or inhibited wound healing, often compounded by nutritional compromise. Extravasation of vesicant agents frequently results in ulcerated lesions. Total or partial alopecia may be common with selected agents. In addition, total body hair (eyebrows, lashes, beard, axillae, genital, and extremity) may be lost. When return growth commences, the hair may be a different color or texture. Prolonged therapy can result in permanent loss of hair.

Drug eruptions common to the cancer population result most often from chemotherapy. Patients receiving simultaneous radiotherapy and actinomycin-D or doxorubicin may have severe desquamative skin reactions at the irradiated site (recall reactions). Skin rashes are common with several agents, notably bleomycin and allopurinol. The use of steroids can produce fragile skin with a tissue-paper consistency. Acnelike eruptions over the back and face are common.

Erythema multiforme is often seen in cancer patients receiving penicillin, although it may occur without apparent cause. It is characterized by scattered cutaneous vesicles and is often widespread. A more severe form of the disorder, Stevens-Johnson syndrome, results in bullous lesions of the eye, oral mucosa, skin, and urethra. Secondary infection of the lesions is common.

In cancer patients, erythema nodosum is a frequent hypersensitivity reaction to penicillin or sulfonamides, although it may be associated with an infectious process or collagen disease. It is characterized by tender, subcutaneous, anterior leg nodules.

Radiation therapy (RT) produces similar impairments in wound repair and temporary or permanent alopecia. Skin damage within the treatment portals may range from erythema or tanning of the skin to dry or moist desquamation. The term dry desquamation refers to flaking or scaling, with pruritus. Moist desquamation describes skin that is painful, weeping, or with tissue sloughing. The Oncology Nursing Society recognizes three levels of radiation impairment: (1) that of potential damage; (2) impaired skin with dry or moist desquamation; and (3) skin that has large, open, purulent skin lesions.

Surgical intervention results in disruption of skin integrity by penetration from surgical scalpels, drains, or sutures. In addition, postsurgical swellings and fluid accumulations (e.g., postmastectomy lymphedema) may also result in cutaneous impairment. Invasive procedures (e.g., catheterization) are known to introduce pathogens as well.

Disease-related causes of skin impairment.   There are numerous rare cutaneous manifestations associated with malignant diseases (Table 9C–2). **Thrombocytopenia** is encountered frequently, however. The presence of petechiae, purpura, or ecchymotic areas often heralds significant platelet deficiency (*see* Chapter 9A).

Cutaneous metastases usually occur late in the course of an illness. Solid tumors of the breast and lung, squamous cell carcinomas of head and neck, malignant melanoma, and lymphomas are the tumors that most often metastasize to the skin.

Primary malignant skin cancers: These include melanoma, basal cell carcinoma, squamous cell carcinoma, and Kaposi's sarcoma. In addition, patients with primary cancer of another system have a high incidence of developing a second skin cancer.

Melanoma represents ~3% of malignant tumors, but it is noted for its explosive and unpredictable potential. Primary lesions are pigmented, flat, elevated, or ulcerated lesions. It is a neoplasm of melanin-producing cells.

TABLE 9C-2
Cutaneous Manifestations of Malignant Disease

Manifestation	Most common associated malignancies
Acanthosis nigricans	Gastric, colon, and pancreatic carcinoma
Acquired icthyosis	Solid tumors, metastases
Anogenital Paget's disease	Adenocarcinomas from skin, urethra, or rectum
Bowen's disease	Solid tumors
Dermatomyositis	Solid tumors
Exfoliative dermatitis	Leukemias, lymphomas
Generalized hyperpigmentation	Metastases, primary tumors of adrenals or pituitary glands
Pachydermoperiostosis	Lung carcinoma in men >40
Thrombocytopenia	Leukemia, multiple myeloma, solid tumors
Thrombophlebitis	Pancreatic carcinoma
Xeroderma pigmentosum	Solid tumors, metastases

Basal cell carcinoma occurs primarily on the head and neck areas and rarely metastasizes. **Squamous cell carcinomas** arise in areas of exposure to the sun. Capable of metastasizing to lymph nodes, the lesions can increase to large, fungating masses.

Kaposi's sarcoma, once relatively rare, has increased in incidence in recent years. It affects persons of Jewish or Mediterranean descent and patients with acquired immune deficiency syndrome (AIDS). The sarcoma manifests as multiple cutaneous and subcutaneous purplish nodules on the extremities.

Mycosis fungoides: A slowly progressive cutaneous T-cell lymphoma, mycosis fungoides ultimately encompasses the lymph nodes and viscera. The initial skin characteristics commonly appear as unsightly, reddened, peeling skin with severe pruritus. This condition progresses to large, painful, ulcerations that exude serosanguinous material. The lesions frequently become infected with bacteria (e.g., *Staphylococcus aureus, Pseudomonas aeruginosa*) or fungal pathogens. The prognosis is poor, with eventual death from septicemia or visceral involvement.

Premalignant lesions: **Actinic keratosis** consists of scaly, hyperkeratoid lesions involving the face, neck, and dorsum of the hands. There may be **subsequent malignant changes** from a much earlier radiation dermatitis. **Leukoplakia** affects squamous epithelial mucous membrane to produce a white, patchy appearance. **Dysplastic nevus syndrome** appears as multiple nevi distributed throughout the body, with malignant potential based upon depth of skin involvement.

Skin complications. The following skin effects of malignancy and/or treatment are the most common problems encountered by patients.

Pressure sores (decubitus ulcers) result from the effects of pressure and shearing forces on the body. Their development and tenacity is aggravated by moisture, poor nutrition, immobility, edema, and poor skin turgor. The most common sites are ischial, sacral, and femoral trochanteric prominences. Secondary sites include the knees, elbows, and heels. The cancer patient at high risk for the development of pressure sores is usually malnourished, incontinent, has limitations in mobility or activity, and/or limited fluid intake. The hypoproteinemia, vitamin C deficiency, and negative nitrogen balance accompanying malnutrition decrease collagen formation and cell production. Other predisposing factors include: tissue wasting, anemia, edema, advancing age, motor and sensory impairments, circulatory impairment, obesity, and certain systemic diseases (e.g., diabetes, neuropathies, vascular diseases). Chemotherapy, steroids, and radiation further compromise skin integrity because of delayed wound healing, nutritional impairment, fragility, and changes in the inflammatory process. Infection and fever increase metabolic demands, thus interfering with the wound-healing process. Altered mental status is often implicated in decubitus formation because the patient is less likely to change position and more likely to be incontinent.

Edema includes ascites, lymphedema, or peripheral edema and results in the distension of tissues and the disruption of cell environment. Patients at high risk for the development of edema are those who are postsurgical (especially mastectomy or lymphatic dissection), or who have primary or metastatic lymphatic disease; primary or metastatic liver disease; concomittant cardiopulmonary deficiencies; malnutrition (e.g., hypoalbuminemia, hypoproteinemia); and/or fluid and electrolyte imbalance (e.g., nausea/vomiting, diarrhea, hormonal impairment).

Infection of the dermis and subcutaneous tissues is called **cellulitis**. The most common pathogens are staphylococcal or streptococcal bacteria. Usually a break in the skin's integrity at a site of edema is followed by bacterial colonization, which leads to redness, warmth, pain, and swelling.

The problem of **alopecia** usually results from treatment of the patient's malignancy. The extent may range from thinning of scalp hair to total body-hair loss. The time when regrowth begins is dependent upon the schedule of treatments and doses of the agents used. Some chemotherapeutic agents and whole-brain radiation affect growth and metabolism of cancer and normal cells. Hair loss occurs as a side effect of this treatment. Chemotherapy can cause constriction of the hair shaft and hair breakage above this level. Partial hair loss results, but the root remains intact and active. Larger doses of chemotherapy or more potent agents and radiation cause the base, or bulb, of the hair root to atrophy, and the entire hair filament is lost. Complete scalp epilation results. (Although some hairs are left untouched, it appears as complete loss). Whole-brain radiation (5,000 to 7,000 rads) commonly results in permanent damage to hair follicles, with no regrowth. Lower levels of brain radiation may permit regrowth after three months.

Pruritus is associated with mycosis fungoides, Hodgkin's disease, liver metastases, jaundice, diabetes, uremia, dry skin, or mechanical irritation (e.g., clothing friction). It can be described as a disagreeable cutaneous sensation creating a desire to scratch, and itching is the major complaint. Internal or external stimulation of nerve ends causes a state of increased excitability. Cycles of increasingly more severe itching and scratching may develop, resulting in disruption of skin integrity. The noxious stimuli can be increased by external or internal heat, capillary dilation, and tissue anoxia.

The pruritic condition **urticaria** may result from allergic response to foods, drugs, infectious agents, or chemicals. Hives may appear as transient wheals or welts and cause the itching sensation (*see* Chapter 15E).

Jaundice usually results from primary or metastatic liver or biliary tree involvement. Increased RBC lysis in cancer patients may be a prehepatic cause of jaundice. Intrahepatic causes, other than carcinomas, include hepatitis, cirrhosis, or drug uptake impairment. Extrahepatic causes include biliary obstruction or primary carcinoma of the pancreas, gallbladder, or biliary tree.

Incontinence of bowel or bladder may result in impaired integument integrity from the effects of constant moisture. The incontinence may be related to sphincter impairment (e.g., spinal cord compression; malignant diseases of bladder, anus, or rectum) or altered mental capacity (*see* Chapter 11).

Immunocompromise. The cancer patient may be predisposed to infections either from treatment-related or disease-related causes.

The varicella-zoster virus is responsible for causing **herpes zoster** and **chickenpox.** First exposure to this virus usually causes the disease known as chickenpox. After exposure and subsequent infection, the body normally produces antibodies that combat varicella-zoster infection. While most viruses are destroyed, some lodge in nerve ganglia and remain dormant until reactivation. When the virus is reactivated, by an unknown mechanism(s), the body attempts to fight with previously acquired immunity. If the varicella-zoster viruses are not destroyed, they will continue to multiply and spread down the sensory nerves to the skin. This subsequent infection is called herpes zoster, or "shingles."

A higher incidence of herpes zoster is found in patients who are immunocompromised, possibly because their immune system is not able to initiate and maintain an effective response when reactivation of varicella-zoster occurs. At highest risk are patients with lymphoma or Hodgkin's disease, those who are undergoing RT or chemotherapy, those with lung cancer, leukemia, multiple myeloma, reticuloendothelial cancers, those who have undergone spinal cord treatment or manipulation, bone marrow transplant, splenectomy, or are taking steroids, and the aged.

Herpes simplex 1 or 2 are usually localized, vesicular lesion(s) in the oral or genital regions. Primary herpetic gingivitis is manifested by numerous painful oral and circumoral lesions.

Systemic bacterial or fungal infections may produce pyogenic cutaneous lesions (*Staphylococcus* and *Candida* most commonly responsible). Immunosuppressed patients frequently suffer from moniliasis.

Anogenital ulcerations, abscesses, and infections are common in neutropenic patients. Pain and discomfort are generally prodromal symptoms. The dermis and epidermis generally are involved. Other risk factors for development include hemorrhoids, diarrhea, constipation, and GI side effects of chemotherapy (see Chapter 9B).

Thrombophlebitis may occur in superficial or deep veins. There is generally a localized area of warmth, tenderness, and intense erythema limited to a very short segment of the vein. A cord is often palpable. Thrombosis and hypercoagulability are associated with most malignancies. The highest incidence is seen with mucinous adenocarcinomas of the pancreas and prostate (see Chapter 15G).

Assessment

Observation of a patient's current skin condition and a history of any impairments constitute the major focus of assessment. General observations include: color, vascularity, evidence of bleeding or bruising (e.g., petechiae, hematoma); lesions (color, grouping, type, size, distribution); areas of edema, moisture; configurations, texture, mobility, turgor; nails; and hair. A complete history should be obtained with special emphasis on allergies, medication use, past and present skin disorders, recent infectious exposure, and associated symptoms.

Nursing assessment for **pressure sores** must include identification of high-risk patients (Table 9C–3) and descriptions of location, date of onset, stage, and complicating factors.

In assessing **edema**, considerations must include awareness of patients at high risk for edema development. Common signs and symptoms are weight gain, ill-fitting clothes, changes in urinary frequency, dyspnea, and changes in BP. Usual weight and recent changes in weight need to be ascertained. Measurements of the affected area (e.g., abdominal or extremity girths) should be documented daily or weekly and compared with prior measurements or with the opposite extremity when possible. Review of current medications and nutritional status may highlight correctable areas. Obtaining a total blood profile for levels of protein, albumin, iron stores, and electrolytes is mandatory. Skin assessment must include inspection for areas of erythema, sloughing, weeping, temperature changes, pulses, broken skin, and infection.

Assessment of the patient with **pruritus** must include identification of high-risk patients (e.g., Hodgkin's disease, jaundice) and factors that affect the desire to scratch (e.g., increase with heat or decrease with cold). Although individual response to the itching sensation is variable, it is generally strongest at night, with fevers, in areas surrounding body openings, and with drier skin.

Assessment and diagnosis of **herpes zoster** is based upon history and physical examination, prodromal characteristics, and the presence of lesions.

TABLE 9C-3

Assessment of Patient's Risk for Pressure Sores

Parameters	0	1	2	3	Score
General state of health	good	fair	poor	moribund	
Mental status	alert	lethargic	semicomatose; confused, uncooperative	comatose	
Activity	ambulatory	needs help	chair-fast	bed-bound	
Mobility	full ROM	limited	very limited with aid	immobile	
Incontinence	none	occasional	usually (urine)	total (urine and feces)	
Oral nutrition intake	good	fair, underweight or overweight	poor (emaciated, obese)	none (cachectic)	
Oral fluid intake	good (2,000 ml/day)	fair (needs encouragement)	poor (<500 ml/day)	none	

Count these as double (bracketing the Activity and Mobility score-2 and score-3 cells: chair-fast / bed-bound / very limited with aid / immobile)

Total score: _____

Predisposing disease: 1 point each for diabetes, neuropathies, vascular diseases, anemias, dermatitis.

High risk = ≥12 points.
ROM, range of motion.
Compiled by Knoll Pharmaceutical Co., Whippany, N. J., for Memorial Sloan-Kettering Cancer Center, New York.

Herpes zoster is characterized by four phases:
1. In the prodromal phase there may be fever, malaise, pain, pruritus, or a change of sensation in body area(s). There are no lesions.
2. During the eruption (exanthem) phase, erythematous patches appear and progress to vesicles, then crust, usually along dermatome(s). This stage is associated with fever, headache, malaise, chills, lymphadenopathy.
3. In the dissemination phase, lesions are scattered over the entire body. There is coalescence of vesicles in large, bullous areas. These may be hemorrhagic and gangrenous; frequently there is visceral involvement.
4. The postherpetic neuralgia phase does not appear in all patients though usually in the aged. There is pain at the lesion sites for an extended time after lesions have disappeared.

The risk of dissemination is highest in immunocompromised patients, and it carries with it the risk of neurological involvement and visceral impairment.

Diagnosis of **mycosis fungoides** is based upon skin biopsy and bone marrow aspirations. Full metastatic workup is warranted (e.g., bone survey, liver/spleen scan). Nursing assessment must include attention to skin integrity as well as comfort (pruritus, pain), nutrition, infection, and coping needs.

Nursing assessment of **cutaneous metastases** involves ongoing inspection of skin for color, vascularity, edema, injuries, palpable nodes, and lesions. Susceptible areas in high-risk patients should be palpated—i.e., the area surrounding and overlying enlarged lymph nodes, breast or abdominal masses, and malignant skin lesions (e.g., melanomas, sarcomas). Any masses or lesions need to be evaluated and documented for:
1. Mobility.
2. Configuration.
3. Size (cm).
4. Location and distribution.
5. Vascularity, bleeding, friability.
6. Depth estimate (cm).
7. Structure (e.g., nodule, scale, erosion, fissure, ulcer).
8. Drainage (color, amount, character).
9. Odor.
10. Infection.

Other areas that are specific to various skin impairments will be addressed as part of the nursing management protocols.

Medical management

Medical management of **edema** is based upon correction of underlying disorders. Control of edema is one goal, often a primary one if the underlying cause is not correctable. Edemas are usually managed by diuretic therapy. Administration of colloids often preceeds diuretics to obtain the maximal diuresis with minimal side effects (lymphedema, however, is refractory to diuretic therapy). Paracentesis is employed to control ascites and its symptoms. This may be accomplished through intermittent or continuous drainage, palliative drainage, or with the addition of sclerosing agent(s) to prevent reaccumulation of fluid. Lymphedema is frequently managed with fitted elastic stockings (e.g., Jobst) and postoperative exercises.

Surgical intervention to remove tissue or tumor and improve drainage is often used. Antibiotics and steroids may be employed to combat infections and inflammation.

Cellulitis is frequently seen in cancer patients with edema, leukopenia, and vascular deficiencies. Medical treatment for cellulitis consists of antibiotic therapy and wound care.

Medical interventions for **pruritus** are aimed at treating the underlying disease. A careful history, noting drug use and recent exposure to infectious diseases or chemicals, and physical examination is necessary to determine etiology. Laboratory tests include CBC and blood chemistries, especially liver function tests.

Medical treatment of **herpes zoster** usually consists of antiviral chemotherapy (FIAC, vidarabine, acyclovir) and discontinuance of any systemic chemotherapy. The use of corticosteroids is controversial. Without treatment, the natural course of the disease leads to disappearance within ~4 wk. Antiviral agents are given to decrease the severity of the outbreak, relieve symptoms, and prevent possible dissemination.

Medical treatment of **mycosis fungoides**, dependent upon lesion characteristics and systemic involvement, consists of topical chemotherapy, systemic chemotherapy, and/or RT. Potent topical preparations of nitrogen mustard, BCNU (carmustine), or CCNU (lomustine) are applied to the skin (avoiding scalp and eyelid), with weaker concentrations to the perineum and axillae. Occasional systemic side effects of the chemotherapy occur from these topical treatments. Systemic chemotherapy usually involves high-dose methotrexate with citrovorum rescue, cyclophosphamide, doxorubicin, vincristine, and prednisone. Often, combinations of intradermal bacillus Calmette-Guérin (BCG) vaccine with bleomycin or cyclophosphamide, vincristine, and prednisone are used.

Mycosis fungoides is very radiosensitive. Remarkable control of the lesions is possible for extended periods of time. Furthermore, radiation is usually necessary for the lesions to heal. The usual schedule is 9 to 12 wk of electron-beam RT in doses of ≤400 rads/wk (total 3,000 to 3,600 rads per lesion). Additional rads are given to the areas of perineum and feet. Shielding of the cornea, lens, nails, and eyebrows is imperative. Side effects of this RT range from mild erythema, edema, and hyperpigmentation to cutaneous bullae. Treatment is limited also by skin tolerance levels.

Medical interventions for **cutaneous metastases** are aimed at treating the underlying tumor with systemic chemotherapy and/or local irradiation to shrink the lesion(s). Topical applications of 5-fluorouracil (5-FU) are occasionally used. Surgical excision or debulking of the tumor may be warranted.

Nursing management

The goal of nursing is to maintain the skin's natural integrity. Nursing management of integument impairment must include identification of high-risk-patients, continuous assessment, planning a preventive and interventive program of care, and ongoing evaluation of the effectiveness of any protocol.

The problems most common to cancer patients are: pressure sores, edema and its corollaries, cellulitis, pruritus, varicella-zoster infections, mycosis fungoides, alopecia, malignant lesions, and the skin effects from RT. For management of the patient with thrombophlebitis, urticaria, and infections, the reader is referred to the extensive coverages in other chapters of this text.

Pressure sores. The formation of a pressure sore follows a predictable pattern. The first, or threatened stage is evidenced by redness from loss of the epidermal layer and results from transitory circulatory disturbances. It is relieved when the source of pressure is removed. The second stage is characterized by definitive superficial tissue damage, with superficial ulcer formation, with the inevitable breakdown. The third stage consists of ulceration, with necrotic tissue extension from the subcutaneous tissues to the fascia. The fourth stage is characterized by penetration of the deep fascia; usually extensive compromise is present. An "iceberg" effect is common, with the scope of outer epidermal damage smaller than the underlying destruction. Spread of necrotic damage and frequent infections can lead to osteomyelitis.

The major forces at work in the formation of pressure sores are pressure, time, friction, and shearing. Blood-flow obstruction occurs when **external pressure** causes elevation of capillary pressure for >1 to 2 hr. Obstruction of the flow leads to tissue ischemia and tissue death. **Time** is the second component in pressure-sore development. More pressure exerted over less time results in a more rapid impairment than does less pressure over a longer time. **Friction** hastens the breakdown process by compromising the integrity of the epidermal and dermal layers. If there is friction, skin compromise may develop with significantly less pressure over a shorter time period. **Shearing** (pushing force) stresses underlying fascial layers and contributes to the development of ulceration. A patient lying supine is exerting pressure on vulnerable areas. Being pulled up to the head of the bed adds the destructive friction and shearing forces. The basic principles underlying nursing management are the relief of forces causing ulcer formation, correction of underlying impairment(s), and meticulous hygiene. Nursing interventions are categorized as preventive and interventive. Table 9C–4 presents detailed management plans.

Edema. The effects of edema, ascites, and lymphedema on skin integrity can be considered similar in terms of nursing management. No matter what the cause, fluid-filled skin becomes fragile and at increased risk for infection because of decreased vascular supply. Common disorders seen with cancer populations include: generalized edema(anasarca); mild to massive peripheral edema(especially lower body); dependent edema (related to gravity); subcutaneous edema; lymphedema; and ascites (fluid accumulation within the peritoneal cavity). Nursing management of impaired skin integrity from edema is based upon a preventive and interventive design (Table 9C–5).

Cellulitis. Basic nursing management is described in Table 9C–6.

Pruritus. The main goal of nursing management is to prevent scratching, with the subsequent impairment of skin integrity (Table 9C–7).

Herpes zoster. The patient with herpes zoster is infectious to any person who has not had chickenpox or who has an impaired immune system. The mode of transmission is by direct contact with lesion drainage or respiratory droplets of a patient with herpes zoster. Second and third bouts of herpes zoster are not uncommon.

Nursing management is based upon minimizing discomfort from pain and pruritus, preventing or minimizing complications, preventing the spread of varicella-zoster virus to others, and supporting the patient and family through the illness(Table 9C–8). Complications arise from secondary bacterial infection of lesions and inadequate food/fluid intake.

Mycosis fungoides. Management includes oral care, pain and pruritus control, nutritional support, and skin care. Sensitivity on the part of the care-giver to the effects of mycosis fungoides on body image and appearance is of paramount importance.

Alopecia. Blood supply, and therefore chemotherapeutic drug supply, to the hair follicles can be diminished by the use of scalp tourniquets or ice packs to the head, and hair loss can *sometimes* be minimized or prevented during administration of chemotherapy. The use of these prevention techniques is controversial. Opponents feel that preventing the access of chemotherapeutic agents to the scalp may result in scalp metastases from the primary site. Therefore, hair-loss prevention techniques are currently contraindicated in patients who may be prone to scalp metastases (e.g., leukemics). Table 9C–9 describes the protocol currently used when situations permit scalp hypothermia/tourniquets.

The stresses involved with anticipating hair loss and the actual loss itself, which usually occurs over several days, need to be addressed in any nursing management plan.

Cutaneous metastases. Metastasis to the skin from underlying malignancy is both distressing for the patient and a nursing management challenge. The lesions are most common with advanced malignancy but may also occur as a result of localized tumor growth. The management of skin metastases is based upon prevention and control of bleeding, odor, secondary infections, and trauma. Nursing management is outlined in Table 9C–10.

RT effects upon skin. Harmful skin effects from RT have decreased in recent years because of the use of more penetrating RT techniques. Smaller treatment areas with less local scatter of radiation have reduced the incidence of serious complications. Still, nursing intervention is necessary to help prevent skin damage through patient education and management of the now infrequent reactions. The major goals of nursing intervention are:

1. To reduce irritation in the treatment area. Heating pads, alcohol, hot-water bottles, and ice caps should be avoided. Sunlight should not be allowed to reach the treatment area. Shaving should be avoided; men should use an electric razor on the beard. Wear cotton clothing over the radiation site. Avoid tape or jewelry in the area of treatment, tight or constricting clothing.
2. Avoid unintentional augmentation of radiation effects on the skin.
3. Continue ongoing assessment of treated areas. Check for changes in color, moisture, scaling, temperature. High-risk areas include skin folds, radiation portals (entry and exit).
4. Teach the patient general skin care. Do not wash off radiation markings; cleanse gently with plain water and pat dry; do not apply any lotions, powders, or ointments to treatment area.

Initial, or acute, reactions of the skin to RT begin 1 to 6 wk after the onset of therapy. Recovery is expected 2 to 3 wk after treatment is completed. Denuding of epidermal layers may result in dry or moist

TABLE 9C-4

Nursing Protocol for the Management of Potential or Actual Pressure Sores

Factor	Intervention
Patients at high risk **General prevention**	**Maintain skin integrity:** Interrupt forces of friction and shearing: use draw sheet on bed; use to raise patient in bed; use footboard; elevate head of bed to maximum of 30 degrees except at meals; have trapeze on bed to assist patient in movement; lift — do not pull — to help patient change positions; use alternating-pressure air mattress on bed. Interrupt time and pressure forces by changing position q 1–2 hr; have a planned, posted schedule. Practice meticulous hygiene: maintain clean, dry skin; pay special attention to skin-fold areas and moist areas.
Cachexia	**If patient is without breakdown areas:** use egg-crate, water, or alternating-pressure mattress; provide nutritional support (*see* Chapter 8); assess high-risk areas daily (bony prominences, ischial tuberosities, trochanters, sacrum, coccyx, heels, etc.); *see* General prevention; use heel pads, sheepskins; apply lotion to bony prominences and pressure areas.

Incontinence	Observe all areas under General prevention and Cachexia.
	Do not use waterproof pads (Chux) or diapers next to patient's skin; layer draw sheet with pads between layers.
	Give perineal care with soap, water, air drying after each elimination.
	Offer bedpan or urinal q 2 hr; allow frequent and adequate time for toileting.
	Odor control; identify and correct causes, when possible.
	Maintain clean, dry environment for patient.
	Evaluate the need for a bladder and/or bowel training program (see Chapter 11).
Immobility	Observe areas under General prevention and Cachexia.
	Perform range-of-motion exercises with all extremities; obtain physical therapy consultation.
Patients with pressure sores	
Stage I	Observe all practices under General prevention.
	Cleanse site daily with water and soap; air dry.
	Avoid: rubbing site, heat lamp, doughnuts.
	Apply lotions to bony prominences and stage I area.
	Take measures to toughen skin and prevent breakdown:
	Apply tincure of benzoin or Skin-Prep to site; let dry thoroughly; do not cover.
	Consider covering threatened sites with Op-Site or Stomahesive.
Stage II	Practice steps under General prevention and Stage I.
	Apply Maalox to site — let dry;
	Cover site with Op-Site or Stomahesive.
	Change dressing when moisture appears underneath or q 48 hr, whichever is sooner.
Stage III	Follow all procedures under General prevention and Stages I and II.
	Proceed with simple debridement as necessary:
	surgical;
	whirlpool;
	manual:
	Use fine mesh gauze for wet to dry dressings; soak gauze in water, NS, or Chloropactin; change q 4-6 hr.

Factor	Intervention
	If eschar present, may need extensive debridement: surgical; whirlpool; manual: Apply Silvadene q 12 hr; flush with NS (Silvadene **contraindicated** with leukopenic patients); After eschar removed, apply Chloropactin (1 g in 500 ml NS) q 12 hr. Obtain plastic surgery consultation if indicated. Assess for secondary infection (frequently bacterial or candidiasis): Culture all ulcerations on first appearance, weekly, or if indications of infection are present (e.g., odor, purulent drainage). Obtain sensitivity report on any positive cultures. Do not use cornstarch (known to support the existence of some pathogens), powders, sugar, yogurt. Dress the site with open wet soaks with water, NS, or Chloropactin, followed by antibacterial/antifungal ointment.

NS, normal saline.

TABLE 9C-5

Nursing Protocol for the Management of Edema, Lymphedema, and Ascites

Factor	Intervention
General prevention	Teach postmastectomy and axillary-dissection patients lymphedema precautions: Avoid all cuts, bruises, scratches, pinpricks, insect bites, burns, chemicals, hangnails, jewelry, venipunctures, heavy carrying, nail-biting, injections, BP readings on *affected* side. Recognize signs and symptoms of infection. Notify physician on appearance of symptoms. Practice hand care: nails, cuticles, hand cream. Avoid prolonged standing and sitting of patient. Elevate affected extremities as much as possible. Consult with physician regarding postoperative exercise program for patient. Practice good hygiene. Obtain nutritional consultation and intervention for high-risk patients.
Patients with edema, lymphedema, ascites	Assess extent of involvement continually: measure girths and extremity circumference; compare to opposite extremity and prior readings; assess respiratory impairment from ascites; weigh patient daily; be alert for signs and symptoms of infection.
	Position patient for maximum drainage: maintain sustained elevation of extremities; use high Fowler's position for ascites.
	Employ planned exercises: obtain occupational therapy and physical therapy consultations as indicated; assist with ambulation as necessary.
	Practice meticulous skin care: keep skin dry, clean; pay particular attention to areas of moisture and intertrigo; turn and position q 1–2 hr; avoid hot-water bottles, heating pads on affected area; use lamb's wool between swollen digits; avoid constricting clothing; provide scrotal support if genitalia affected. Allow no venipunctures, IV therapy, parenteral medications, chemotherapy in area of involvement.
	Consider dietary restriction of sodium and water; add protein supplements.
	Administer colloids, antibiotics, diuretics in accordance with medical regimen.

TABLE 9C-6

Nursing Protocol for the Management of Cellulitis

Factor	Intervention
General prevention	Identical to Table 9C-5 except: avoid lotions, powders, creams near site; avoid further impairment of skin integrity by preventing trauma to affected site.

Cellulitis	Monitor temperature.
	Administer antibiotics.
	Care for skin:
	  practice meticulous hygiene;
	  elevate affected extremities.
	Care for wound:
	  cleanse with water and povidone-iodine (Betadine), half-strength;
	  flush area with water, do not rub;
	  pat dry;
	  cover with dry sterile dressing;
	  if necessary, debride manually with wet to dry sterile dressings (water and povidone-iodine).
	Culture area upon appearance of signs of inflammation and weekly:
	Observe wound and skin precautions with positive cultures.
	If tissue is weeping:
	  practice would care as above: cleanse, flush, and obtain cultures;
	  if cultures positive, observe wound and skin precautions;
	  cover with dry, sterile, nonadhering (Telfa) dressing.
	Protect area from further damage:
	  avoid hot-water bottle, heating pads next to area; constricting clothing, elastic stockings;
	  venipunctures, IV therapy, chemotherapy, and parenteral medications in area;
	  use bed cradle in bed.
	Monitor for signs and symptoms of septicemia:
	  elevated temperature, decreased BP, change in affect, shortness of breath, chills;
	  abnormal laboratory values — especially WBC and differential.

TABLE 9C-7

Nursing Protocol for the Management of Pruritus

Factor	Intervention
Discomfort	Administer systemic medications per physician's orders to relieve sensations of itching, e.g., oral cholestyramine resin, anabolic steroids, systemic corticosteroids, antihistamines (e.g., diphenhydramine, cyproheptadine, hydroxyzine).
	Use diversion to assist patient to focus thoughts on subjects other than the desire to scratch.
	Evaluate the need for alleviation of elevated anxiety levels.
	Maintain normal body temperature; administer antipyretics as needed.
	Use topical measures to relieve sensations:
	gentle firm pressure (if sensation localized);
	soft brush (e.g., infant type) for stroking area;
	soothing baths (e.g., oatmeal, soybean, oil); if infection is cause of pruritus, use povidone-iodine or potassium permanganate;
	topical steroids (e.g., hydrocortisone);
	antipruritic lotions (e.g., phenol, hydrocortisone, shake lotions, emulsions); use only if patient not leukopenic;
	local anesthetic creams;
	tepid or cool wet compresses/soaks;
	soaps made for sensitive skin (e.g., Aveeno);
	lubricants or bath oils to prevent dryness.
Potential skin breakdown	Take measures to prevent skin trauma (e.g., cut fingernails short).
	Use old, soft bed linens; no starch.
	Use cool, light cloth/cotton bedclothes.
	Avoid actions causing perspiration.
	Assess for allergic responses to medications.

TABLE 9C-8

Nursing Protocol for the Management of Herpes Zoster

Factor	Intervention
Communicability of disease	Prevent the spread of herpes zoster to other patients and staff: assess early and continually for prodromal signs and appearance of lesions in high-risk populations; practice strict isolation of suspected or confirmed patients; be sure care-givers have adequate varicella titers and are not pregnant.
Painful lesions	Minimize discomfort of pain and pruritus: assess involved area and characteristics of the discomfort; administer systemic analgesics, antihistamines, and antipyretics as necessary; avoid narcotics if possible; achieve local relief through cool-water compresses and topical steroids; cover lesions with sterile, occlusive dressings; explore use of relaxation, biofeedback, distraction.
Potential superimposed infections	Prevent secondary infections: Look for signs/symptoms of infection (e.g., increased temperature, purulent drainage). Culture lesions, nasopharynx, sputum, blood, rectum, urine, and parenteral sites with every febrile episode. Avoid introduction of pathogens by: meticulous hand-washing and skin care; avoiding urinary catheterization; changing IV sites q 48 hr; perineal care with povidone-iodine and water (half-strength) after each elimination.

	Avoid breaking lesions:
	keep fingernails short or mitted;
	use padded bedrails;
	cover lesions with dressings.
	If there are coalescent areas:
	maintain dry, sterile dressings;
	weigh dressings to determine output;
	monitor electrolytes, protein, fluid, and laboratory values.
Systemic involvement of disease	Seek immediate attention of opthamologist for any lesions of head or face. Be alert for signs of widespread dissemination: evaluate neurological status daily; evaluate and document pulmonary status.
Decreased oral intake	Maintain adequate food and fluid intake: if oral lesions: use cool, saline mouthwashes, analgesics (*see* Chapter 9B); check for swallowing difficulty; make dietary adjustments (e.g., soft, non-spicy foods).
Immobility	Perform range-of-motion exercises with all affected extremities.
Need for information	Teach disease characteristics and sequelae of disease/treatment.

TABLE 9C-9

Nursing Protocol for the Management of Patients at Risk for Alopecia

Factor	Intervention
Stress of alopecia	Identify risk of alopecia to patients: discuss agents and usual pattern of loss; identify places to obtain toupees, wigs, and scarves prior to expected loss so patient is able to prepare; instruct patient in use of ice cap or scalp tourniquet if indicated; stress possibility of hair regrowth.
Local trauma to hair/scalp	Minimize hair loss: discourage the use of harsh shampoos, hair coloring, permanent waves.
Supply of blood to hair/scalp	Minimize hair loss in chemotherapy patients by mechanical means, if indicated. Scalp hypothermia: start IV line first; hypothermia may cause peripheral vasoconstriction and difficult vein access; apply ice cap 10 min prior to start of infusion; ice cap to be maintained in place during infusion and for 30 min after; monitor for side effects of hypothermia (e.g., dizziness, headache, cold complaints). Scalp tourniquet (e.g., pneumatic cuff): pressure of scalp sphygmomanometer to be above systemic systolic BP; time on to be: 10 min before infusion, during infusion, and 10 min after infusion; monitor for side effects of tourniquet (headache, nerve damage).

desquamation after 3 to 4 wk of therapy. After ≥6 mo, a delayed skin response may appear as fibrosis, atrophy, telangiectagia, or tanning of the area. Nursing management of skin impairment from RT is specific for the type of desquamation or ulceration.

Dry or moist desquamation: Precautions against irritation to the treatment area and unintentional augmentation of radiation effects should be observed. Ongoing assessment of the irradiated area should be performed. Skin may be cleansed with warm water by irrigation or cotton and patted dry with soft material. As much exposure to air as possible is beneficial. If **dry desquamation** occurs, cornstarch may be dusted on the area between treatments. If **moist desquamation** occurs, the skin may be cleansed with saline or water. Rinses with half-strength peroxide and water may be used 1 or 2 times/day and patted dry. If the area is to be covered by clothing, a nonadherent dressing can be used; otherwise the area should be exposed to air. Culture of the drainage should be obtained weekly and prn.

Large, draining lesions: Ongoing assessment of large, draining lesions includes notation of characteristics and drainage, measurement of the size of the impairment, and monitoring of electrolytes. Observe precautions and control of odor (*see* Table 9C–10). Prevent trauma to lesions and supply systemic analgesics as necessary. If lesions become infected, they may be irrigated with a half-strength solution of water and peroxide. Antibiotic ointments may be applied. Drainage should be cultured weekly and prn.

Bibliography

1. Couillard-Getreuer, D. L. Herpes zoster in the immunocompromised patient. *Cancer Nursing* (October 1982). 361–370.

   Article provides overview of pathophysiology, clinical course, and medical management of immunocompromised patients with herpes zoster. Includes detailed protocols for care of mild to severe herpes zoster infections.

2. Dean, J. C., and S. E. Salmon. Symptom management: alopecia. *American Cancer Society Proceedings of the Third National Conference on Cancer Nursing.* American Cancer Society, Inc., Atlanta, Georgia. 1981. 130–136.

   Review of literature on methods of preventing chemotherapy-induced alopecia by scalp tourniquets and hypothermia. Comprehensive bibliography with concise discussion of growth of hair and effects of chemotherapy upon it.

3. Hilderly, L. Skin care in radiation therapy: a review of the literature. *Oncology Nursing Forum* (Winter 1983). 51–57.

TABLE 9C-10

Nursing Protocol for the Management of Cutaneous Metastases

Factor	Intervention
Nonulcerating lesions	Gentle skin care, no rubbing: wash daily with tepid water, pat dry; apply dry dressing (occlusive if topical medications used). Limit environmental insults to area: avoid pressure/friction; make sure clothing is nonirritating, nonconstricting; cover with dressing to limit irritants and mechanical trauma; consider use of protecting shield if in area of frequent trauma.
Ulcerating or draining lesions	Follow steps above for nonulcerating lesions. Consider use of irrigating syringe to cleanse lesion. If indicated debride eschars: wet to dry dressings with hydrogen peroxide (half-strength), proteolytic enzymes, or Dakin's solution. Use nonadhering dressing next to ulcer; cover with dry sterile dressing; change dressing as often as necessary for odor or saturation; if drainage profuse, consider use of ostomy appliance and referral to enterostomal therapist.
Bleeding lesion	Irrigate gently with sterile water or NS via syringe. Apply direct, mild pressure to site with nonadherent dressing to stop bleeding; consider use of pressure dressing or elastic bandage to maintain pressure if bleeding not stopped. Apply Gel-foam to small areas of bleeding. Consider cautery (silver nitrate or electrocautery). Change dressing only as often as necessary for odor control and drainage; do not disturb Gel-foam or eschars; *no* debridement.

Massive, malignant, fungating lesions or large surface area	Follow procedures for nonulcerating or ulcerating lesions; hemostatic control as for bleeding lesions; odor control as below; prevention and management of infections as below.
Odor control	Cleanse lesions with mild soap and water or NS to remove exudate or prior medication applications; solutions should be at room temperature.
	If lesion *shallow:*
	apply plain, fresh yogurt (room temperature) to lesion and surrounding skin;
	wait 5–10 min and rinse off yogurt with NS;
	apply thin coat of petroleum jelly;
	repeat process q 6–8 hr; control of odor usually can take 2–4 days with regular schedule;
	dress area with clean, soft, absorbent dressing.
	If lesion *deep:*
	follow entire process for shallow lesions **except** substitute fresh buttermilk at room temperature for yogurt and omit petroleum jelly.
	Explain all processes and rationales to patient.
	Balsam of Peru or activated charcoal may be used on top of layered dressing (**not** wound) (Hollister & Co. manufactures an activated charcoal dressing); then cover with 4 × 4-in. dressing.
	Culture lesions weekly and prn.
	Deodorize room:
	use activated charcoal on tray in room corner;
	place cotton balls saturated with deodorizer in room;
	change dressings frequently and seal used dressings in plastic bag; discard from room promptly.
Risk of secondary infections	Culture exudate weekly and prn.
	Use aseptic technique for all dressing changes.
	Employ topical antibacterial agents, irrigations, or systemic antibiotics prn.

NS, normal saline.

302   Handbook of Oncology Nursing

Includes historical perspective of changes in radiation equipment and techniques, past and current patterns of skin care. Covers terminology and definitions of degrees of impairment, with recommendations for use.

4. Olsen, E., R. E. Edmonds, B. J. Johnson, J. McCarthy, L. M. Schroeder, L. F. Thompson, and M. Wade. The hazards of immobility. *American Journal of Nursing* (April 1967). 779–797.

   Classic nursing articles on immobility effects, still not outdated. Section on skin remains basic to understanding and preventing skin impairments with complex patients.

5. Oncology Nursing Society, Clinical Practice Committee. Guidelines for nursing care of patients with altered protective mechanisms. *Oncology Nursing Forum* (Spring 1982). 83–91; (Summer 1982). 115–118.

   Comprehensive nursing guidelines for herpes zoster, malignant skin lesions, and skin care during radiation therapy. Suitable for quick reference.

6. Price, R. W. Herpes zoster, an approach to systemic therapy. *Medical Clinics of North America* (September 1982). 1105–1118.

   Medical article outlining epidemiology and pathogenesis of a herpes zoster infection; pertinent for understanding current medical research and practice. Therapeutic strategy for various immunocompetent or deficient groups is addressed, including treatment of postherpetic neuropathy.

7. Sibrack, L. A. Cutaneous signs of internal malignant disease. *Primary Care* (June 1978). 263–280.

   Medical article describing skin manifestations associated with various malignancies, dermatoses commonly and uncommonly associated with malignant disease, and non-specific skin changes of internal neoplasms. Skin markers representing specific malignancies are cited.

8. Staab, M. A. Mycosis fungoides: a rare cutaneous malignant lymphoma with multifaceted nursing challenges. *Cancer Nursing* (February 1980). 17–25.

   Nursing overview of mycosis fungoides including clinical appearance, course, and epidemiology, and extensive description of medical treatment. Basic nursing management indicated in table format.

9. Torrance, C. Pressure sores: pathogenesis, prophylaxis, and treatment. *Nursing Times* (March 19, 1981). 9–12.

   Third article in a four-part series on pressure sores. Focuses on current medical management and surgical intervention.

10. Winkelmann, R. K. Pharmacologic control of pruritus. *Medical Clinics of North America* (September 1982). 1119–1131.

    Comprehensive article outlining pathogenesis and medical treatment of pruritus (not specific for cancer patients). Research results of effective agents are cited.

CHAPTER 10

MOBILITY

Glee I. Wahlquist

Standard: The client and family maintain an optimal mobility level of the client consistent with the disease and therapy.

Outcome criteria: The client and family
1. state the cause of the immobility, the treatment, and the outcome of the treatment.
2. describe an appropriate management plan to optimally integrate the alteration in mobility into life-style.
3. describe optimal level of activities of daily living in keeping with disease state and treatment.
4. identify health services and community resources available for managing changes in mobility.
5. use measures to aid or improve mobility.
6. demonstrate measures to prevent the complications of decreased mobility.

Mobility, the ability to move from place to place, is a concept related to but not limited to ambulation. Prosthetic or orthotic devices may increase a patient's mobility although he remains nonambulatory. Environmental factors, too, such as stairs or expense, may limit mobility for an otherwise ambulatory person. A decrease in mobility for any reason generally leads to a decrease in interaction with the environment and necessitates an increase in dependence on others for daily activities.

For the person with cancer, there are many factors that affect mobility. This chapter focuses on mobility problems created by neuromuscular dysfunction, bone metastases, and fatigue. Included is a description of upper motor neuron (UMN) and lower motor neuron (LMN) problems (*see also* Chapter 14B), peripheral neuropathy, and methods of assessment of functional status and ambulatory potential. Mobility is presented as an integral part of rehabilitation, which is briefly discussed.

Pathophysiology

The ability to walk is under voluntary muscle control, primarily, and requires an intact nervous system to complete the movements from the point of one heel strike to another. Therefore, an understanding of both the sensory and the motor processes involved will facilitate evaluation of mobility status.

Neuromuscular dysfunction.   The act of walking depends upon a constant interaction of sensory and motor function. Because the major tracts for sensation and movement are separate, their functions may be altered independently.

Sensation: Sensory loss alone may account for problems with mobility. The sensory fibers involved in walking are located primarily in the joints and skin. The principal sensation in joints is **proprioception**, which involves both position and vibration senses. Afferent fibers convey sensations to the spinal cord and up to the medulla, where the fibers cross and extend to the anterior cerebral cortex. CNS tumor involvement of these areas may result in inability to judge (1) shapes, textures, or forms of objects and (2) body parts in relation to each other, or degree of pressure against a body part.

The skin senses **pain, heat,** and **cold**. Afferent fibers carry these sensations via spinal nerves to the cord, where the fibers cross and are transmitted up the lateral spinothalamic tracts. Fibers then end in the thalamus, where a synapse occurs and the impulse travels to the cerebral cortex.

Sensory fibers emerge from the spinal cord at the dorsal spinal root and supply various areas of the body in known pathways called dermatomes. Table 10–1 lists some of the more important anatomical landmarks associated with the dermatomes. Cancer patients experience

TABLE 10–1

Important Anatomical Landmarks Associated with Dermatomes

Dorsal spinal root	Region innervated
C-2	posterior head
T-1	upper thorax, inner arm
T-4	nipple line
T-10	waist
L-1	inguinal area
S-3 and -4	sacral area

root distribution of pain in herpes zoster and spinal cord compression. The segmental or radicular pain of herpes zoster is caused by inflammation of spinal nerves and/or dorsal root ganglia.

Compression and irritation of dorsal roots by tumors also cause segmental sensory changes such as paresthesias, hyperalgesia, or impairment of pain and touch sensations. The pain sensation radiates segmentally along the path of nerves extending from dorsal spinal roots and is usually intensified by any act that increases intraspinal pressure (coughing, sneezing, straining). More detailed discussions of these conditions can be found in Chapters 9C and 14D.

Motor function: Motor impulses are converged primarily by upper motor neurons (UMN) and lower motor neurons (LMN). Technically, the term upper motor neuron refers to any neuron conveying impulses from the cerebral cortex to the anterior horn cell of the spinal cord; by far the most important UMN is known as the corticospinal (pyramidal) tract. This tract conveys motor impulses. It begins in the motor strip of the cerebral cortex, passes through the internal capsule, pons, and then crosses low in the medulla. From the medulla it travels down the spinal cord until it makes a synapse with an anterior (ventral) horn cell. Interruption of the corticospinal pathway above the level of the medulla, e.g., because of primary or metastatic brain tumors, results in paralysis of the opposite side of the body (hemiplegia) or weakness (hemiparesis). The face may or may not be involved.

Corticospinal tracts can also be interrupted in the spinal cord, on one or both sides, by primary or metastatic tumor involvement, radiation myelitis, or surgical trauma. This interruption results in paraplegia, monoplegia, and, if high enough in the cord, quadriplegia (*see* Chapter 14D). Two important concepts to keep in mind are that (1) upper motor neuron refers both to brain and to spinal cord motor fibers and (2) whenever an interruption occurs suddenly, as in stroke or sudden cord compression, the resulting paralysis will be flaccid because of a condition known as **spinal shock,** in which there is absence of reflex activity at and below the level of the lesion for a period of time.

The lower motor neuron (LMN) includes efferent and afferent pathways from the anterior horn cell of the spinal cord to the muscle by way of the peripheral nerves. Included in this tract is the reflex arc. Damage to the LMN occurs from tumor infiltration or compression of (1) the spinal cord or (2) peripheral nerves. Clinical signs differentiating UMN and LMN lesions are presented in Table 10–2. These signs may vary in configuration and degree; for example, a negative Babinski sign does not necessarily rule out UMN dysfunction.

TABLE 10–2

Clinical Differentiation of Complete UMN and LMN Dysfunction

Indicator	LMN	UMN
Paralysis	Flaccid	Spastic: increased resistance to passive movement
Deep tendon reflexes (patellar, Achilles)	Absent	Hyperactive and may be associated with clonus
Plantar reflexes	Flexor	Extensor
Clonus	Absent	Present: rhythmic contraction of a muscle after stimulation. Ankle clonus is elicited by strong dorsiflexion of the foot with the knee held in flexion
Muscle atrophy	Rapid	Slow (because of disuse)
Trophic changes	Brittle nails, loss of hair, tendency of the skin to ulcerate	None
Babinski sign	Absent	Present

LMN, lower motor neuron; UMN, upper motor neuron.

Bone metastases. The principle cause of decreased mobility for the patient with bone metastases is pain. A detailed discussion of the problem is provided in Chapter 7A. This chapter focuses on the mobility problems imposed by metastases to weight-bearing bones with the resulting risk of pathological fracture.

Cancer commonly metastasizes to bones, especially the vertebrae, pelvic bones, proximal femur, and ribs. Other sites include the humerus, scapula, sternum, skull, and clavicle. Almost half of all patients with cancer of the lung, breast, or prostate will develop bone metastases, accounting for 80% of the total incidence.

Bone metastases may be osteolytic, osteoblastic, or mixed lesions. Osteolytic lesions result from increased bone resorption because of substances such as osteoclast-activating factor, or prostaglandins, thought to be secreted by the tumor. Multiple myeloma and cancer of the thyroid, breast, or kidney are examples of tumors most likely to cause osteolytic bone metastases. The increased bone resorption associated with these lesions places the patient at high risk for hypercalcemia and bone fractures.

Osteoblastic metastases result in increased bone formation at the site of bone disease. These lesions appear dense by radiography and may cause hyperphosphatemia and hypocalcemia. Tumors most often associated with osteoblastic disease include cancer of the prostate or breast, lymphoma, and carcinoid tumors.

Tumor metastases to bone indicate disseminated disease and therefore shortened survival. Patients may, however, live for months to years with bone metastases and thus comprise a large group of persons with chronic problems of pain and decreased mobility.

Peripheral neuropathy.   For persons with cancer, peripheral nerve involvement may occur because of treatment effects, direct compression of the nerve by tumor or hemorrhage or, less frequently, from the remote effects of cancer.

The peripheral nervous system includes all nervous system structures outside of the brain and spinal cord. Axons of the sensory (afferent) nerve fibers originate in the skin and joints and enter the dorsal (posterior) horn of the spinal cord, where they merge into the dorsal(posterior) columns. The motor(efferent) fibers emerge from the spinal cord and terminate on muscles. The fatlike myelin sheath that covers the axons of the peripheral nerve is most susceptible to damage, and myelin degeneration may occur with or without involvement of the underlying axon. When the axon is preserved, recovery of function may be rapid, because all that is needed is remyelination. If the axon is destroyed, however, a new axon must grow and reconnect to the appropriate muscle before function can begin — a lengthy process.

Symptoms of peripheral neuropathy vary in degree and kind. Muscle weakness is most severe in the hands and feet, as the longest and most distal nerves are affected. Atrophy of the muscles is less rapid than in instances of acute LMN damage and is proportional to the number of axons involved. Degree of patellar and Achilles reflex loss tends to be out of proportion to the amount of muscle weakness. Alteration of sensation usually involves pain, vibration, and position senses and is associated with paresthesias (persistent burning, "pins and needles" tingling) and numbness. The mechanism for paresthesias is not understood. When there is loss of proprioceptive functioning, the individual's gait is incoordinated, or ataxic. When the hands and feet are insensitive to pain, they become more susceptible to burns, injuries, and development of sores.

Motor and sensory manifestations associated with administration of **chemotherapy** resemble other neuropathies. The area of sensory loss tends to be bilaterally symmetrical and associated with varying degrees of reflex and motor loss. Usually, the feet are more involved than the hands. Although this type of polyneuropathy is often described as "glove and stocking," the line of demarcation associated with sensory change is gradual rather than sharp.

Of the drugs used in chemotherapy today, vincristine remains the most toxic, regularly producing effects on the nervous system that constitute the dose-limiting effect of this drug. Initial symptoms occur between the second and third week of administration and include loss of Achilles reflex, sensory alterations (particularly paraesthesias), and muscle weakness. Generally, weakness is maximal distally so that the extensor muscles of the fingers and wrist and dorsiflexors of the feet are involved first. Weakness may progress rapidly and involve proximal muscles of the limbs if the dose of the medication is not reduced. Reduction in dose is followed by a gradual return of functional loss. Involvement of cranial nerves or the autonomic nervous system, resulting in bladder and bowel atonia, has been known to occur (*see* Chapter 11). Procarbazine and cisplatin have also been known to produce peripheral neuropathy.

Table 10–3 presents the numerous causes of polyneuropathy in the population at large. Although cancer-related neuropathies dominate the list, the two principal causes in the adult population are those associated with alcoholism and diabetes.

Disorders of neuromuscular transmission. Eaton-Lambert syndrome is a disorder of neuromuscular transmission, most commonly encountered in patients with oat cell carcinoma of the lung. The clinical pattern is diverse: some individuals are asymptomatic, some have slow movements, and some have pronounced weakness. This condition resembles myasthenia gravis except that the weakness is seldom as severe, and there tend to be aching muscles and fewer fluctuations in symptom severity. Nevertheless, patients' mobility may be severely compromised. Reflexes are depressed, and there is no definitive response to cholinergics. The condition may be demonstrated clinically by having the patient grasp the clinician's hand and noticing increase in the strength of grasp.

Fatigue. Fatigue and weakness may account for decreased mobility, even in the absence of neurological impairment or bone metastases. Other factors responsible include protein-calorie malnutri-

TABLE 10–3
Conditions Resulting in Polyneuropathy

Status	Bilaterally symmetrical	Nonsymmetrical
Chronic	Nutritional deficiency associated with alcoholism	—
Subacute/ acute	Chemotherapy	Diabetic neuropathy
	Remote effects of cancer, principally of the lung	Brachial neuropathy associated with axilla radiation
	Lymphoma	Tumors of nerves: ganglioneuroma, neurofibromas
		Less common tumors: glomus, Kaposi's sarcoma
		Metastatic tumor involving the spinal cord or brachial plexus
		Herpes zoster (may also be bilateral)

tion (*see* Chapter 8), disuse atrophy of trunk, neck, and leg muscles, and depression. In addition to the fatigue generally experienced by patients undergoing chemo- and radiotherapy (RT), fatigue may be a result of anemia associated with chronic or acute blood loss or other effects of treatment on the bone marrow (*see* Chapter 9A). Determination of the underlying mechanisms causing fatigue or weakness will assist care-givers in constructing a plan that will both minimize the causes of fatigue and maximize the patient's mobility potential.

Assessment

Inasmuch as optimal mobility depends upon intact sensory and motor systems, assessment is based upon a complete neurological examination. The nurse should be familiar with the most commonly used functional assessment tools for attempting measurement of overall rehabilitation potential and performance status.

The sensory system.   The sensory assessment is not only difficult to conduct, but the results of the examination are often questioned because the patient needs to be alert, moderately intelligent, and willing to respond for the examination to be valid. In addition, instruments used to elicit sensation are crude and rudimentary, as are the guidelines for interpretation. A further difficulty arises when the patient describes "numbness," "pain," or other sensory symptoms, but the clinician is unable to elicit objective evidence of dysfunction. The following guidelines should be employed when conducting the sensory assessment:

1. First obtain the history, including loss of feeling, tingling, burning or other unusual sensations in the extremities.
2. Determine how the symptom relates to functioning in activities of daily living. For example, is the patient falling, tripping, frequently burning his fingers, unable to find his keys in his pocket?
3. Avoid suggesting symptoms to the patient.

The procedure for assessment of the sensory system is outlined in Table 10–4.

The motor system.   The functional unit of the musculoskeletal system is the joint and its associated structures. After taking the history, the examination consists of a series of tests shown in Table 10–5.

In recording of findings, muscle strength is graded according to the criteria listed in Table 10–6. In most instances the 0-to-5 scale is used, but some facilities prefer the normal-good-fair or the percentage format.

The Achilles.   To elicit the reflex:

1. Have the patient relax.
2. Position the ankle so that the foot can be dorsiflexed.
3. Strike the Achilles tendon briskly with a loosely held reflex hammer.
4. If there is no foot movement, use reinforcement by asking the patient to grasp both hands together tightly.

Reflexes are graded in the following standard manner: 0 for no response; 1, diminished; 2, normal; 3, brisk; 4, hyperactive and may be associated with increase in tone and clonus.

Conditions such as diabetes, alcoholism, obesity, nutritional disorders, and old age may suppress the Achilles reflex. In addition, reflex activity may be diminished by certain antineoplastic agents, particularly vincristine.

Gait.   Assessment of gait is based upon the sensory/motor assessment. Gait requires integration of sensory and motor aspects of the nervous system as well as an intact musculoskeletal system. As

TABLE 10–4

Sensory Examination

Sensation	Method
Touch	Stroke dermatome areas briefly with wisp of cotton. Areas with hair will require less stimulation.
Temperature	Touch dermatome areas with hot- and cold-water-filled test tubes and ask patient to identify sensation.
Pain	Touch dermatome areas with point or dull end of safety pin; ask patient to report feelings of "sharp" or "dull."
Vibration	Starting with fingers and toes, place a vibrating tuning fork on the most distal joint of the extremity; place finger under the joint to feel the loss of vibration at the same time as the patient. If no vibration is felt by the patient, move the tuning fork proximally to the next bony prominence.
Position	Gently hold the tip of the toe between thumb and first finger. With the patient's eyes closed, move the joint slightly up or down. Ask the patient to report which way the joint has been moved.

mentioned earlier, mobility is not limited to ambulation, so that if a person uses a wheelchair, crutches, cane, or orthotic equipment, it is important to make certain that the patient is able to use it efficiently and effectively. It is a nursing responsibility to see that barriers that preclude mobility both in and outside of the home are identified. Sample questions used in the initial history will help the nurse determine if there is a problem in ambulation:

1. Can you walk independently. If "yes," how far can you walk?
2. Do you use any equipment to walk, i.e., walker, cane, crutch, brace, wheelchair?
3. Can you leave your home at will?
4. Do you have falls?

TABLE 10–5
Motor Examination

Test	Method
Inspection	Observe the muscles of the limbs for asymmetry, atrophy, or involuntary movements.
Muscle tone	With the patient supine, take all joints through range of motion, noting increase or decrease in movement resistance.
Muscle strength	Test flexion and extension of the hip, knee, ankle, and foot bilaterally and with maximal examiner resistance.
Reflexes	Test patellar and Achilles reflexes.
Babinski sign	Stroke the lateral aspect of the foot beginning at the heel. Positive response is an upward movement of the great toe.
Gait	Have the patient walk. Normal gait is 60 strides/min with an 8-cm width and heel-to-toe pattern. Observe strides, trunk posture, arm swing, abnormal lifting, dropping, or swing of the leg, circumduction of the hip, inversion or eversion of the foot.

TABLE 10–6
Grading of Muscle Strength

Score			Performance standard
5	N	100%	complete range of motion against gravity with full resistance
4	G	75%	complete range of motion against gravity with some resistance
3	F	50%	complete range of motion against gravity
2	P	25%	complete range of motion with gravity eliminated
1	T	10%	evidence of slight contraction, no joint motion
0		0	no evidence of contractility

N, normal; G, good; F, fair; P, poor; T, terrible.

5. Do you have stairs to climb, and can you climb them?

6. What types of activities do you engage in outside the home?

Mechanism of walking.   If motor and sensory systems are intact, the patient is asked to stand, then shift weight back and forth, and then walk. A belt around the waist will help stabilize the unsteady patient.

The walking cycle is a pattern involving flexion-extension of the hip, knee, and ankle. Disruption of the cycle results in a limp. The walking pattern can be broken down into a swing cycle, consisting of hip flexion, knee extension, and ankle dorsiflexion, and stance consisting of hip extension and foot placed flat.

In addition to hip extension, the other two requirements for walking are sufficient balance to maintain a vertical posture and adequate intellectual capacity to comprehend and follow instructions. Sensory loss, particularly loss of position sense, will require the patient to keep observing where his feet are placed.

The major muscles involved in walking are the quadriceps (hip flexion), tibialis (heel strike and toe swing-through) and gastrocnemius (toe push-off), all of which are tested in the motor and sensory examination.

The caloric requirement in walking is about 0.5 calorie/meter/kg body weight. Whenever normal ambulation is disturbed, as in problems with muscle weakness, this figure becomes markedly elevated. Although it may seem obvious that energy requirements increase as speed in walking does, it may be less obvious that a slow gait is not so efficient in energy use. Weight of the patient is also a factor. The greater the patient's weight, the greater the amount of energy needed to ambulate. The use of crutches will also increase energy requirements by as much as 3 or 4 times normal requirements.

Common problems noticed in gait patterns include: (1) short, guarded steps to avoid heel strike in persons experiencing pain upon weight-bearing (e.g., bone metastases); and (2) broad-based gait, common when there is general unsteadiness in walking. The patient raises the center of gravity to compensate for incoordination or unsteadiness.

Functional assessment.   Functional assessment is the method by which the patient's abilities in performing skills of daily living (including vocational and social pursuits) are described, coded, and given numerical value.

Rehabilitation specialists have identified four components of the functional evaluation: (1) medical status; (2) performance status; (3) social status (ability to perform role behaviors); and (4) support of significant others.

Functional assessment, then, is an outgrowth of the initial assessment and provides a systematic means for identifying patients' problems and evaluating programs. Gathering data about functional status may also help in the area of nursing staffing.

Medical rehabilitation involves an interdisciplinary approach to the improvement in the patient's functional ability. Considerable physical effort is generally required. For this reason, not all persons with mobility problems resulting from cancer will be suitable candidates for rehabilitation. For example, the person with lower-spinal-cord metastasis resulting in paraplegia would be suitable for rehabilitation only after the medical condition has stabilized. In this situation, the spine must be stable and the patient relatively free of pain and wanting to learn self-care activities.

Instruments used in functional evaluation. Two rehabilitation scales commonly employed in cancer care are the PULSES profile and the Karnofsky scale. The acronym PULSES derives from P for stability of *physical condition*, U for independence in *upper extremity* functioning, L for independence in *lower extremity* functioning, S for *sensory* intactness (communication, vision, hearing), E for *excretory* control, and S for *social support* and role behaviors (Table 10–7). Each of the variables is graded from 1 (total independence) to 4 (total dependence) and then all are summed. Patients are evaluated prior to intervention, during rehabilitation, and at the conclusion of therapy.

In 1949, Karnofsky and Burchenal recommended that four criteria guide in the evaluation of "new" chemotherapeutic agents. The resulting Karnofsky scale is based on:

1. Subjective improvement: indications that the patient feels better, including less pain, better sleep, and better appetite.
2. Objective improvement: blood constituents have improved or tumor size has decreased.
3. Performance Scale: a scale of independence and nursing care needs. (Best score 100. Worst score 0, equals death.) (Table 10–8)
4. Length of remission and prolongation of life.

The authors felt that effective treatment would accomplish one of these objectives. The performance scale criterion continues to be widely used as a means of defining functional capabilities and areas for rehabilitation, although, because it was developed for the purpose of evaluating chemotherapeutic agents, its application is limited.

Management

The effects of prolonged bed rest and immobility are well known: pulmonary compromise, skin breakdown, osteoporosis and hypercalcemia, depression, and further weakness and immobility. For the person with advanced cancer, these problems may be compounded by malnutrition, pain, and fatigue. The primary management goal is to optimize patient activity and mobility while minimizing stress, fatigue, and pain.

Effective medical or surgical treatment of the underlying malignancy affecting mobility is an initial management concern. Surgery or RT may provide curative or palliative relief for the patient with spinal cord compression caused by tumor (*see* Chapter 14D).

Metastatic bone lesions may respond dramatically to systemic chemotherapy for the primary tumor, especially breast cancer and multiple myeloma. Local RT to the affected bone is useful both for its antitumor effect and for pain relief. The dose and schedule of RT vary according to the specific tumor type.

When the patient fails to respond to these measures, and when the lesion exists in a weight-bearing area (long bones, vertebrae), the patient is at high risk for pathological fracture. Added risk factors are: (1) lytic lesion >3 cm in diameter; and (2) ≥50% destruction of bony cortex as visualized radiographically.

Support may be provided by way of a lightweight external orthotic device or by internal fixation. Intramedullary nailing or prosthetic replacement provides rigid fixation of the involved bone and joint, and methyl methacrylate cement may be used to fill bone spaces resulting from lytic lesions.

Table 10–9 describes a nursing management protocol for persons with limitations in mobility. The importance of collaboration with physical therapists in the care of these patients cannot be overemphasized. A program of gradual, goal-directed mobilization that provides for muscle strengthening, assistance devices, and nutritional and pharmacological support requires the coordination of various professionals as well as that of the patient and family.

Problems not related to cancer may be a factor in mobility. For example, patients receiving analgesics or sedatives may feel their energy level is reduced. This problem should not be confused with actual motor impairment. For this reason, the history should include all medications taken by the patient. Other pathological conditions, specifically alcoholism and diabetes, can cause peripheral nerve problems as well.

Health education is a therapeutic intervention that can be used to promote mobility. Not only should patients and family receive suitable instruction related to chemotherapeutic agents and their potential reactions in the peripheral nervous system, but individuals with documented mobility impairment may also need instruction regarding new walking patterns and nutrition (*see* Chapter 8).

A physical therapy consultation may prove quite useful, particularly if the individual has monoplegia, or foot drop, secondary to peripheral neuropathy. Patients with a mono- or hemiplegia will need to learn new

TABLE 10-7
PULSES Profile

Assessment criteria	Variable
P Physical condition: Includes diseases of the viscera (cardiovascular, GI, urologic, endocrinal), psychiatric, and neurologic disorders	1. Health problems sufficiently stable that medical or nursing monitoring is not required more often than at 3-mo intervals.
	2. Medical or nurse monitoring is needed more often than 3-mo intervals, but not each week.
	3. Health problems are sufficiently unstable as to require regular medical and/or nursing attention at least weekly.
	4. Health problems require intensive medical and/or nursing attention at least daily (excluding personal care assistance only).
U Upper limb functions: Self-care activities (drink/feed, dress upper/lower, brace/prosthesis, groom, wash, perineal care) dependent mainly upon upper limb function	1. Independent in self-care without impairment of upper limbs.
	2. Independent in self-care with some impairment of upper limbs or able to direct own care.
	3. Dependent upon assistance or supervision in self-care with or without impairment of upper limbs.
	4. Dependent totally in self-care with marked impairment of upper limbs.
L Lower limb functions: Mobility (transfer to chair, toilet, tub, or shower; walk; use stairs; wheelchair) dependent mainly upon lower limb function	1. Independent in mobility without impairment of lower limbs.
	2. Independent in mobility with some impairment in lower limbs, such as needing ambulatory aids, a brace or prosthesis, or else fully independent in a wheelchair without significant architectural or environmental barriers, or able to direct own care.
	3. Dependent upon assistance or supervision in mobility, with or without impairment of lower limbs, or partly independent in a wheelchair; or, there are significant architectural or environmental barriers.
	4. Dependent totally in mobility, with marked impairment of lower limbs.

S Sensory components: Relating to communication (speech and hearing) and vision

1. Independent in communication and vision without impairment.
2. Independent in communication and vision with some impairment, such as mild aphasia, dementia, psychological dysfunction, or need for eyeglasses or hearing aid, or needing regular eye medication.
3. Dependent upon assistance and interpreter, or supervision in communication or vision.
4. Dependent totally in communication or vision.

E Excretory functions (bladder and bowel)

1. Complete voluntary control of bladder and bowel sphincters.
2. Control of sphincters allows normal social activities despite urgency or need for catheter, appliance, suppositories, etc. Able to care for needs without assistance.
3. Dependent upon assistance in sphincter management or else has accidents occasionally.
4. Frequent wetting or soiling from incontinence of bladder or bowel sphincters.

S Support factors: Consider intellectual and emotional adaptability, support from family unit, and financial ability

1. Patient and family are able to fulfill usual roles and perform customary tasks.
2. Must make some modification in usual roles and performance of customary tasks.
3. Patient is dependent upon assistance, supervision, encouragement or assistance from family, a public or private agency because of any of the support factors.
4. Family/patient is dependent upon long-term institutional care (chronic hospitalization, nursing home, and excluding time-limited hospital for specific evaluation, treatment, or active rehabilitation).

PULSES Total: Best score is 6. Worst score is 24.

Adapted from Granger, C. V., G. L. Albrecht, and B. B. Hamilton. Outcome of comprehensive medical rehabilitation: measurement by PULSES profile and the Barthel index. *Archives of Physical Medicine and Rehabilitation* (April 1979). p. 145–154.

TABLE 10–8
Performance Scale

Condition	Percentage	Comments
A. Able to carry on normal activity and to work. No special care is needed.	100	Normal, no complaints, no evidence of disease.
	90	Able to carry on normal activity, minor signs of symptoms of disease.
	80	Normal activity with effort, some signs or symptoms of disease.
B. Unable to work. Able to live at home, care for most personal needs.	70	Cares for self. Unable to carry on normal activity or to do active work.
A varying degree of assistance is needed.	60	Requires occasional assistance, but is able to care for most of own needs.
	50	Requires considerable assistance and frequent medical care.
C. Unable to care for self.	40	Disabled, requires special care and assistance.
Requires equivalent of institutional or hospital care. Disease may be progressing rapidly.	30	Severely disabled; hospitalization is indicated although death not imminent.
	20	Hospitalization necessary, very sick, active support treatment necessary.
	10	Moribund, fatal processes progressing rapidly.
	0	Dead.

Reprinted with permission from Karnofsky, D. A. and J. H. Burchenal. The clinical evaluation of chemotherapeutic agents used in cancer. *In* MacLeod, C. M., editor. Evaluation of Chemotherapeutic Agents. Columbia University Press, New York. 1949. p. 196.

ambulatory patterns and should receive every possible assistance in learning a new method of walking. Persons with foot drop should wear an orthotic device (ankle-knee orthosis) to prevent tripping over the toes.

If the patient has generalized weakness, it is appropriate to increase his center of gravity with the use of a cane. Depending upon the degree of weakness and resulting instability, the individual may select a single-tipped or broad-based quad cane. To measure the cane, hold it about 6

TABLE 10-9

Nursing Protocol for the Management of Altered Mobility

Factor	Intervention
Comfort	Alleviate pain (*see* Chapter 7A).
	Schedule ambulation/exercise according to patient comfort.
Endurance	Obtain base-line VS, CBC.
	Provide nutritional support (*see* Chapter 8).
	Schedule ambulation activities according to patient tolerance.
	Provide assistive devices that impose minimal stress: walker or cane to decrease weight-bearing on long bones, corset for vertebral support.
	Obtain physical therapy consultation for gait training.
	Evaluate continually for changes in tolerance, VS, CBC.
Balance	Observe sitting, standing, and gait balance.
	Obtain physical therapy consultation for muscle-strengthening exercises; to provide assistive devices that raise center of gravity and provide adequate support.
Ambulation	Plan activities of daily living according to ambulatory ability.
	Collaborate with physical therapist to teach new ambulatory patterns if necessary.
	Use properly measured assistive devices.
Sensation	Consult with MD regarding need for orthotic device, e.g., patient with foot drop or with bone metastases.
Proprioception	Teach safety for potential falls.
	Obtain physical therapy consultation.
Peripheral neuropathy	Provide assistive devices for activities of daily living.
	Teach safety to avoid potential extremity injury.
	Obtain occupational therapy consultation.

MD, physician; VS, vital signs.

inches from the side of the foot; the patient's elbow should be slightly flexed. Canes are particularly useful if weakness is unilateral. The cane should be used on the unaffected side. If the weakness is bilateral, a walker may be helpful in maintenance of balance. Select a walker that is lightweight and can be folded to transport in a car. Crutches may be useful for the person with bilateral weakness. Crutches require a great deal of physical stamina to use, however, and therefore may not be appropriate for many patients. If gait training is indicated, a physical therapist should be consulted.

When the proprioceptive sense is absent, the patient will not know where his feet are unless he is looking at foot placement. He will need education in the prevention of falls, including learning to always walk in a lighted area. If sensation is absent, the patient's feet will be particularly likely to develop sores and other wounds. Instruction in foot care, including inspection and the wearing of appropriate shoes, is needed.

Problems in mobility have traditionally been a large concern of those involved in rehabilitation. Although not all cancer patients will be able to profit from a very active program of physical rehabilitation, a cancer-care nurse who thinks in terms of rehabilitation and gathers data by means of a functional evaluation tool will, in the long run, be able to offer patients a vastly superior type of care.

Bibliography

1. Abeloff, M. D. Complications of Cancer. Johns Hopkins University Press, Baltimore. 1980.

    Includes chapters on physical rehabilitation and surgical management of bone metastases.

2. Adams, R. G., and M. Victor. Principles of Neurology. McGraw-Hill Book Co., New York. 1981. Second edition.

    A basic comprehensive neurology text, useful in understanding clinical situations.

3. Mauch, P. M. The treatment of metastatic cancer to bone. In DeVita, V. T., S. Hellman, and S. A. Rosenberg, editors. Cancer: Principles and Practice of Oncology. J. B. Lippincott Co., Philadelphia. 1982.

    Provides a concise and comprehensive discussion of the pathophysiology, clinical presentation, and management of bone metastases. Surgery, radiotherapy, and chemotherapeutic treatment options are described.

4. Minna, J. D., and P. A. Bunn. Paraneoplastic syndromes. In DeVita, V. T., S. Hellman, and S. A. Rosenberg, editors. Cancer: Principles and Practice of Oncology. J. B. Lippincott Co., Philadelphia. 1982.

    Discusses the neurological manifestations of cancer within the broader context of paraneoplastic syndromes. Pathophysiology, diagnosis, and treatment of neurological syndromes that occur as remote effects of cancer are described.

5. Weiss, H. D., M. D. Walker, and P. H. Wiernik. Neurotoxicity of commonly used antineoplastic agents. New England Journal of Medicine (July 1974). 127–133.

    This article describes neuropathies and other neurotoxic effects of chemotherapeutic agents.

6. Wood, C. A., J. Anderson, and J. W. Yates. Physical function assessment in patients with advanced cancer. Medical and Pediatric Oncology (March/April 1981). 129–132.

    Three scales were used, in conjunction with the Karnofsky scale, to measure physical activity, and authors found a high correlation between traditional physical functioning measures and the Karnofsky scale. These scales were the ambulation capability, activity, and time up.

CHAPTER 11

ELIMINATION

Standard: The client and family manage alterations in elimination (which may include fecal and urinary diversions, fistulas, diarrhea, constipation, bladder insufficiencies, incontinence, or fecal or urinary obstruction) to be consistent with activities of daily living.

Outcome criteria: The client and family
1. state appropriate actions if changes in elimination patterns occur.
2. describe the relationship between adequate elimination and physiologic integrity.
3. identify and manage factors that may affect elimination, such as diet, stress, physical activity, and neurogenic conditions.
4. develop a plan for managing an altered elimination route within personal life-style.

A: ANATOMICAL ALTERATIONS
Alice Basch

FECAL DIVERSION

Framework

The surgical alteration of the GI tract is commonly undertaken when a tumor invades the system or a mechanical blockage occurs. After the initial physiologic recovery from the surgical procedure and anesthesia, functioning of the remaining alimentary system returns to what was previously normal for the individual. Fecal consistency is dependent on the site of intervention, the amount of intestine removed, and whether additional treatments or medications are needed for symptom management or control of disease.

Most frequently the stoma, or opening, will be matured (i.e., the inner lining of the intestinal tract is turned over onto itself, as one would turn up a cuff on a sleeve) at time of surgery. This creates a surface that is moist, pinkish-red in color, and closely resembling other healthy mucosal tissue. The color is due to the high numbers of blood vessels found in the mucosa, which account for the occasional drops of blood seen when wiping with a cloth or tissue. The stoma is unaffected by digestive materials found in the stool and will move slightly, consistent with peristalsis.

The descending, or sigmoid, colon, located in the lower left quadrant, is the most common site for colostomy placement. Stomas located at this site are usually 1 to 2 in. in diameter and slightly protruding from the skin surface. Effluent from the sigmoid colostomy will return to the stool consistency normal to the individual prior to disease.

Fecal output becomes softer and contains higher concentrations of enzymatic material the higher in the colon the surgical intervention is performed. A left transverse colostomy may produce stool of peanut-butter to semiformed consistency and be mildly irritating to skin surfaces. Transverse colostomies, usually placed at waist level, are 2 to 3½ in. in diameter and are often unmatured at the time of surgery, creating a moist, light-red to pink cauliflower-shaped structure. Because of positioning, effluent consistency, and size, these colostomies are the most difficult to manage in terms of maintaining a seal and protecting peristomal skin.

The ascending colostomy is an intervention higher in the colon and is located on the right side of the abdomen. Effluent seen at this location will be primarily liquid and highly enzymatic to surrounding skin, i.e., the effluent digests the skin and is therefore a potential source of skin breakdown.

Small-bowel ostomy output, occurring with an ileostomy or jejunostomy, is primarily liquid in nature and extremely enzymatic. Skin breakdown from fecal contact can occur within several hours when ostomies are located in the small bowel. Stoma diameter is usually small, 1 to 1½ in., and will be seen in the right lower quadrant. For improved pouch seal, the stoma will protrude ½ to 1 in. (Fig. 11A–1).

Management

During the first several days after creation of a stoma, all types of ostomies should be managed in a similar manner. Appropriate

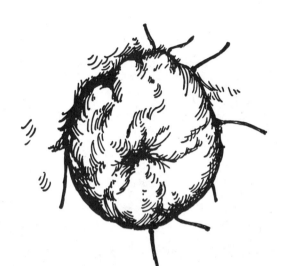

Figure 11A–1.   Healthy ileostomy, protruding ~1 in. from abdominal wall.

pouching systems should include an open-ended, odor-proof pouch and some type of skin barrier to be used between the pouch and skin. Individual institutions may choose a particular manufacturer according to availability of products and the hospital's ability to maintian a varied inventory. The general management of the new colostomy should include procedures and equipment that protect the skin from the fecal material, provide an odor-proof material for patient, staff, and visitor comfort, and provide an opening in the bottom of the bag for the emptying of waste material.

Pouching procedures.   Pouching procedures need to be given to the new ostomate. Following are two sample procedures. The first is for changing the **drainable appliance** with karaya washer. Necessary supplies include (1) the correct appliance with an opening of ⅛ to ¼ in. larger than stoma diameter (Hollister); (2) skin sealant (e.g., United Skin-Prep wipes #4204 or Skin-Prep spray, Hollister skin gel, Bard Protective Barrier Film); and (3) warm water, washcloth, and towel.

1. Remove old appliance. Be careful to support the skin as you gently remove the adhesive area.
2. Wash area around the stoma with warm water. *Do not use soap,* which can leave a film on the skin, causing irritation or

poor appliance adherence. *Do not rub.* Do not be concerned if small amounts of karaya do not come off the skin. They will not interfere with the new appliance. If you have difficulty removing a large amount of the karaya, soak a tissue with water and hold it on the karaya. The karaya will soften and can be removed easily.

3. *Pat area dry — do not rub.*
4. Measure stoma, using a measuring guide, and be sure you have the correct opening in your appliance.
5. Wipe area to be covered by appliance adhesive with skin sealant, or spray with skin sealant spray.
6. Allow skin sealant to dry thoroughly.
7. Remove cellophane covering from karaya and paper backing from adhesive.
8. Place opening in appliance over stoma.
9. Apply gentle pressure over skin barrier to ensure that it seals to the skin.
10. Smooth adhesive backing carefully to eliminate wrinkles.
11. Apply clamp to end of pouch.

Next, are instructions for use of a **two-piece, open-ended appliance.** Necessary supplies include (1) 2-piece, open-ended appliance (Hollister 2-piece or Squibb Sur-Fit); (2) skin sealant (Skin-Prep), (3) Stomahesive or Hollihesive paste (optional); and (4) warm water, washcloth, and towel.

1. Remove old appliance.
2. Cleanse gently with warm water and pat dry.
3. Cut opening in adhesive to fit stoma.
4. Apply skin sealant to peristomal area and allow to dry well. Apply Stomahesive paste around stoma (optional).
5. Remove paper backing from wafer.
6. Center appliance over stoma. Press gently around opening to ensure seal. It may be helpful to start at the bottom and evenly press as you move toward top.
7. Snap bag onto flange. You will hear a snap or click when it is secured. You may also attach bag to flange before securing the appliance over the stoma.
8. Frame with paper tape. Apply tape around four sides of appliance, half on skin and half on wafer.
9. Apply clamp to end of pouch.

Irrigation. After several days of bowel functioning and regular dietary intake, instruction in irrigation can begin for the appropriate patient with a sigmoid colostomy (Table 11A–1). Proper height of the irrigation fluid is important to obtain a thorough irrigation and fluid

TABLE 11A–1

Considerations for Irrigation in Patients with Sigmoid Colostomy

Positive	Negative
Regular bowel movements prior to current disease and surgery	History of irregular bowel movements
Motivation	Lack of motivation
Full mental and emotional capacities	Poor orientation or depression
Full dexterity	Severe arthritis, amputation, or other factors affecting dexterity
Appropriate bathroom facilities, including running water	Lack of appropriate bathroom facilities, including lack of running water
	Blindness
	Frequent travel
	Frequent changes in daily schedule
	Diarrhea (radiation, chemotherapy, virus, etc.)
	Terminal status
	Temporary colostomy

return. A bag held too high may cause water to flow high in the colon, causing a more liquid return lasting over several hours. If the patient is standing or sitting, the bag should hang between shoulder and nipple level. If the patient is supine, the bottom of the irrigation bag should hang 18 in. above the stoma. An irrigation that takes longer than 1½ hr from time of start of fluid to final return should be evaluated for proper technique. Instruction for an appropriate colostomy irrigation is shown below.

1. Choose a convenient time for irrigation.
2. Fill irrigation bag with 1,000 ml (1 quart) lukewarm tap water.
3. Let some water run through the tubing to clear it of air.
4. Hang irrigating bag so that the bottom of the bag will be between breast and shoulder level. (If patient is supine, nurse or care-giver will perform procedure. Bag will hang 18 in. above stoma.)
5. Remove old appliance carefully, supporting your skin as you pull off the adhesive.
6. Place faceplate of irrigating sleeve over stoma and secure with belt. It is usually easiest to sit on the toilet for irrigation.

7. Direct open end of irrigating sleeve into the commode or other receptacle. Irrigating sleeve will be open at the top for insertion of cone into stoma.
8. Observe for opening from which stool is being discharged. With a double-barrel colostomy, a second opening may be present. It will not harm you to insert solution into this opening, but the water will probably be eliminated from the rectum.
9. Lubricate the cone with water-soluble lubricant (K-Y Jelly, Lubafax).
10. When the cone is in front of the stoma, in position to insert, begin slow water flow as you insert the cone.
11. Insert cone until there is no backflow of water. It is *not* necessary to insert all the way to the flat edge. Never force the cone into the stoma.
12. Allow water to flow in quickly. If cramps develop, slow the flow of the solution; also, check to see if the water is too hot or too cold.
13. When most of the water has gone in or if a full feeling occurs, stop the water flow.
14. Remove the cone from the stoma and the irrigating sleeve.
15. Clip the top of the irrigating sleeve closed, so that fluid return will not escape.
16. Allow irrigation to return. Results may take from 20 to 45 min. While waiting for the return, you may continue with regular morning routine by cleaning the bottom of the irrigation sleeve and folding or clipping the end of the sleeve. You may feel a slight cramping with the return or a feeling of warmth as the water and stool is eliminated. If the return takes longer than 25 to 45 min, contact the enterostomal therapist.
17. When the return is complete, remove the faceplate and the irrigating sleeve.
18. Cleanse area around the stoma with warm water (*no soap*).
19. Apply new appliance.

The first irrigation should be done with not more than 500 ml warm water to evaluate patient tolerance to the procedure. To determine direction of the colon, the stoma may be gently dilated prior to beginning the procedure. With few exceptions, a cone tip or shield should always be used for irrigations. A cone tip will prevent too high a water infusion or possible bowel perforation if the catheter is forced. Because the colon lacks nerve endings and the patient cannot feel the catheter against the wall of the bowel, caution must be used to avoid perforation. An experienced nurse or enterostomal therapist may be consulted to determine when a catheter can be used.

When a person with a sigmoid colostomy achieves bowel regulation (no stool leakage during 24- to 48-hr period between irrigations), he may feel comfortable pouching the stoma with a small, closed-ended pouch or gauze covering. The patient should be reminded to keep a supply of open-ended pouches for use during travel and when diarrhea may occur because of changes in medication, treatment for disease, and viral illness.

Regularity cannot be achieved for stomas not located in the sigmoid colon. If a patient is not regulated within 6 wk of initiating proper irrigations, the likelihood of future bowel regulation is minimal.

Common problems

Stoma complications.   Most stoma complications occur within the first year of surgery. Stoma viability and functioning should be assessed with each appliance change and recorded for future reference.

The first assessment for any stoma is to determine viability. A healthy stoma is a deep-pink to red color. A **compromise in the blood flow** to the stoma from trauma, edema, or other causes will appear as a purplish-to-black stoma. If not reversed or surgically altered, the stoma will become necrotic and sluff off, leaving an opening that may be difficult to pouch.

Stricturing, or narrowing, of the stoma opening is another frequently seen complication. Unless the condition causes symptoms of obstruction, intervention is not required. Occasional dilation of the stoma is recommended, but it seems to have little effect on the stricturing and may cause formation of additional scar tissue if performed too rigorously.

Stoma **retraction** which creates an opening below skin level, will cause effluent to undermine the appliance, creating skin breakdown and leakage. An appliance with a flexible faceplate or increased convexity may aid in adherence.

Visually, stoma **prolapse** (Fig. 11A–2) may be one of the most distressing of complications to the patient. Stomas matured and not having fixation of the mesentery internally seem to prolapse more frequently, but the causes of prolapse are not clear. Occasionally a stoma will prolapse and spontaneously retract, with no further problems. If the prolapse recurs or remains extended over long periods of time, a feeling of pressure and abdominal discomfort may occur. A mild support, such as panty hose or a manufactured prolapse belt, and avoidance of injury can help relieve symptoms. Surgical revision can be made if the prolapse compromises blood flow or if abdominal discomfort occurs.

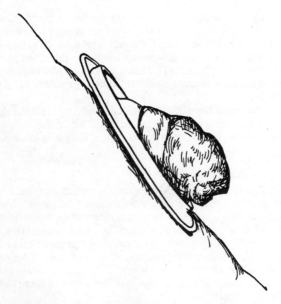

Figure 11A–2. Prolapsed colostomy.

Dysfunction in consistency/volume/odor. The nature and volume of colostomy and ileostomy effluent is determined by normal physiology and location of the stoma. A change in the individual's normal output may result from a variety of causes (Table 11A–2).

Diarrhea in the regulated or sigmoid colostomy presents as frequent, soft-to-liquid stools. The colostomate should switch to an open-ended appliance, if not already using one, and empty fecal material prn. If the colostomate is to begin therapy that may result in diarrhea, such as abdominal radiation or chemotherapy, he should stop irrigation until treatment is concluded and bowel functioning returns to previous condition. On occasion, after radiation treatment, a formerly regulated ostomate will be unable to achieve beneficial results from irrigation. He should then be encouraged to stop the procedure and manage the colostomy like a higher colonic stoma.

When transverse colostomy, ascending colostomy, or ileostomy patients develop diarrhea, severe complications can result from dehydration and changes in electrolytes. Fluids, electrolytes, and skin integrity should be carefully monitored and any alterations treated. A bland, low-roughage diet, which may include rice, toast, applesauce,

TABLE 11A-2

Potential Sources of Alteration in Consistency/Volume/Odor of Effluent

Causative factor	Constipation	Diarrhea	Odor	Gas
Food	apple juice and sauce carrot juice celery corn bananas Chinese food mushrooms nuts popcorn milk products	beer fried and greasy foods excessive fruit milk products nutritional supplement rich sauces spicy foods	asparagus beans broccoli cabbage cheese fish eggs garlic and spices onions	beer carbonated beverages cabbage family dairy products legumes onions
Drugs	chemotherapy: vincristine iron antibiotics aluminum hydroxide β-adrenergic blockers codeine and opiates tricyclic antidepressants	chemotherapy: busulfan doxorubicin fluorouracil methotrexate mithramycin mitotane antibiotics antihypertensives sulfasalazine (Azulfidine) digitalis lithium carbonate vitamin D	antibiotics vitamins	
Other	decreased fluid intake inactivity tumor blockage	emotional upset infection virus	bacterial colonization poor hygiene stricture, dysfunction, or obstruction of intestine	chewing gum improper colostomy irrigation talking or swallowing air while chewing

bananas, yogurt, and other foods that can help create bulk, will aid in controlling the high-liquid-volume output. Fluids containing sodium and potassium should be provided. Examples include tea, coffee, strained orange juice, bouillon, Gatorade, cola, and other sodas.

With severe or chronic diarrhea, oral medication may be of benefit in treating symptoms. Nonprescription oral agents may include Kaopectate, Pepto-Bismol, and aluminum-hydroxide-containing antacids. Prescription medications include diphenoxylate with atropine (Lomotil), loperamide (Imodium), tincture of opium, and codeine derivatives.

Continued diarrhea may indicate changes in the mucosal lining, stricture, mechanical blockage, or viral disease, and a physician's examination should be made to rule out pathologic causes. Cases of severe fluid-and-electrolyte depletion may require IV therapy for replacement of lost nutrients.

Constipation in the ostomate and the nonostomate often arises from the same causes. Fluid loss, inactivity, diet, and medication may all contribute to constipation. As with the nonostomate, diet changes, stool softeners, mild laxatives, and retention enemas or irrigation can be used to treat bowel problems. Paralytic ileus, bowel stricture, adhesions, tumor, and kinks in the colon may be other causes of constipation and should be treated medically.

Blockage in the ileostomate can occur from consumption of a diet high in roughage. Common offenders include corn, mushrooms, popcorn, coconut, and Chinese foods. Thorough chewing of food can help eliminate problems from blockage. If blockage occurs and is unrelieved with gentle stomal dilation and oral fluids after 24 hr, an ileostomy irrigation can be performed by a qualified professional.

The newly formed stoma will produce large amounts of flatulence and strong odors, a result of increased bacterial colonization during the first days after surgery, when anesthesia and mechanical manipulation have decreased peristalsis of the colon. With increased activity and normalization of diet, gas and odor will decrease. Continued problems with gas and odor could result from diet, medication, treatment, or disease (*see* Table 11A-2). Odor can be effectively controlled with a variety of commercially prepared pouch deodorants, odor-proof bags, and oral agents, such as parsley, charcoal, and bismuth subgallate, in moderation.

Alterations in skin integrity. The peristomal skin, although often exposed to a variety of irritations, will maintain integrity if properly protected. Irritated and even severely excoriated skin will heal rapidly when promptly and properly treated. Basic principles to follow in skin care of the ostomate include protecting the skin from irritating fluids and chemicals; maintaining a clean and moisture-free environment; and treating irritations early. If skin under appliance becomes irritated from fecal discharge, the following procedure should be used as soon as possible. The supplies for this procedure are karaya or Stomahesive powder and skin sealant (e.g., United Skin-Prep spray/Skin-Prep wipes #4204).

1. Remove old appliance, clean and dry peristomal skin, sprinkle irritated area with powder (it may sting slightly).
2. Brush off excess powder, using a tissue.
3. Spray with skin sealant spray or wipe with skin sealant wipes to seal powder to irritated area.
4. Allow sealant to dry completely. (It will go through 3 stages: wet, sticky, and completely dry).
5. Apply appliance in usual manner.
6. If irritation does not improve, assess skin or consult with enterostomal therapist for skin allergy, *Monilia* infection, or change in application procedure.

The patient with an ileostomy or a transverse colostomy is highly susceptible to skin breakdown from a variety of causes. A skin barrier (e.g., Hollister Premium Skin Barrier, Squibb Stomahesive, karaya washers) should always be used to prevent problems from developing. Choice of barrier will be determined by availability, cost, and effectiveness. A skin sealant (e.g., United Skin-Prep, Sween Prep, Hollister skin gel, and Bard Protective Barrier Film) will provide added protection from mechanical irritation when adhesives are removed and from irritating fluids and chemicals.

Assessment of skin irritation requires consideration of location of irritation in relation to barriers and appliance, skin exposure to effluent, description of irritation, and the patient's subjective complaints (Table 11A–3). Examining a recently used appliance and barrier for patterns of erosion is another useful means of determining etiology of irritation. A patient history of allergic reactions and sensitivity will also assist in documenting and eliminating irritants. A final assessment can be made by observing the patient's pouching procedures, which may indicate a need for modification of application, such as a longer drying period for skin sealants or adhesives.

Once the cause of the irritation is determined, a remedy can be easily determined, and the skin will usually heal within several days. In most cases, simply eliminating the irritant or adding a sealant or barrier to the pouching procedure will reverse the skin damage. Severe excoriation or infection may require additional treatment or prescription medication, such as systemic antibiotics or topical antifungal agents (Table 11A–4). Repeated excoriation because of badly placed

TABLE 11A–3

Assessment of Alteration in Skin Integrity

Irritant	Signs	Symptoms
Fecal	Irritation will be seen in areas of skin that have contact with fecal effluent. There may be slight erythema to denuded, bleeding, or weeping skin. Most commonly seen in ileostomy, ascending, or right transverse colostomies.	Itching, burning, or stinging. Mild to severe pain intermittently or continually. Stinging with application of alcohol- or acid-containing products.
Urine	Irritation seen on stoma or peristomal area in contact with urine. Skin may be erythemic, lacerated, or bleeding, and encrustations may be seen on the skin, stoma, or old appliance (white sandpaper-textured particles). Excessive skin growth (hyperplasia) may develop on stoma or skin.	Itching or burning. Patient will complain of poor appliance adherence and urine leakage. Also may complain of strong urine odor.
Chemical soap detergents skin cement or solvents	The peristomal area in which the barrier or appliance adheres may or may not follow pattern of adhesive. Irritated areas may be erythemic or edematous.	Itching or burning.

Mechanical	Irritation will be seen in areas of adhesives and under belt tabs or edges of faceplates. Irritated areas will be erythemic, eroded, or abraded. Areas of bleeding or patches and crusts may develop.	Mild to severe pain will be felt on skin. Cuts or abrasions to the stoma will have no associated pain because of lack of nerve endings.
Infection/fungus *Candida albicans* *Staphylococcus aureus*	Irritation does not follow a pattern. It may extend beyond the pouch or barrier and frequently will be seen in skin folds. Lesions will show up as patchy dry or scaly areas. They may also present as moist erythema or white papular lesions.	Severe itching will be the major complaint. A few individuals will complain of stinging.
Allergy	Irritation will follow a distinct pattern, corresponding to the suspected allergen. Skin area will appear erythemic, edematous, and may have a rash.	Itching.

TABLE 11A-4

Management of Alteration in Skin Integrity

Irritant	Medical intervention	Nursing intervention
Fecal	Chronic severe fecal excoriation may be caused by poor stoma placement. Surgical revision may be required if pouching procedures are inadequate for skin protection.	Add or change type of skin barrier to protect the skin from fecal contact. A seal of ≥3 days will aid in skin healing. Follow procedure for treatment of mild to severe exocriation.
Urine	*See* above.	Maintain a urine pH of 5.5–5.6. Use vinegar-and-water soaks 1:2 for 15–30 min daily to treat skin. If irritation chronic, use disposable appliance to prevent crystal buildup, antireflux valve, and night-drainage hookup. Maintaining a leak-proof appliance seal will prevent further skin damage.
Chemical	Not applicable.	Discourage use of soaps. If using soap, rinse thoroughly and use only oil- and fragrance-free soaps (Ivory). Allow cements or solvents to dry completely. If irritant isolated, eliminate, or use barrier or skin sealant between irritant and skin.

Mechanical	Severe lacerations to the stoma may require assessment for reconstruction.	Maintain pouch seal for 3–5 days to decrease abrasions from tape removal. Use push/pull method to remove the old pouch. Use skin sealants for friable skin and gauze padding under belt tabs. Measure opening in appliance for proper fit and center appliance over stoma.
Infection/fungus	Prescription of nystatin powder for *Candida*, topical or systemic antibiotics for *Staphylococcus*.	Areas not covered by an appliance will heal spontaneously if kept clean and dry. Lesions will need to be cultured if etiology unknown.
Allergy	Antihistamines if severe.	Remove or substitute for the source of irritation. Include a skin sealant or barrier between the skin and irritant. Skin may be tested if source of irritation is uncertain: 1. Place a 3–5-cm patch of the suspected item on the forearm or abdomen. 2. Cover with a clear adhesive film (Op-Site). 3. Observe in 24 and 48 hr for reaction.

or poorly constructed stoma may require evaluation for surgical reconstruction.

The person with a regulated colostomy will have very few skin problems associated with his diversion. Effluent from a sigmoid colostomy is usually firm, with little remainder of digestive enzymes. Because the individual may often use only a gauze pad to protect clothing from mucous discharge, allergic reactions are minimal. When skin irritation does occur, it should be assessed and treated in the same manner as for other fecal diversions.

Alterations in appliance adherence.   An appliance is expected to maintain a seal for 3 to 7 days. A decrease in adherence should alert the ostomate to the need for reassessment of application procedure or equipment. Aging, changes in hormones, weight, and in activity and environment can affect ostomy management.

Aging, pregnancy, and other **hormonal alterations** may affect the texture of the skin and oil production of skin pores. Oily skin will interfere with adhesive adherence. Dry skin promotes adherence. A particularly oily skin may benefit from a denaturing agent (e.g., UniSolve Adhesive Remover) after removal of the old appliance and prior to application of any powders, sealants, barriers, or adhesives.

A **change in weight** of >10 pounds will likely alter stoma size. Significant weight changes can also change abdominal contours, thus affecting adherence. Using a convex faceplate may increase wearing time on protruding bellies. Changes in abdominal contours may also occur after additional surgery for other causes, and a change in appliance or procedure may then be beneficial.

Other considerations include **weather** and **activity**. Humidity and hot weather will often affect the normal wearing time of an appliance, and appliances may require more frequent changes. Hot moisture, as found in saunas and steam rooms, can also loosen adhesive and melt skin barriers.

Increased activity may affect adherence of the appliance if the person perspires much. In most cases, an acceptable wearing time of ≥3 days can be achieved by adding adhesive or by substituting barriers that may disintegrate less rapidly on that individual (e.g., Squibb Stomahesive, Hollister Premium Skin Barrier, Colly-Seel).

The formation of **abdominal hernias** also alters adherence. A girdle with an opening cut for the stoma or a hernia belt manufactured for the ostomate can be used for patient comfort. A faceplate with a flexible adhesive area is usually adequate. A surgical repair of the hernia may be required or elected for some individuals.

All stoma, skin, or contour changes should be assessed by a qualified enterostomal therapist, nurse, or physician to determine comfort, safety, appropriateness of the pouching procedure, and need for surgical revision.

Another type of drainage pouch is the continent ileostomy (Fig. 11A-3). This type of ostomy has a stoma located low in the right quadrant, and fecal material is drained 3 to 4 times a day with a 28 French catheter. A surgically created nipple valve is designed to prevent gas, odor, or stool leakage between intubations. This nipple valve remains closed by the pressure of the contents of the ileal pouch and is opened by insertion of the catheter. Construction of the reservoir is limited to a select group of patients and medical centers because of the complexity of the surgery. Specific information on care of the continent ileostomy should be obtained from the patient if possible, an enterostomal therapist, or a surgeon experienced in caring for this type of ostomy.

URINARY DIVERSION

Framework

The construction of a urinary diversion bypasses the bladder, the storage area of the urinary tract. After bypass, urine drains continually,

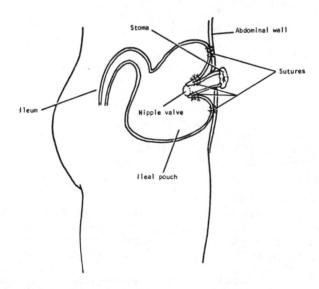

Figure 11A-3. Schematic drawing of a continent ileostomy.

requiring a collection pouch in place at all times. Normal urine is clear yellow, has no odor, and averages 1,500 ml/day.

The most common type of diversion created is the ileal or colon conduit, which is usually located in the right lower quadrant. Figure 11A–4 illustrates the construction of the ileal conduit, in which the surgeon will take a 6- to 8-cm segment of the ileum (or segment of the colon if a colon conduit) to use as a conduit between the ureters and the skin surface. With the peristalsis moving toward the outside, backflow of urine to the kidneys is decreased. Other common diversions are the ureterostomy, in which one or both ureters are brought directly to the skin surface; the vesicostomy, in which the bladder is brought to the abdominal wall and an opening is constructed in the suprapubic region; and the nephrostomy, in which an opening is made directly in the kidney on one or both sides in the lower flank area. Another type of diversion is the continent vesicostomy. This surgery creates an internal urine reservoir that can be emptied by intermittent catheterization during the day. Only a small, select group of patients, those with a completely areflexic bladder, are candidates for this type of surgery.

Management

Proper management of urinary output includes pouching of the stoma for ≥3 days without leakage (*see* procedures for changing appliances outlined above). A pouch containing an antireflux valve will prevent backflow of urine and decrease skin or urinary problems. The opening in the pouch or barrier should be 1/16 to 1/8 in. larger than the stoma so as to avoid skin problems associated with urine contact on skin. Skin barriers (e.g., Bard Coloplast ReliaSeal and Squibb Stomahesive) will aid in adherence and not melt as quickly as karaya in the urinary diversion. Many urinary ostomates can also achieve excellent seals without the use of a skin barrier.

Use of a leg bag during the day and straight drainage at night will prevent urine buildup in the pouch. A bag >1/3 full of urine is more likely to leak and create skin problems or provide a medium for bacteria growth.

Common problems

Dysfunction in consistency/volume/odor.   A change in volume, consistency, or odor of urine may be indicative of problems. A decrease in urine production will be seen when inadequate quantities of fluid are consumed. Urine will appear darker, more concentrated, and have a stronger odor.

Odor in urine can be a result of dietary intake, bacteria, or urine pH. Asparagus is known to cause a distinct urinary odor in the ostomate and nonostomate alike. Infection and an increased number of bacteria

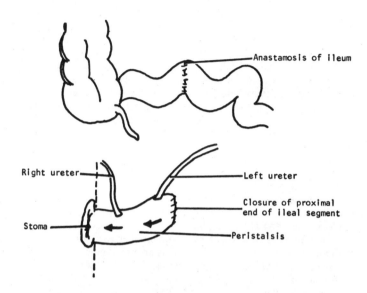

Figure 11A–4. Schematic drawing of the formation of an ileal conduit.

will result in changes in odor and appearance of urine. Because bladder and nerve endings are lacking, the usual signs of urinary tract infections, such as pain, burning, and frequency, will not be present, and the ostomate needs to assess urine periodically for change in odor and appearance. Sterile cultures should be performed to prevent misdiagnosis of infection. As in the case of the nonostomate, if infection is determined, medications will be prescribed.

The following is the procedure for the collection of a sterile urine specimen using the ileal conduit, single-lumen method. Necessary supplies include (1) a standard catheterization kit (14 or 16 French straight catheter); (2) K-Y Jelly and antiseptic solution if not found in kit; (3) warm water, soap, washcloth, and towel; and (4) clean urinary diversion (urostomy) appliance.

1. Gently remove urostomy appliance. (If appliance is permanent, it is not necessary to remove faceplate).
2. Wash stoma and area around it to remove mucus and traces of adhesive.
3. Rinse well with clear water.
4. Open catheterization kit. Proceed to cleanse stoma and skin using sterile technique.

5. Wait for peristalsis of ileal conduit to force urine out of the stoma. This will wash the antiseptic from the stoma.
6. Lubricate catheter.
7. Gently advance catheter 1½ to 2 in. into the stoma and collect urine into a sterile container. (Note: wait for the stoma and conduit to relax before advancing catheter to desired distance).
8. Adhere clean urostomy appliance or pouch according to procedure above or other preferred procedure.

Alkaline urine is a common cause of urine odor and may create a host environment for bacteria growth. Urine pH should be tested periodically and should measure 5.5 to 6.5. Phenaphthazine paper (Nitrazine paper) is used to measure the pH of urine as it falls on the skin, not while on the stoma or in the pouch. Methods for acidifying urine include: ingestion of cranberry juice, administration of 2 to 10 g ascorbic acid (vitamin C) in divided doses during the day, providing an acid-ash diet, and increasing fluids.

Alterations in skin integrity. Skin problems are often associated with alkaline urine and may show up as encrustations or hyperplasia (an overgrowth of skin). Along with acidification of the urine and treatment of infection if present, skin should be treated with daily vinegar-and-water 1:2 soaks of 15 to 30 min. A similar solution can be instilled through the bottom of the pouch to decrease bacterial count in the pouch.

Other skin problems seen in the urinary ostomate are caused by factors similar to those affecting the fecal ostomate, and assessment is made in a similar manner (*see* Table 11A–3).

Urinary appliances should maintain a leak-free seal for ≥3 days. When applying a urinary pouch, the skin should be thoroughly dry, or the seal will not hold. Other considerations involve skin barrier breakdown caused by urine and a poorly fitting appliance. Alterations in adherence also may result from the same causes, described above, as for fecal diversions.

MANAGEMENT OF OTHER DRAINING WOUNDS

Draining wounds, other than those described previously, are managed according to the same concepts. As with fecal diversions, skin protection, odor containment, and drainage collection are the expected outcome of all wound management.

Small draining openings, such as fistulas or Penrose drain sites, may be managed using the techniques described above. As with other fecal diversions, skin should be protected from irritating discharge or chemicals.

Large draining wounds, such as wound dehiscence or abscess, which are not contained with conventional pouches, may require specialized care and creative management from an experienced nurse or enterostomal therapist. Several products for wound containment are available; these provide access to wounds for irrigation or connection to active or passive draining techniques.

Drainage sites located in skin folds or creases, such as suprapubic catheters, can become management problems. The use of additional pastes (karaya, Stomahesive, etc.,) and skin cements may increase adherence and protect surrounding skin.

Bibliography

1. Broadwell, D. C., and B. S. Jackson. Principles of Ostomy Care. C. V. Mosby Co., St. Louis. 1982.

    A complete guide to ostomy and wound care. Contributing authors cover areas related to the role of enterostomal therapy, pathology, and medical management of ostomy-related disease, anatomy and physiology, nursing management, psychosocial issues, age-related issues, and future trends.

2. Goligher, J. C. Alternatives to conventional ileostomy in the surgical treatment of ulcerative colitis. *Journal of Enterostomal Therapy* (May/June 1983). 79–83.

    A descriptive article explaining 4 methods of surgical treatment of ulcerative colitis. Pros and cons of each procedure are presented for the reader.

3. Hill, G. Ileostomy: Surgery, Physiology and Management. Grune & Stratton, New York. 1976.

    A surgical textbook on ileostomy construction. Presents common complications and medical management.

4. Jeter, K. F. Hyperplasia or what? *Journal of Enterostomal Therapy* (September/October 1983). 181–184.

    This article presents and defines common urinary ostomy skin conditions. Using case-study methods, 2 classic situations are presented and appropriate therapy discussed.

5. Kretschner, P. The Intestinal Stoma. Major Problems in Clinical Surgery. Volume 24. W. B. Saunders Co., Philadelphia. 1978.

    A textbook on pathology and surgical procedures involving ostomies. Discusses common postoperative complications and solutions.

6. Taylor, S. V. Meeting the challenge of fistulas and draining wounds. *Nursing '80* (June 1980). 45–51.

A case-study approach to difficult drainage problems. Products are not up-to-date, but the article does contain helpful ideas for a smaller hospital, which may not stock a large variety of equipment.

7. Thielman, D. E. Patient teaching guidelines. *Journal of Enterostomal Therapy* (September/October 1983). 166–168.

The author has provided 4 concise, one-page guidelines for patient teaching after ostomy surgery. Included are colostomy, ileostomy, urinary diversion, and a general guideline for all types of ostomies.

8. Watt, R. Colostomy irrigation yes or no? *American Journal of Nursing* (October 1974). 1806–1811.

A complete article on irrigation including the pros and cons of colostomy irrigation.

9. Watt, R. Ostomies; why, how and where: an overview. *Nursing Clinics of North America* (September 1976). 427–444.

A classic article that provides a general overview of ostomy management.

B: FUNCTIONAL ALTERATIONS — BOWEL
Jody Gross

Constipation and diarrhea are alterations in bowel function that frequently occur in hospitalized patients, including certain groups of cancer patients. As diarrhea most commonly has an adverse effect upon the nutritional status of the patient, it has been discussed in detail in Chapter 8; this section will focus on constipation. Methods usually employed to treat constipation are inconsistently implemented and are geared to episodic rather than prophylactic management. No standard accepted regimen or protocol is used in practice, with the result that many patients suffer discomfort, take numerous laxative doses, and may require enemas or other invasive procedures to reestablish normal bowel habits. Patients prone to constipation are easily identified, and measures should be instituted to prevent changes in bowel habits, because resolution of constipation is a more difficult task — time-consuming and uncomfortable for both the patient and the nurse.

Pathophysiology

Defecation is a complex process that involves several intrinsic and extrinsic reflex mechanisms and the action of both voluntary and involuntary muscles. Activities such as food ingestion initiate, via the myenteric plexus, the gastrocolic reflex. This reflex, and others at various GI tract junctures that are intrinsic to the GI tract — such as the duodenocolic and jejunocolic reflexes — result in a mass movement that propels fecal matter into the rectum. Mass movements, peristaltic waves that arise in the colon, occur 3 to 4 times a day and are strongest during the first hour after eating breakfast. When enough stool has collected in the rectum to exceed the threshold of stimulation, receptors in the rectum initiate the defecation reflex by transmitting afferent impulses through the myenteric plexus and to the spinal cord and the brain. The myenteric plexus initiates further peristaltic waves, and spinal cord reflexes intensify these peristaltic motions — which are weak without CNS augmentation — and cause contraction of the rectal musculature and relaxation of the internal anal sphincter. The impulses to the brain arouse awareness of the urge to stool and lead to voluntary contraction of the external anal sphincter. If the individual does not allow defecation to proceed, there is a decrease in the intensity of the urge, the reflex dies out, and it will usually not return until more feces have entered the rectum. Continual ignoring of the call to stool will result in diminished sensitivity of the rectum, so the arrival of more feces or further peristaltic mass movements fail to initiate defecation. As feces remain in the colon and rectum, water is continually absorbed across the wall of the gut, so that the stool is further compacted and hardened. Though more stool is required to initiate defecation, the stool already present in the rectum has become hard, dry, and small.

When defecation is allowed to proceed, the most physiologically comfortable position is squatting, with hamstring muscles in the thigh contracted. The glottis is closed, the diaphragm and abdominal muscles contracted, and voluntary cortical inhibition of the external anal sphincter ceases. These actions serve to increase intra-abdominal and intrathoracic pressures and relax the anal sphincter, allowing stool to pass. This process normally occurs between 3 times/day and 3 times/wk in 98% of the population.

Assessment

Constipation may be defined as the passage of hard, dry stools, associated with an undue amount of straining, which may be decreased in frequency and may leave the patient with a sensation of incomplete evacuation. Consistency of stool and the degree of difficulty in defecation are objective signs of the constipated state, and both should be in evidence when patients are diagnosed as constipated. Decreased frequency of bowel movement is subjective and probably irrelevant because the range of normal frequency is so great. Frequency and feelings of rectal fullness are issues of great concern to patients, however, and should be dealt with as part of treatment. Rectal fullness may also indicate underlying disease, such as hemorrhoids, prolapsed rectal mucosa, or tumor, and should be investigated. Constipation can be classified by physiologic and pathologic causes.

Primary constipation. This condition exists without any underlying organic disease. It may be self-induced by a decreased intake of food or dietary fiber; lack of exercise; or ignoring the call to stool. Decreased stool bulk from decreased intake may contribute to constipation by two mechanisms: by decreasing the GI motility and peristalsis associated with a full gut, and by lack of stimulation of sensory receptors in the rectum and initiation of the defecation reflex. Lack of exercise leads to a decrease in GI tract motility and in the muscle tone needed to generate adequate intra-abdominal pressure for defecation. Environmental factors may also cause the individual to ignore the urge to defecate; these factors include poor or inaccessible toilet facilities, conditions that prevent answering the call to stool, and hospitalization, which interrupts normal routines and affects activity and food and fluid intake.

Motility disorders. Diverticular disease, irritable bowel syndrome, idiopathic slow transit, and other conditions that may cause hypomotility may be the cause of constipation.

Psychiatric conditions. Emotional states can have a profound effect upon the GI tract. Disorders in which constipation is often a presenting symptom include anorexia nervosa and depression, because these conditions are associated with decreased mobility, food intake, and muscle tone.

Known organic disease. This condition is not as common as primary constipation. Constipation may occur as a presenting symptom of bowel carcinoma. Hemorrhoids, anal fissures, and perianal abscesses cause pain or difficulty with defecation, so the individual suppresses the call to stool. Other GI or pelvic diseases may interfere with defecation reflexes. Neurologic conditions, such as spinal cord or cerebral injuries, tumors, or metastases, may give rise to severe constipation by interfering with the extrinsic innervation of the gut. Hypercalcemia, by disturbing the electrophysiology of colon muscle; dehydration, by causing hardened feces and decreased fecal mass in the rectum; fluid and electrolyte imbalances, which interfere with absorptive processes and gut musculature; and debility associated with impaired metabolism and nutrition and generalized weakness may all contribute to constipation.

Medical and surgical treatment. Constipation may be related to drugs, including aluminum- and calcium-containing antacids, because these ions are constipating; narcotics, which bind to receptors in the myenteric plexus as well as in the CNS and prevent peristaltic waves; and anticonvulsants, antidepressants, anesthetics, and other drugs that act on the CNS or affect transmission of nerve impulses. Furthermore, patients receiving cytotoxic therapy with vinca alkaloids, particularly vincristine, may experience constipation or obstipation as well as peripheral neuropathies.

Other iatrogenic causes include fluid depletion and decreased food intake resulting from treatment for disease, such as chemotherapy, radiation therapy (RT), and diagnostic procedures. Lack of physical activity because of immobilization and hospitalization or surgical trauma, which may halt peristalsis, also interferes with maintenance of normal bowel function. Bedpan use may contribute to constipation because the patient may suppress the urge to defecate if a bedpan is not readily available. Evacuation on a bedpan is a difficult and uncomfortable process, because the patient cannot assume the normal squatting position. Attempting the passage of a normal bowel movement on a bedpan is usually unsuccessful, increasing the tendency toward constipation as well as exhausting the patient and endangering his cardiovascular status. Oxygen consumption increases when a bedpan is used rather than a commode or toilet, and intrathoracic pressure may be raised enough to be classified as a Valsalva maneuver (>40 mmHg for >8 sec). If a patient is already constipated, attempts to defecate using a bedpan may result in Valsalva maneuvers in $>50\%$ of straining episodes.

The presence of thrombocytopenia and leukopenia enhances the dangers of constipation for the patient. In the patient prone to bleeding, Valsalva maneuvers performed while straining at stool may increase intracranial pressure, and this may be the causative event in producing a retinal or potentially fatal cerebral hemorrhage. Perirectal abscesses account for ~25% of infections in patients with acute leukemia and can occur in patients who are leukopenic as a result of cytotoxic therapy. The presence of any abnormality of bowel function — whether diarrhea or constipation — that increases the likelihood of rectal mucosal tears or irritation increases the risk of infection at this site. These risks are compounded for the patient suffering from mucositis as a result of cytotoxic therapy.

Medical management

Many agents exist to treat constipation. Currently, >700 different over-the-counter laxative preparations are available in the USA. The majority of preparations are divided into four categories of laxatives. Table 11B-1 lists common agents, doses, and onset of action.

TABLE 11B–1

Laxative Dosages and Onset of Action

Agent	Usual dose	Onset of action (hours)
Bulk producers		
Bran	10 g/1 tb	12–24
Cellulose derivatives	1–3 tb, 1–3 times/day	
Calcium polycarbophil	1–4 tablets, 1–4 times/day	
Saline laxatives		
milk of magnesia	15 ml	3–6
magnesium citrate	200 ml	
Epsom salts	15 g	
lactulose	15–60 ml	24–48
Stimulant laxatives		
bisacodyl	10 mg	6–10
senna		
powder	2 g	6–10
syrup	8 ml	6–10
cascara extract	300 mg	6–10
bisacodyl suppository	10 mg	¼–1

tb, tablespoon.

Bulk producers. Bulk producers are hydrophilic agents that absorb significant quantities of water in the gut, consequently softening as well as increasing the size of the stool. Peristaltic waves, though initiated by intrinsic reflexes, are also stimulated by adequate quantities of fecal matter in the bowel lumen. The best source of bulk is dietary fiber, most commonly bran, a substance often lacking in the diet of many Americans. A decrease to approximately half the former number of laxative doses after an increase in dietary fiber has been noted among geriatric patients on regular diets. The inclusion of anywhere from 10 to 20 g of bran in the daily diet has been shown to have a positive effect on evacuation, though it remains difficult to establish the minimum amount of dietary fiber to treat constipation. Fiber content of foods is determined as either crude or dietary. Crude fiber content in food is determined by measuring the cellulose and lignin content of foods remaining after boiling in acid and alkaline solutions. Dietary fiber consists of the cellulose, lignin, and other polysaccharides that are not digested by the small intestine; 20 g of crude fiber $\cong$ 60 g of dietary fiber. There are a multitude of high-fiber foods from many sources including whole wheat bread (9.5 g fiber/100 g of food), all-bran cereals (26.7), peanuts (9.3) and peanut butter (7.5), unpeeled pears (8.6), and peas (7.9).

If bran in therapeutic quantities is unpalatable, polysaccharides and cellulose derivatives, such as psyllium (Metamucil) or calcium polycarbophil (Mitrolan), may be employed. The dosage range of psyllium is 1 to 3 teaspoons, 1 to 3 times/day, adjusted to the individual's needs. Metamucil contains dextrose as a dispersing agent so there is little danger of bolus formation in the gut if it is taken with adequate quantities of fluid. Fluid intake must be sufficient to deal with the increase in bulk, or water will be pulled across the colonic mucosa from the extracellular fluid. Intake of fluids in all forms should be ~3,000 ml/day. Occasionally, bulk producers may cause flatulence or abdominal cramping. These side effects may be decreased or avoided by the gradual introduction of these agents into the diet and by use of divided doses. Dietary fiber should be ingested at every meal and other bulking agents given therapeutically 1 to 4 times/day.

Stool softeners and lubricants. These agents, the most common being mineral oil and dioctyl sodium sulfosuccinate (DSS), lubricate and soften the stool. Mineral oil is infrequently used, because it results in unpleasant seepage from the rectum and may cause lipid pneumonia, especially in a debilitated and bedridden patient. If mineral oil is used, for example in resolution of fecal impaction, the patient should be instructed to sit up for several hours after ingestion of the oil. DSS is a surface-active agent with detergent properties that allows water to penetrate the feces and increases the permeability of the gut mucosa. DSS may affect intestinal absorption adversely and is best used as a temporary measure in patients with hard stools. These agents do not increase GI motility, and bulk producers are probably as effective in softening stool. DSS has been shown to be ineffective in altering the incidence of constipation among elderly medical patients.

Osmotic or saline laxatives. Saline laxatives, including Epsom salts, milk of magnesia, and other sodium, magnesium, and potassium salts, are unabsorbed solutes that retain water in the small bowel and increase the flow of fluid into the colon. Their cathartic effect is unpleasant and may lead to excessive absorption of cations by the bowel. These agents do not encourage a return to normal bowel function and are most useful as preparative agents for diagnostic tests and in prophylaxis of hepatic coma.

Lactulose is a synthetic disaccharide for which no corresponding disaccharidase exists in the small bowel, so lactulose enters the colon unmetabolized. It is acted upon by colonic bacteria to produce an osmotic catharsis. It is effective in the treatment of vincristine- or narcotic-induced constipation that has not been resolved with use of other agents or interventions.

Chemical stimulants.   These agents include castor oil — whose violent cathartic action should preclude its use — and the anthraquinone and polyphenolic compounds. The most common anthraquinones are senna (Senokot) and cascara. The polyphenolics are usually represented by bisacodyl (Dulcolax). These compounds are effective but should be used with caution because they are habit-forming, can lead to electrolyte disturbances and histiologic changes in the bowel, and can cause myenteric plexus degeneration after prolonged use. Bisacodyl is active only in the colon, where it increases peristalsis by stimulating sensory nerves. It must not be administered with alkali, such as antacids, which cause activation of the agent in the small intestine. Senna and cascara are also active only in the colon after interaction with colonic bacteria. Because of their specific site of action these agents are recommended for general use as a temporary measure, in the minimal effective dose. Both substances are available as oral and rectal agents. Prunes contain a phenolic substance and should be considered as therapeutic agents for their laxative effect.

Suppositories and enemas.   Agents that are administered per rectum have not been discussed here because it is felt their use should be avoided in cancer patients. Many cancer patients receive treatments that cause myelosuppression, a condition that precludes the use of enemas and suppositories because of the risk of perirectal infection or hemorrhage. An effective method of treating constipation should incorporate agents that may be used at any time, with as little ill effect as possible. It should be noted, however, that suppositories may act mechanically by stimulating sensory receptors in the rectum. If indicated, glycerine suppositories may be a useful stimulus to defecation when no further laxative action is warranted.

Nursing management

A comprehensive bowel program for cancer patients susceptible to constipation is presented in Table 11B-2. This program advocates a preventive approach as the best method of treating constipation, which may be a long-term problem.

The protocol should be applied with caution to patients who have GI disease, bowel obstruction, or who are unable to tolerate a significant amount of bulk-producing agents. Program modifications may be made for patients with disease involving the spinal cord. Patients with a history of constipation should first embark upon a retraining program that may include mineral oil and judicious use of enemas and suppositories and that can be based on the format presented in Table 11B-2. Once the patient is retrained, the prophy-

TABLE 11B–2

Nursing Protocol for Prophylactic Bowel Management

Problem	Intervention
Maintenance of adequate bulk and softness of stool	Provide a high-fiber diet; include approximately 5–10 g of dietary fiber daily. Ensure adequate fluid intake of ~3 liters daily. If needed, administer other bulk producers, such as cellulose derivatives or calcium polycarbophil, in recommended dosages.
Encouragement of normal bowel function	Ensure adequate physical activity to maintain abdominal and other muscle tone and promote GI tract motility: consult with physical therapist in development of program of light exercise; if patient is bedridden, schedule bed exercises. Use toilet or bedside commode for all bowel movements; avoid bedpan use. Provide footstool if raised toilet seat is necessary. Plan bowel movements for same time each day. Provide hot drink approximately ½ hour before planned defecation to stimulate gastrocolic reflex.
Ensuring bowel movement q 3 days	Add prunes to diet; give in evening for laxative effect in morning, in morning for laxative effect in evening. Provide laxative agents for patients who do not establish or maintain routine habits: magnesia, bisacodyl, or senna; lactulose for patients receiving vincristine or high doses of narcotic analgesics.

lactic approach of the program should prevent recurrence of constipation. Cancer patients previously identified as being at risk for
constipation or whose condition is threatened by leukopenia or
thrombocytopenia and who are not in the excluded categories listed
above may all use this program.

Monitoring patients on a prophylactic bowel program includes
assessing daily dietary fiber, calorie, and fluid intake, medications,

performance status, frequency and consistency of stools, and the number of laxative doses given.

Successful implementation of the program should result in decrease in the need for laxatives and other interventions, easy passage of a soft, formed stool ≥q 3 days, and fewer complaints of discomfort or constipation.

Though developed for hospitalized patients, this protocol can easily be used by the patient for home management of constipation. All therapeutic agents used, with the exception of lactulose, are available without a prescription. As an aspect of preventive self-care, this program presents an excellent opportunity for nurses to engage in patient teaching.

Bibliography

1. Avery-Jones, F., and E. Godding, editors. Management of Constipation. Blackwell Scientific, London. 1972.

    A comprehensive discussion of constipation, including colon physiology, etiology, and management of constipation.

2. Benton, J., H. Brown, and H. Rush. Energy expended by patients on the bedpan and bedside commode. *Journal of the American Medical Association* (December 23, 1950). 1443–1447.

    Interesting study that documents increased energy consumption during bedpan usage.

3. Fingl, E. Laxatives and cathartics. *In* Goodman, L. S., and A. Gilman, editors. The Pharmacological Basis of Therapeutics. Macmillan, Inc., New York. 1980. Sixth edition.

    Excellent review of therapeutic agents used in management of constipation.

4. Guyton, A. Textbook of Medical Physiology. W. B. Saunders Co., Philadelphia. 1976.

    Sections contain discussions of normal bowel physiology and pathophysiology of constipation.

5. Halpern, A., N. Shaftel, D. Selman, H. Shaftel, P. Kuhn, S. Samuels, and H. Bird. The straining forces of bowel function. *Angiology* (October 1960). 426–436.

    Another study that documents effects of constipation, specifically the increase in intrathoracic pressures during straining.

6. Klein, H. Constipation and fecal impaction. *Medical Clinics of North America* (September 1982). 1135–1141.

    A short review of etiology, symptomatology, and medical management of constipation and impaction.

7. Pollman, J., J. Morris, and P. Rose. Is fiber the answer to constipation in the elderly? A review of the literature. *International Journal of Nursing Studies* (No. 3, 1978). 107–114.

A survey of articles on constipation in the elderly and various interventions used to manage this problem.

C: FUNCTIONAL ALTERATIONS — BLADDER

Glee I. Wahlquist

Persons with a urinary dysfunction deviate from cultural norms and may suffer shame, embarrassment, depression, and isolation. The significance of this problem to the patient and family warrants a total approach to the symptoms associated with urinary dysfunction and their related sequelae. Urinary dysfunction, including incontinence, is not a normal state and should not be treated as such by the nurse. Careful assessment and development of an appropriate care plan based upon predetermined goals result in sound management.

Framework

Voiding is incompletely understood. It is a complex reflex that is controlled by the bladder and the spinal cord. The bladder, consisting of smooth muscle, fills passively until it contains ~150 ml. As the bladder continues to fill with urine, its intrinsic tone is exceeded. When the increased pressure exceeds a threshold value, stretch receptors in the bladder wall are stimulated and initiate the micturition reflex via parasympathetic nerve fibers. The parasympathetic afferent (sensory) fibers enter the sacral cord segments at S–2, S–3, and S–4. Efferent (motor) fibers pass from S–2, S–3, and S–4 as preganglionic fibers to the hypogastric plexus, from which they emerge to innervate the bladder. The micturition reflex causes a contraction in the wall of the bladder. If urination does not occur, the contraction will die out, and bladder pressure will drop. The reflex may not occur again for a few minutes to ~1 hr. Strength and frequency of contractions increase as the bladder continues to fill, however. The trigonal muscle of the bladder, which maintains tonic closure of the urethra, allows urine to pass when bladder pressure is high enough to overcome the pressure of the muscle. For this reason, this muscle is referred to as the internal sphincter of the bladder.

The micturition reflex is an automatic cord reflex, but numerous feedback loops in the cortex and brainstem provide facilitation and inhibition of micturition. The micturition reflex is partially inhibited by these higher centers until urination is desired. This inhibition is accomplished by maintenance of the tonic contraction of the external urinary sphincter, the urogenital diaphragm. When voiding is appropriate, cortical fibers facilitate sacral nerves to initiate a micturition reflex and inhibit the tonic contraction of the external sphincter, allowing relaxation of the sphincter and related perineal musculature and emptying of the bladder. Voiding should be in a steady stream and last ~1 min. The adult bladder empties ~q 4 to 6 hr, with the average 24-hr volume being 1 to 2 liters. The total 24-hr volume should not fall <500 ml.

Voluntary urinary function may be prevented by one of three types of pathophysiologic processes: total incontinence, failure to fill, and failure to empty.

Total incontinence. Associated with an uninhibited bladder, this is the most common type of urinary dysfunction, resulting in uncontrollable urination. The condition is caused by cortical or brainstem damage that interrupts the inhibiting neurons that prevent micturition. Because the sacral nerves are continually excited, the smallest amount of urine that stimulates the micturition reflex will cause urination. This problem may be seen in cancer patients with brain metastases with bilateral hemispheric involvement.

Failure to fill. This condition is caused by a reflex, or upper motor neuron, bladder. Here, the reflex arc to and from the spinal cord remains intact, but voluntary control is lost because of cord dysfunction (upper motor neuron lesions) above S–2, S–3, and S–4. As a result, micturition is uncontrolled by inhibiting and facilitating impulses from the brain, and the patient voids small amounts with moderate residual volumes.

Failure to empty. Flaccid bladder occurs when the sensory or motor nerve fibers leading to and from the bladder and the spinal cord are destroyed (lower motor neuron lesions). As micturition reflexes are not initiated, the bladder does not empty but continues to fill.

Overflow dribbling: The bladder may overflow small amounts of urine through the urethra. This occurs in cases of spinal cord compression, or after radiation (RT) or surgery that involves sacral segments or nerves leading to and from the bladder.

Abdominal surgery, RT, spinal cord tumor, and primary or metastatic tumor are variables frequently associated with voiding dysfunction. In some cases, the actual voiding problem may be the first indication of a lesion.

Assessment

When the patient has urinary incontinence, inability to void, dribbling, or frequent urinary tract infection, a careful assessment is indicated. The assessment involves three areas: factors that are likely to affect rehabilitation, careful history, and bedside examination.

Rehabilitation potential.   Because a great deal of teaching is involved in bladder retraining, the patient's ability and motivation to learn must be assessed and an evaluation made of the home situation, including the ability and willingness of the family to become involved in a bladder management program. Assessment is made of the patient's physical condition, especially whether he possesses the coordination and strength necessary to maneuver to the toilet or manipulate a catheter. The prognosis of the underlying disease will affect the feasibility of embarking upon a rehabilitation effort.

History.   A history, concentrating on those areas of concern in evaluating urinary dysfunction, should be elicited from the patient. These areas include:

1. prior incidence and pattern of urinary tract infection;
2. problems associated with incontinence, i.e., urgency, frequency, urge incontinence, nocturia;
3. present method of managing any existing urinary dysfunction including catheter, appliance, or padding;
4. present method of voiding, i.e., normal, strain, sitting, standing, manual abdominal pressure (Credé);
5. past medical history that may be involved in the present bladder problem.

Bedside examination.   Bedside examination should focus on establishing bladder and related neurologic functioning. Intactness of sensation in the sacral segments (perianal and posterior leg area) should be tested using a wisp of cotton and gentle pressure with a sharp pin. All areas should be tested. The patient should be able to feel sensation on the posterior portion of both legs and in the sacral area. Insertion of a gloved, lubricated finger into the patient's rectum should produce a motor "grab" response as the muscle contracts around the finger. A flaccid anal sphincter indicates interruption in reflexes from the cord. In the presence of some cord lesions, it is possible to have sensation intact and motor component absent. In this case, the patient would have the desire to void but be unable to empty. To make an accurate measure of residual urine volume, the patient should be asked to void. Catheterization immediately after voiding will establish the amount of urine left in the bladder. If possible, the head of the bed should be elevated. When urine flow ceases, the catheter is then removed slowly, pausing every few cm to allow urine remaining in the bladder to be collected. Both voided and catheterized amounts should be measured separately and the percentage of residual urine determined as well. The catheterized specimen may be sent to the laboratory for urinalysis, culture and sensitivity, and cytology, if appropriate. Table 11C–1 presents a useful format for summarizing assessment.

TABLE 11C–1
Bladder Dysfunction History Guide

Name	Age	Sex	Hospital number	Date
History				
Medications		Method of voiding		

Presence or lack of symptoms

— nocturia	— enuresis	— impotence
— frequency	— retention	— burning
— urgency	— intermittency	— hematuria
— incontinence	— hesitancy	

Urinalysis Cytology (as indicated)	Culture	Residual volume

Examination
  Mental status:

  Sensation perianal:

Reflexes:		BC	KJ	AJ	Bab
	R				
	L				

CMG:	IVP
Impression	Plan

AJ, ankle jerk; Bab, Babinski's sign; BC, biceps contraction; CMG, cystometrogram; IVP, IV pyelogram; KJ, knee jerk.
Adapted from Krane, M. J., and M. B. Siroky, editors. Clinical Neuro-Urology. Little, Brown & Co., Boston. 1979. p. 54.

Medical management

If residual urinary volumes are >70 to 100 ml, the patient is prone to develop bacteriuria. Evaluation of the nervous system control of bladder function is made by cystometrogram, which measures the strength of the muscular contraction initiated by the micturition reflex. The bladder itself will be examined by cystoscope, and in males, the prostate will be palpated. Because patient cooperation is needed to perform the cystometrogram test, the patient does not receive a general anesthetic. After testing, mild hematuria, burning, and urgency caused by instrumentation may occur. The patient should be instructed as to the symptoms of urinary tract infection (i.e., frequency, burning, urgency at urination) in the unlikely event that this occurs. An IV pyelogram may be performed to assess kidney and ureter function.

Nursing management

Regardless of the cause or nature of the urinary dysfunction, there are two goals for nursing care of persons with voiding dysfunction: to restore or maintain urinary continence or develop socially acceptable alternatives; and to prevent the development of urinary tract infection (Table 11C–2).

Continence.   For patients with uninhibited bladder, retraining using timed voidings, in which the nurse monitors fluid intake and at scheduled times toilets the patient, and reduction of fluid prior to sleep may succeed in maintaining dryness. In patients incontinent because of brain metastases, padding for both male and female are acceptable alternatives. For the male, condom catheter drainage may also be employed, especially during sleep. Those patients experiencing failure to fill may achieve continence through treatment with anticholinergic agents, such as oxybutynin chloride (Ditropan) or propantheline bromide (Pro-Banthine), which decrease bladder spasticity. In others with upper motor neuron bladder, dryness is achieved by using anticholinergic medication in combination with intermittent catheterization. In these patients, continence is achieved by anticholinergic administration until the patient cannot void, and he then catheterizes himself as would the patient with flaccid bladder. For some, padding— or a condom catheter for males — will still be required.

For patients with flaccid bladder, intermittent catheterization is the recommended choice for maintaining dryness. Other methods, including straining or Credé (manual pressure above the bladder), should not be conducted unless approved by a physician, because these techniques tend to force urine into the ureters and may leave unacceptable residual volumes.

TABLE 11C–2

Nursing Protocol for Care of the Patient with Urinary Dysfunction

Factor	Intervention

Maintenance or restoration of continence	Utilize techniques appropriate to type of dysfunction:
	    total incontinence (uninhibited): timed voidings; use of condom catheter or padding; decreasing of HS fluid.
	    failure to fill (reflex): administration of anticholinergic agents; use of intermittent catheterization; use of condom catheter or padding.
	    failure to empty (flaccid): intermittent catheterization.

Prevention of infection	Make certain the bladder empties completely.
	Provide frequent times for bladder emptying.
	Maintain an intake-and-output record.
	Maintain acid urinary pH (<7):
	    avoid foods producing alkaline urine or urinary residue, i.e., citrus fruits;
	    measure urinary pH $\geq$ q day.
	Avoid the use of indwelling catheters whenever possible.

HS, at bedtime.

Infection.   Complete emptying will remove 99.9% of bacteria present in urine; however, 0.1% will theoretically remain. These small numbers of organisms are diluted by a fresh flow of urine, so that numbers decrease rapidly if the bladder is emptied frequently and completely. Some authorities also postulate that overextension diminishes the bladder's blood flow and, ultimately, leads to the development of bacteriuria.

Bacteria multiply logarithmically, and with 100 ml of residual volume, the bacterial doubling time will be ~1 hr. Thus, in 2 hr the rate of growth has exceeded inflow of urine and by 4 hr the growth is almost 4 times that of inflow, so that the patient will not be able to remove bacteria by voiding.

Catheters.   **Indwelling catheters** should be avoided in the long-term management of urinary dysfunction. The use of these devices is associated with bacteriuria, febrile urinary tract infection, and sepsis.

For each day the indwelling catheter remains, the chance of bacteriuria increases 5 to 10%. In addition, indwelling catheters may lead to the development of renal calculi, penoscrotal fistulas, and hematuria. In spite of complications arising from the use of indwelling catheters, there remain instances in which this method of treatment is useful. These include situations where (1) intermittent catheterization is not feasible (e.g., for the patient who has impairments of upper extremities, memory, or motivation and whose family is not able to assist); (2) surgery to relieve obstruction is contraindicated; (3) measuring output accurately is essential and the patient is not able to assist in this task; and (4) bladder filling is not desired (e.g., in certain postoperative situations). In the event the patient requires an indwelling catheter, a nursing care plan is presented in Table 11C-3.

TABLE 11C-3
Nursing Protocol for Care of the Patient with an Indwelling Catheter

Factor	Intervention
Prevention of trauma	During procedure: use generous amounts of lubricant; do not force catheter; use smallest size catheter possible.
	Secure catheter to the abdomen in males to prevent rubbing of the penis at the scrotal junction, thereby preventing fistula formation; to the thigh in females so it does not pull when taped.
Prevention of infection	Keep the drainage system closed at all times. Obtain specimens using the needle aspiration port. Change entire system if opened. Keep the drainage bag below the level of the bladder at all times. Ensure adequate fluid intake; keep accurate intake-and-output record. Keep the urinary meatus clean. Maintain urine acidity. When crystals form in the drainage tube, change the entire system. Remove the catheter as soon as is possible.

Intermittent catheterization is preferred to the use of the indwelling urinary catheters because it is associated with a reduction in the incidence of urinary tract infection and other sequelae. Nursing actions associated with use of this method of catheterization are presented in Table 11C–4.

If the patient's potential for rehabilitation is good, he should be taught to catheterize himself. Providing self-care in urinary elimination encourages independence and inclusion in normal daily activities. Because incomplete emptying, rather than introduction of a catheter, is believed to lead to bacteriuria, self-catheterization does not require sterile technique; it is therefore easily accomplished at home by patients with adequate coordination and motivation. Table 11C–5 describes the necessary steps in teaching clean catheterization.

A printed self-catheterization guide can be prepared for patients. In addition to particulars about the catheterization procedure and care of equipment, information about purchase of catheters, times of catheterization, medications, fluid balance sheets, and indications for calling the nurse or physician should be included.

TABLE 11C–4

Nursing Protocol for Care of the Patient
Using Intermittent Catheterization

Factor	Intervention
Maintenance of continence	Monitor intake and output. Catheterize q 4–6 hr depending on volume obtained. Monitor intake. Do not let bladder become overdistended (>300 ml).
Prevention of infection	Institute bacterial surveillance: Obtain a dip slide or a sterile specimen for culture and sensitivity q wk. (Dip slides are inexpensive [~$1.00] in comparison to cultures [~$10.00].)
Promotion of independence	Teach patient to catheterize himself. Use protective garments as necessary, especially during sleep.

Discharge planning.   Health teaching prior to discharge, regard-less of the type of bladder dysfunction, should include (1) the importance of regular, frequent emptying of the bladder; (2) accurate planning of intake and output; (3) the signs of bacteriuria and urinary tract infection, which should be reported to care-givers; and (4) the correct use of appliances or treatments.

Bibliography

1. Felder, L. Neurogenic bladder dysfunction. *Journal of Neurosurgical Nursing* (June 1979). 94–105.

   Provides a clear, concise review of related physiology, commonly employed diagnostic studies, classification of dysfunction, and nursing care.

2. American Association of Urology Allied. Intermittent self-catheterization (procedure for teaching). *AAUA Journal* (January-March 1982). 18–22.

   Explicitly describes the method for teaching self-catheterization to males and females.

3. Krane, R. J., and M. B. Siroky, editors, Clinical Neuro-Urology. Little, Brown, & Co., Boston. 1979.

   Probably the most thorough text dealing with these problems. Chapters are written by well-known experts; bibliographical material is extensive.

4. Lapides, J., A. Diokno, F. Gould, and B. Lowe. Further observations on self-catheterization. *Journal of Urology* (August 1976). 169–171.

   Presents results of a study using clean intermittent catheterization for a variety of courses. Procedures developed in conjunction with nurse Betty Lowe are presented here and earlier studies cited.

5. Platt, R., F. Polk, B. Murdock, and B. Rosner. Mortality associated with nosocomial urinary-tract infection. *New England Journal of Medicine* (September 9, 1982). 637–642.

   Excellent description of serious complications arising from catheter-associated urinary-tract infections.

6. Stamm, W. E. Guidelines for prevention of catheter-associated urinary tract infections. *Annals of Internal Medicine* (March 1975). 386–389.

   Contains Center for Disease Control guidelines for care of patients with indwelling urinary catheters.

7. Wahlquist, G. Intermittent catheterization: can it be used with persons experiencing cancer? *Oncology Nursing Forum* (Winter 1980). 16–19.

   Discusses the rationale for the use of intermittent catheterization, with a case study.

TABLE 11C-5
Procedure for Clean Catheterization*‡

Female[§]	Male
1. If possible, wash your hands. (Catheterization should *not* be postponed because you cannot wash your hands or your perineum; the risk of infection from retained urine is too great.)	1. If possible, wash your hands. (Catheterization should *not* be postponed because you cannot wash your hands or your penis; the risk of infection from retained urine is too great.)
2. Sit on a table, with your feet on the table and your knees flexed apart.	2. Sit on a chair or toilet with your feet on the floor. If you are uncircumcised, retract your foreskin for the rest of the procedure.
3. With a well-lighted mirror, identify your vagina, clitoris, and urethral meatus (Fig. 11C–1).	3. Using a washcloth, soap, and water, thoroughly wash the end of your penis.
4. Separate your vaginal folds. Using a washcloth, soap, and water, thoroughly wash the exposed area with downward strokes.	4. Place some lubricant on a paper towel and use this to lubricate the first 7–10 in. of the catheter.
5. Place some lubricant on a paper towel and use this to lubricate the first 3 in. of the catheter. With the hand you normally use for skilled tasks, hold the catheter as you would a pencil or a dart. Hold the catheter on the unlubricated part.	5. With the hand you normally use for skilled tasks, hold the catheter as you would a pencil or a dart. Hold the catheter on the unlubricated part.
6. While using the index and ring fingers of your other hand to separate your labia, press (locate) your urethral meatus with the middle finger.	6. Hold your penis at a right angle to your body and slowly insert the catheter 7–10 in., until urine begins to flow steadily (Fig. 11C–2).

[Continued on p. 362]

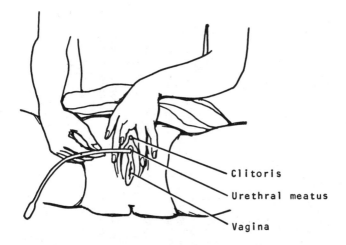

Figure 11C–1.   Self-catheterization — female.

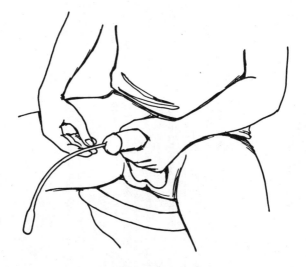

Figure 11C–2.   Self-catheterization — male.

[Continued from p. 360]

7. Raise your middle finger and insert the catheter ~3 in. into your urethra until urine begins to flow steadily (see Fig. 11C–1).

8. After all urine has drained, carefully and slowly remove the catheter.

9. Wash and soak the used catheter in warm, soapy water. Then rinse it inside and outside, dry it, and place it in a clean plastic bag for future use.

7. After all urine has drained, carefully and slowly remove the catheter.

8. Wash and soak the used catheter in warm, soapy water. Then rinse it inside and outside, dry it, and place it in a clean plastic bag for future use.

* This table is intended to assist the nurse with teaching the patient clean catheterization. It is suggested that the nurse (1) perform the procedure, explaining the various steps to the patient, (2) have the patient perform the procedure, in the nurse's presence, explaining the various steps to the nurse, and (3) once the patient demonstrates competence, allow the patient to perform the procedure in private.

‡ This procedure should be performed in a well-lighted area. Necessary equipment includes rubber catheter, water-soluble lubricant, paper towel, plastic bag for used catheter, and receptacle (e.g., toilet) for urine collection. Optional equipment includes washcloth, soap, and water.

§ If the female patient lacks perineal sensation, she should probably always perform this procedure with a mirror reflecting her perineum. If perineal sensation is present, and if the patient is proficient at self-catheterization, she can use the touch technique, which provides more freedom and flexibility because mirrors and lights are not necessary.

CHAPTER 12

SEXUALITY

Susan Gross Fisher

Standard: The client and partner can identify aspects of sexuality that may be threatened by disease and can enumerate ways of maintaining sexual identity.

Outcome criteria: Client and partner
1. identify potential or actual alterations in perception of sexuality or sexual function.
2. identify alternate methods of expressing sexuality.

Throughout history, sexual attitudes and sexual behaviors have engendered social and political controversy. Sex has been associated with procreation, morality, love, homosexuality, pleasure, sin, marriage, aggression, and money. Governments, churches, and individuals have attempted at various times to deny and/or control the sexual practices of others. Cyclic struggles between sexual repression and expression have resulted in widespread ambivalence and conflict within society.

Recently, however, there has been systematic scientific inquiry into human sexuality. Society's increasing sexual awareness and tolerance has led to increased sexual knowledge, a less judgmental approach, and greater sexual satisfaction among individuals. Sexuality remains, however, a very personal issue, often involved with religious belief and philosophical tenets. Sexual expression, therefore, continues to reflect human individuality in this contemporary world.

Sexuality, now considered an integral aspect of people in states of illness as well as health, may greatly affect the quality of life. In the field of oncology, health-care providers now realize that sexual health care must be investigated and integrated into the care of cancer patients. Increasingly, successful antitumor therapy offers both longer survival and improved quality of life for oncology patients. Health-care providers must look to the patient for direction in establishing priorities of goals and objectives. The significance of sexual issues will vary with each individual, and therefore a unique approach is required for each patient's care.

Many illnesses affect sexuality. The diagnosis of cancer, however, imposes a special threat because of its complex impact on the physical, emotional, and social aspects of the individual as a sexual being.

Pathophysiology

Human sexuality is the complex dimension of maleness or femaleness in personality; it develops from and is nurtured by biologic and psychosocial phenomena. Sexuality is expressed in every human act by a unique blend of physical attributes and emotional responses. Sexual beliefs, attitudes, and behaviors — the components of sexual expression — are interwoven with sexuality.

Prenatal biologic occurrences result in the development of obvious sexual determinants present at birth. These external organs are the basis for sexual "assignment," which stimulates gender-specific responses from the environment to the newborn child. These sociocultural responses combine with many biologic and psychologic forces to mold the individual's sexuality throughout the life cycle. Sexual behavior, the externalized expression of sexuality, therefore becomes quite individual and, in effect, inseparable from the personality.

The sexual response, a physiologic pattern linked to sexual expression, is relatively similar in most individuals. It encompasses a series of vasocongestive and myotonic reactions controlled by neurologic and hormonal channels. It occurs within four phases: excitement, plateau, orgasm, and resolution (Table 12–1). This response is strongly dependent on sexual drive (libido) and strongly influences sexual gratification. Gratification, an important key to the significance of sexuality to the individual, in turn affects sexual drive. This response loop varies dramatically among individuals and even within the same individual at different times. Multiple organic and/or psychogenic factors are responsible for this variability.

Factors related to sexuality. The normal **growth and development** of the human organism is an excellent example of the complex interplay among biologic, psychosocial, and cultural factors. These interactions usually occur in a predictable pattern that increases in complexity in a hierarchical manner. Within each developmental stage the individual has specific psychosocial and sexual milestones that must be accomplished before he is able to advance successfully to another stage (Table 12–2). The eventual ability to express mature love and share intimacy is dependent upon this natural progression. A number of factors, both internal and external to the individual, can

TABLE 12-1
Sexual Response Cycle

Phase	Male	Female
Excitement	Penile erection Testes draw up toward body Nipple erection Increased cardiac and respiratory rate	Vaginal lubrication Increased size and sensation of clitoris and labia minora Neuromuscular tension Increased cardiac and respiratory rate Breast enlargement and nipple erection Upward movement of uterus Expansion of vaginal walls "Sex flush" over body parts
Plateau	Increased circumference of penis Enlargement of testes Secretions of lubricating fluid from Cowper's glands	Uterus draws up further Vagina expands Clitoris retracts Labia minora turn bright red Vagina contracts to form "grasping" orgasmic platform
Orgasm	Ejaculation Pelvic thrusts with general muscular contractions	Uterine contractions "Tenting" phenomenon: distension of deeper portion of vagina
Resolution	Genital swelling subsides and organs return to preexcitement phase Loss of erection	Congestion of organs subside Tension release Uterus and vagina return to preexcitement phase

TABLE 12-2
Developmental Stages

Stage	Basic psychosocial task	Sexual task
Infancy	Acquiring basic trust, learning to walk, talk.	Gender identity.
Childhood	Acquiring a sense of autonomy vs. shame and doubt; entering and adjusting to school.	Pleasure-pain associated with organs and eliminative functions: masturbation takes place with resulting shame or acceptance; secondary sex characteristics become evident.
Adolescence	Acquiring sense of identity vs. role confusion.	Mastery over impulse control; acceptance of conflict between moral proscriptions and sexual urges; handling new physiologic functions (menses for girls and ejaculation for boys).
Young adulthood	Acquiring a sense of intimacy vs. isolation; vocational effectiveness, interpersonal security, "sexual adequacy."	Sexual adequacy and performance plus fertility concerns and questions related to parenting.
Middle adulthood	Acquiring a sense of self-esteem vs. despair; adjusting to diminution of one's energy and competence; "empty nest syndrome," plus care of aging parents or their death; adjusting to change in physique and evidence of aging.	For the female, menopause and resulting vasomotor changes, atrophy of breasts, reduction of clitoral size, and loss of vaginal lubrication; for the male, delay on attaining an erection, a reduced compulsion to ejaculate, episodic impotence, possible prostatitis.
Old age	Adjusting to loss of friends, family; confrontation with old age and dying; painful joint conditions; reduced hearing and visual acuity; adjustment to social stigmatization of being "old."	Reduced vitality, fear of incompetence or injury (coital coronary); fear of being viewed as "dirty old person"; unavailability of a partner (widowhood); limited physical capacity and reduced options.

Adapted from Schain, W. Sexual problems of patients with cancer. *In* DeVita, V. T., S. Hellman, and S. A. Rosenberg, editors. Cancer: Principles and Practice of Oncology. J. B. Lippincott Co., Philadelphia. 1982. p. 281.

impede this process, causing slowing, regression, or arrest. Chronologic age is often, though not always, correlated to developmental age. Ego strength and coping abilities are closely associated with the resolution of conflicts occurring within each stage. The current status of an individual's developmental process is, therefore, often predictive of his response to an upcoming life event.

Three aspects of an individual's personality are closely associated with sexuality and must be considered when providing health care.

Psychologic factors comprise the first aspect. Body image and self-concept are two characteristics that are interdependent and quite subtle in nature, so that to focus on them individually is somewhat artificial. *Body image* is the sense of physical self that is derived from four sources: an individual's actual appearance and body function, an individual's perception of himself, others' perception of the individual, which then influences their response to that individual, and the individual's perception of the "ideal" body. Conflicts arise when there are significant differences among these perceptions. *Self-concept* is an individual's sense of identity and worth. Sexual adjustments required by illness may be particularly difficult for those individuals having a very strong gender-specific identity that is vested in physical attributes. The literature shows these preillness psychologic factors to be highly correlated with a patient's adaptation to illness. A female who is insecure about her appearance will tend to have more difficulty adjusting to the loss of a breast than a woman who is secure in her marital relationship and confident of her attractiveness.

Sociocultural factors constitute the second aspect. These include: race, religion, socioeconomic class, family traditions, and geographic location. These characteristics — outside the control of the individual — often significantly influence and delineate his sexual attitudes and experiences. They are particularly influential in the young person.

Finally, **sexual factors** must be included in any consideration of personality and sexuality. An individual's physical sexual experiences will strongly influence sexual adaptation. Masturbation, sexual intercourse, and nonconventional sexual practices are examples of such experiences. A history of previous sexual dysfunction will also influence a person's response to sexual problems. Personal sexual relationships are a second factor within this category. The availability of a regular partner, the stability, duration, and importance of sexual relationships, the supportive nature of the partner, and the nature of the relationship (homosexual or heterosexual) are characteristics that mold sexuality. The personal feelings of the individual, often known only to him, are the most significant consideration within this framework. These include the individual's private fantasies, his true sexual preference, and the emotional satisfaction he derives from the sexual aspects of his life.

Cancer-related factors affecting sexuality. These factors can be divided into the general and the specific.

General: Cancer, like other diseases, is accompanied by a complex "illness process," the elements of which compromise the patient's sexuality through physical and psychologic insults. These elements are described below.

1. The **diagnosis of cancer** can have a traumatizing effect on the individual. It is often accompanied by fears of mutilation, cachexia, pain, and death. A sense of vulnerability because of the potential loss of body control may aggravate these worries. Such fears can monopolize the patient's thoughts and may obliterate his desire for and capability of participating in a personal sexual relationship. Anxiety, depression, and insecurity may cause decreased libido.

2. The **biologic process of cancer** may bring on symptoms of weakness, fatigue, and malaise. Gradual incapacitation and debilitation may occur. The physical acts of sexual expression demand energy, which may be at a minimum for the patient. Necessary hospitalizations force separation of patient and partner. Usual patterns of communication and the sharing of affection are terminated in the nonprivate atmosphere of the hospital.

3. The **side effects of therapy**, including anorexia, hair loss, nausea, vomiting, and sterility, can alter body image and thereby create a psychosexual problem. Many side effects of therapy are permanent and therefore place a high cost on potential cure.

4. **The family process of accepting and living with the diagnosis of cancer** can be extremely difficult. Family members must deal with many unknowns related to their loved ones. Depression and anticipatory grieving may alter the family/patient interaction. The roles of family members may change as they assume more responsible, independent, and caretaker roles in response to the increasing physical dependency of the patient. Remissions and exacerbations of the disease mandate constant interruptions and alterations in the patient's life-style. Persistent emotional stress, additional home responsibilities, and tiring hospital visits precipitate fatigue in the partner. Sexual expression may therefore decrease. The less-affectionate response of the sexual partner may support and reinforce the patient's perception of himself as "asexual."

Specific: The physiologic effects of cancer on sexuality are dependent on disease type, site involvement, and therapy. Structural changes in the sexual organs may yield alterations in sexual functioning. Tumor invasion into the vulva, peritoneum, and breast of the female or the urinary tract, testes, or penis of the male can interrupt normal sexual functioning. Sexual sensations may be altered by neurologic tumor involvement. Brain tumors, spinal cord involvement, and tumor pressure or invasion into nerve tracts may decrease tactile responsiveness. Vascular compromise because of tumor pressure may also decrease sexual sensation and cause physiologic dysfunction, such as poor lubrication in the female and impotence in the male. Tumors affecting hormone production and balance will also impede normal sexual functioning, because these substances are often essential to libido and sexual response.

The aggressive therapies now offered for cancer often cause multiple side effects. These vary from short-term to permanent. With the emphasis on potential cure, the side effects are frequently minimized by health professionals; however, for the individual who survives the initial insult of cancer, these side effects become a more present reality. Side effects will be discussed according to treatment modality, but it should be emphasized that the nurse must realize that combination therapies will precipitate a variety of side effects, each of which may affect sexual adjustment.

Surgical treatment provides the most obvious and dramatic insult to the patient, and therefore, it often receives the most attention. Much research has documented the presence of sexual problems and the need for sexual adjustments in these patients. Problems frequently stem from changes in appearance and permanent alterations in body functions. The significance of the affected organ(s), either external or internal, to one's body image is a major factor in the individual's ability to adjust to the surgical change. Changes in normal physiologic functioning may occur after surgical removal or alteration in body organs, or because of the interference with the autonomic innervation of organs involved in the sexual response. Common procedures known to affect sexuality are: mastectomy, head and neck surgery, abdomino-peritoneal resection with colostomy, limb amputation, hysterectomy with or without oophorectomy, vulvectomy, prostate or bladder surgery, and removal of testes.

Many effects of **chemotherapy** either directly or indirectly affect the patient's sexuality. The cytotoxic effect of chemotherapeutic agents is not limited to malignant cells. The simultaneous destruction of healthy cells causes negative physiologic effects, some of which are obvious to the patient. Because drugs are frequently given in combination, it has been difficult to estimate the adverse effects of specific agents. Variables such as total drug dose, schedule and duration of therapy, patient age, and disease stage complicate the expected degree of toxicity.

Anorexia, weight loss, nausea, and vomiting can produce a very dramatic change in appearance. The addition of weakness, pallor, and hair loss produces a major insult to the patient's body image and his ability to participate in a sexual relationship. **Hormonal imbalances** brought on by chemical agents may result in impressive personality changes. **Spermatogenesis** in the male patient may be decreased or absent; **sterility** may be temporary or permanent. Similarly, the female often experiences **amenorrhea** and **premature menopause**, accompanied by the usual symptoms of this phenomenon. **Impotence** and **gynecomastia** in males, **poor lubrication** and **dyspareunia** in females, and **decreased libido** in both sexes are common complaints from those receiving chemotherapy.

Radiation to any part of the body can affect sexuality indirectly, in that it can produce weakness and fatigue that make sexual relations difficult. Loss of body hair in the irradiated areas may affect body image, as may the red markings that act as a constant reminder of the diagnosis. Pelvic irradiation may produce permanent sterilization in the male. In the female it may cause: (1) cessation of menses, a symbol of femininity to many; (2) resultant infertility; and (3) pelvic fibrosis, resulting in painful intercourse.

Assessment

To assist the patient and his partner in addressing sexual problems related to cancer, the nurse must be comfortable with her own sexuality, sexual knowledge level, sexual attitudes, and counseling skills. This comfort is imperative for optimal communication between the patient and the nurse. An exploration of personal feelings about such controversial issues as extramarital relationships, homosexuality, masturbation, and abortion will broaden the nurse's awareness of her own value system and her biases toward the values of others. She should be appropriately objective about explicit sexual topics and terminology. A nonjudgmental attitude is vital when assisting these patients. A negative reaction from any health-care provider toward a patient's expression of sexual concern or inquiry for sexual information may overwhelm the patient with feelings of shame and guilt. The nurse needs to be informed, accepting, and supportive of the sexual practices and philosophies of patients.

When caring for patients with cancer, the nurse must be sensitive to the occurrence of sexual problems. Three important guidelines for assessment of these patients are:

1. Be informed about the sexual implications of all therapies that patients are receiving.
2. Assess the patient's sexuality in a structured, specific manner to attain the most complete and useful information, just as any other health history is solicited.
3. Respond to a patient's expressions of concern with consideration of his level of knowledge and his social and sexual value system.

A sexual assessment should be conducted in a setting conducive to the sharing of intimate information. Privacy is mandatory; available time needs to be ample for a lengthy discussion. The nurse should appear interested and avoid such judgmental terms as "normal," "frigid," "impotent," and "unresponsive." These labels too often communicate negative values and biases to the patient. Language should be understandable to the patient, and personal values should be avoided.

A sexual assessment should be structured upon specific objectives: (1) The patient's feelings about his own sexuality and sexual practices should be determined; (2) the patient's usual patterns of sexual expression, including frequency and quality, should be determined; (3) recent changes in sexual feelings or behaviors should be identified; (4) the nature of sexual problems and probable cause should be identified; and (5) the patient's and partner's motivation to remedy the situation should be determined.

A few specific questions will often stimulate a discussion in which the nurse can not only obtain the information necessary for the assessment but may also formulate the foundation for much freer, constructive interaction with the patient. A formal sexual-assessment tool may be detrimental in some cases, because the nurse feels all the questions must be covered, and thus the normal flow of discussion is interrupted. A few key questions will frequently be all that is needed to initiate discussions from which necessary information can be obtained. These questions might include:

1. How do you feel about yourself as a man/woman?
2. How was sexuality viewed within your family?
3. What kinds of relationships have you had with others that have been particularly satisfying to you?
4. What kinds of sexual behaviors/practices have you participated in? How often?
5. Have your sexual experiences been satisfying to you?
6. Has your disease/treatment altered your sexual patterns?

Patients very often need only to be offered the opportunity to discuss sexual concerns. They are frequently quite relieved to know that their sexual problems are viewed as legitimate and that assistance with them is available.

The identification of the patient's developmental stage and psychologic, sociocultural, and sexual personality factors are important steps in the sexual assessment process.

The actual cause of the sexual problem may be a physiologic effect of cancer or cancer treatment, or it may actually be a physiologic expression of a psychologic problem. The following schema may be helpful in categorizing sexual problems, thereby easing the problem-clarification process.

Body image. The cancer patient or his partner will often identify a specific dysfunction as a sexual problem (Table 12–3). Body-image disturbances, however, are frequently the real source of the problem. If the patient's body image is strongly dependent on the affected organ or general appearance, then the alterations caused by cancer and cancer treatment may have an awesome effect on body image. Loss of body function (amputation, colostomy, oophorectomy), value of physical appearance (weight loss, head and neck surgery, mastectomy, alopecia), and loss of independence (hemipelvectomy, laryngectomy) may affect an individual's image of himself, which may, in turn lead to conscious or unconscious sexual alterations.

Inability to have sexual intercourse. This problem becomes a particularly difficult one when the patient is also unable to establish satisfying alternatives for maintaining a sexual relationship. Many

TABLE 12–3
Problematic Sexual Dysfunctions by Sex

Dysfunction	Male	Female
Decreased libido	x	x
Inability to maintain erection	x	
Inability to ejaculate	x	
Inability to lubricate		x
Inability to achieve orgasm	x	x
Lack of satisfaction from sexual experience	x	x
Increased libido	x	x

individuals value conventional sexual intercourse ending in mutual orgasm as the "ideal" sexual act. For many, penile penetration of the vagina is the only physical sexual act that is practiced. For the cancer patient and his partner with this set of values, limited knowledge, or lack of imagination, treatments that render him incapable of achieving orgasm or of having sexual intercourse may produce serious and persistent emotional crises. Radical prostatectomies, abdominoperineal resections, vaginal irradiation, and chemotherapy can cause organic sexual dysfunctions. Clinical investigations, however, have shown that these patients continue to experience sexual desires. Patients may also consciously desire sexual relations because of an unmet need to conceive, an increased wish to give and receive affection, or a need to confirm their self-worth and desirability. For such patients, maintenance of a sexual relationship may be possible if alternative sexual practices are employed.

Infertility/sterility. The ability to bear children is a major element of self-respect for many individuals. The fear of— or actual— interruption of this capability because of cancer and cancer treatment creates feelings of hopelessness and inadequacy. Infertility may have other psychosexual repercussions such as depression, increased desire for sexual intercourse, and seductive behavior. Such patients need to be reassured of their masculinity/femininity and desirability.

Abandonment. Although patients frequently allude to concerns about their marital/personal relationships, the ultimate fear of abandonment is seldom verbalized. The problems of accepting and living with cancer and cancer treatment may well tax a relationship beyond its endurance. The quality of the preillness relationship has been demonstrated to be an important factor in this situation. Even a strong relationship, however, may be unable to survive the stresses of fear, lack of understanding, and inability to cope with cancer on the part of the patient or the partner. This fear of abandonment may be actualized by an increased desire for affection and sexual relations or by a decrease in sexual expression, a form of anticipatory grieving.

Medical management

Advances in the medical management of sexual problems have been receiving much more attention and support in recent years. The morbidity of cancer therapy is now a major consideration in the acceptance of new treatments, and serious efforts are being made to minimize side effects. The following is a brief description of medical interventions developed in response to cancer effects:

Reconstructive mammoplasty. A surgical reformation of the breast, using an artificial implant, is a relatively new procedure that has the potential therapeutic benefit of rebuilding mastectomy patients' self-esteem. Careful screening of the patients for this procedure is important to avoid disappointment in those with unrealistic expectations of surgical outcome. Prospective studies are now in progress to provide guidelines concerning the benefits of this procedure on the patient's body image and sexual functioning.

Vaginal reconstruction.   This rehabilitative surgical procedure in which a functioning vagina is created by means of peritoneal placement of split-thickness skin grafts, offers the patient the option of reestablishing the ability to have sexual intercourse. Reports about this procedure are very optimistic, with an average satisfaction rate of 85% among properly screened patients and partners.

Implantation of a penile prosthesis.   This is a surgical means for reestablishing erectile competence. Two types of penile implants are available at present. The first device is the semirigid rod, which is a nonmechanical implant that simulates the male erection. The degree of flexibility in these types of prostheses varies. The newer type of implant is the inflatable penile prosthesis, which includes a reservoir, tubing, cylinder pump, and expandable rods that are implanted into the corpora cavernosa. Through a controllable hydraulic mechanism, this prosthesis provides the patient with the option of having an erection or a natural-looking flaccid penis. Reports from the Mayo Clinic indicate a successful implantation rate of 90 to 95%, with only an 8% mechanical dysfunction rate over 3 yr. Satisfaction with this new prosthesis is reported by 89% of the patients and their partners.

Sperm banking and artificial insemination.   The cryopreservation of semen and the instrumental introduction of semen into the female genital tract to induce pregnancy are possible options for the couple facing infertility. Sperm banking, for later use in artificial insemination, can be employed before cancer therapy is begun if the semen is of good quality; this is often not the case, however, depending on the type and stage of disease. Sperm motility can also be reduced by 25 to 50% in the freezing process. Therefore, this procedure offers no guarantees to the patient. If sperm banking is unsuccessful, artificial insemination by a donor is a newer alternative that the couple may wish to consider.

Hormone replacement.   The medical supplementation of the production of hormones in the body may be prescribed for the female experiencing premature menopause because of surgery or ovarian suppression. Because of the documented stimulation of some tumors by hormones, however, this therapy is not always available. For the female with vaginal stenosis, the use of hormone creams is sometimes an alternative that greatly enhances the elasticity of the vagina.

Vaginal dilation. Intermittent expansion of the vaginal canal may prevent stenosis caused by radiation. This can be accomplished most naturally by the patient's continued participation in vaginal intercourse with a partner. If this is not appropriate, then the vagina can be dilated on a regular basis by the patient's use of a mechanical vibrator or vaginal dilator. The frequency of prescribed dilation varies from daily to a few times each week. Success of this technique is strongly dependent on patient compliance. Because many individuals link manual dilation with masturbation, patients may be reluctant to carry out this technique.

Nursing management

Preventive. Usually the physiologic effects of cancer and cancer treatment on sexuality cannot be avoided. By being prepared early in the disease or treatment course, however, the patient/partner may be better able to cope with the problems and the adjustments necessitated by them. Sometimes the psychosexual problems of cancer, such as alterations in body image, fear of abandonment, and difficulty accepting infertility, can be minimized by preventive nursing interventions. Frank, informative discussions with the patient facing sexual adjustments arising from cancer is the key to his being able to cope. The sexual assessment is the foundation for the nursing process aimed at preventing, as well as treating, sexual difficulties. The acceptance of sexuality as a significant component of health, and therefore a legitimate concern during illness, should be communicated to the patient early in the illness process. This acceptance can be positively and continually reinforced by providing care aimed toward supporting the patient as a sexual being. Specific examples include: encouraging the replacement of the unisex hospital gown with more masculine or feminine garments; respect for the patient's privacy, especially when physical care is involved; actively participating with the patient in discussions about his changing role within the family and community because of illness; and taking into consideration the sexuality of the patient when offering suggestions for dealing with treatment side effects, such as alopecia and malaise. By integrating the patient assessment data and the available information about the sexual effects of the particular cancer and therapy, the nurse can predict potential problem areas. Counseling of patients in advance should center on the provision of information similar to that given the patient who actually has the problem. The amount of information and the time for it to be provided need to be carefully judged.

The patient's partner often knows and understands the patient best; therefore, he is often a source of irreplaceable support and assistance to the patient. The nurse should attempt to facilitate and encourage this relationship. Adjustment periods will vary for each patient and couple. With time and experimentation, the patient can often deal with the sexual issues brought on by cancer.

Supportive. The nurse need not fear that the initiation of a discussion on sexuality will anger or embarrass the patient. He will quickly communicate his wish to continue or terminate the discussion. A termination by the patient should always be followed by an offer from the nurse to participate in such discussions with the patient in the future. Many patients view the nurse as a caring professional with whom they are quite comfortable. The nurse has the responsibility to offer information and to initiate educational discussions with the patient. Identified sexual problems can be dealt with through an honest, realistic, and creative approach. Table 12–4 outlines some nursing measures that may be useful when caring for cancer patients with sexual problems. Patients will frequently have a blend of these problems, so that several interventions are applicable. For very specific problems, such as managing an ostomy during sexual intercourse or selecting clothing after a mastectomy, the nurse may be instrumental in resolving the issues. Many helpful hints for dealing with such problems are available in literature provided by the Ostomy Association and the Reach to Recovery program. Having representatives of these groups visit the patient can be helpful, and the nurse may find such a visit informative as well.

The PLISSIT Model, developed by Annon in 1974, is a form of brief sexual therapy that can easily be integrated into the nursing process framework subsequent to assessment and problem identification. The first step in the counseling model is giving the patient permission to discuss sexual issues of concern to him. Frequently, all the patient and partner need is permission to resume sexual activity. This resumption is often delayed because of fears of giving cancer to the partner, harming the patient, etc. The nurse should listen carefully to the patient's and partner's feelings about the problem and acknowledge these as valid and appropriate. The second step is to provide the patient with a limited amount of information about the potential effects of cancer and cancer treatment on his sexual functioning, both physical and psychologic. This is the time to deal with the patient's misconceptions, fears, and concerns. The third level of intervention consists of specific suggestions. The patient is provided with defined tasks on which to work, often with the partner, to prevent or solve sexual difficulties. Written material, behavioral modification, and communication techniques are examples of interventions that may be appropriate within this level. Specific methods of foreplay and mutual pleasuring may be discussed. The final level of the PLISSIT model is intensive therapy; this is appropriate with individuals having long-term unresolved sexual problems or severe psychologic disturbances arising from sexual conflicts. The need for intensive therapy should be referred to appropriate professionals such as a psychiatrist, psychologist, or certified sex therapist.

Sexual problems require ongoing monitoring to determine the intensity of the difficulty over time and the occurrence of improvements. The continued interest and involvement of the nurse in the patient's sexual adjustment is an important element in the cancer patient's total rehabilitation.

Bibliography

1. Annon, J. S. The Behavioral Treatment of Sexual Problems. Harper & Row, Publishers, Inc., New York. 1974. Volume 1.

    Very useful synopsis of sexual problems with detailed presentation of PLISSIT counseling model. Includes excellent examples of patient interactions with counselors and specific recommendations to health professionals for dealing with such situations.

2. Burkhalter, P. K. Sexuality and the cancer patient. In Burkhalter, P. K., and D. L. Donley, editors. Dynamics of Oncology Nursing. McGraw-Hill Book Co., New York. 1978.

    Excellent overview of the components of human sexuality, role of cancer and illness in sexuality, and patient care related to sexuality. Includes useful suggestions for sexual history and counseling.

3. Schain, W. Sexual problems of patients with cancer. In DeVita, V. T., S. Hellman, and S. A. Rosenberg, editors. Cancer: Principles and Practice of Oncology. J. B. Lippincott Co., Philadelphia. 1982.

    Chapter offers a useful synopsis of human sexuality and the physical and psychologic effects of cancer on sexuality. Emphasis is placed on surgical treatments and methods for avoiding sexual problems.

4. Vaeth, J. M., R. C. Blomberg, and L. Adler, editors. Frontiers of Radiation Therapy and Oncology. S. Karger A.G., Basel, Switzerland. 1980. Volume 14.

    An invaluable resource for any professional caring for cancer patients, this volume brings together the philosophies and research of many specialists in cancer, human sexuality, and sexual counseling.

TABLE 12-4

Nursing Protocol for the Management of Sexual Problems in Cancer Patients

Factor	Intervention
General	Allow patient time to assimilate information regarding disease and therapy.
	Emphasize positive aspects of sexuality (beautiful hair, slender figure, handsome appearance, prestigious job).
	Allow patient and partner time to grieve for the loss (body part, normal function, usual appearance).
	Encourage patient/partner to express/share concerns and fears.
	Provide general atmosphere of hopefulness.
	Allow time for privacy alone and with partner.
	Emphasize positive aspects of longer survival or cure with treatment.
	Demonstrate awareness and acceptance of patient's sexuality throughout delivery of care.
	Provide educational material related to potential and real sexual problems.
Body image	Encourage care of appearance (makeup, clothes, etc.).
	Assist patient in redefining self-image based on physical alterations.
	Encourage patient to resume career, family and social activities to regain sense of self-worth.
	Involve patient in decisions concerning care.
	Encourage verbalization of positive feelings toward patient by partner.
	Assist partner in adjusting to negative aspects of disease/treatment.
	Educate male patients as to specific meaning of sterility, impotence, and inability to ejaculate.
	Discuss with physician the appropriateness of hormone replacement in females with premature menopause.
	Encourage distractions from disfigurement (use of glamorous underwear, handsome robe, a new moustache).
	Assist patient in obtaining and utilizing appropriate health aids and prostheses, e.g., wig for alopecia, breast prosthesis for mastectomy, artificial limbs for amputations, ostomy supplies for ostomate, facial prosthesis for head and neck surgery.

	Arrange for visit from representative of appropriate support group, e.g., Reach to Recovery, Ostomy Association, Make Today Count (*see* Appendix D). Teach patient specific techniques for concealing disfigurement and managing changes in bodily functions.
Inability to have sexual intercourse	Encourage use of vaginal dilator to maintain patency of vagina. Suggest hormone replacement or lubricants to physician for patients with dyspareunia. Suggest alternate positions to increase patient/partner comfort. Encourage open discussions about sexual problems, likes, dislikes. Emphasize importance of patience, understanding, and communication. Provide patients with information regarding medical interventions, e.g., penile implant, vaginal reconstruction. Provide specific suggestions for alternative methods of arousal and coitus: autoerotic activities — masturbation, mutual masturbation with partner, sexual fantasizing; mutual arousal techniques — caressing, kissing, oral-genital stimulation, manipulation of surgically created orifice; coital alternatives — oral-genital sex, anal intercourse, other nonvaginal approaches.
Infertility	Provide contraceptive information to fertile couples in whom pregnancy is not recommended/desirable. Assist patient in redefining sexuality without procreation. Provide information to patient/partner concerning opportunities for adoption, sperm banking, artificial insemination. Emphasize self-worth independent of parenting. Encourage parenting alternatives (foster care, volunteer in nursery school).
Abandonment	Involve and explain medical treatment and importance of it to partner. Encourage optimal communication between patient and partner. Provide information regarding available resources for counseling and support in the community. Involve partner in health-care decisions as much as possible. Support couple in earliest possible resumption of sexual activity.

CHAPTER 13

OXYGENATION AND VENTILATION

Linda Celentano Norton

Standard: The client and family recognize factors that may impair ventilatory function and can intervene with measures that may enhance optimum ventilatory capacity.

Outcome criteria: The client and family
1. state plans for daily activity that demonstrate maximum conservation of energy.
2. list measures to reduce or modify pulmonary irritants from the environment, such as smoke, dry air, powders, and aerosols.
3. describe the effect of environmental extremes on ventilatory function and oxygen utilization.
4. state effective measures to maintain a patent airway.
5. identify reasons for altered ventilation, such as decreased hemoglobin, infection, anxiety, effusion, and obstructed airway.
6. identify an appropriate plan of action should altered ventilation occur.
7. develop a plan for managing an altered airway.

Perhaps the most challenging aspect of prevention, diagnosis, and management of cancer patients is in the area of pulmonary problems. Most cancer patients are at risk for developing pulmonary problems either by virtue of their disease or from a treatment-related cause. Cancer of the lung, pleural effusions, pneumonia, radiation and drug effects, and respiratory failure are the most common pulmonary problems in cancer patients.

Pathophysiology

Primary carcinoma of the lung accounts for 25% of all cancer deaths and 5% of all deaths in the USA. Furthermore, the lung parenchyma is the most common site for tumor metastases, particularly from cancers of the breast and prostate. Tumors of the pleura, chest wall, diaphragm, and mediastinum often present with respiratory symptoms. Malignant effusions are most often caused by lung cancer, breast cancer, and lymphoma; 50% of diagnostic thoracenteses performed demonstrate a malignancy.

The combined effects of immunosuppression, malnutrition, and cancer place the patient at grave risk for pneumonia. Pneumonia may occur in as many as 80% of patients with acute leukemia during periods of bone marrow relapse, and 50% of acute leukemics will die of unresolved pneumonia. Opportunistic organisms (Table 13–1), fulminant disease, and immunosuppression are factors that increase mortality. Mortality from fungal infections in immunocompromised patients is as high as 90%. For these reasons, clinicians seek prompt diagnosis and treatment for new pulmonary infiltrates, particularly those accompanied by fever. Not uncommonly, pulmonary infiltrates are labeled as either noninfectious or nonspecific, and only at autopsy is a diagnosis confirmed. Some of the noninfectious causes of pulmonary infiltrates are tumor, pneumonitis, intrapulmonary hemorrhage or edema, and radiation- or drug-induced lung disease.

The effect of radiation on the normal lung is an area of increasing knowledge and concern. The larger the lung volume irradiated, the greater the risk of radiation pneumonitis. Approximately 10% of patients with breast or lung cancer treated with radiation therapy (RT)

TABLE 13–1

Pathogens Causing Pneumonia in Cancer Patients

Classification	Organism
Bacteria	*Staphylococcus*
	Pseudomonas
	Escherichia coli
	Klebsiella
	Nocardia
	Mycobacterium tuberculosis
Fungi	*Aspergillis*
	Mucoraceae
	Cryptococcus
	Histoplasma capsulatum
	Coccidioides immitis
	Candida
Virus	Cytomegalovirus
Protozoa	*Pneumocystis carinii*

experience acute symptomatic radiation pneumonitis. Cellular injury from radiation usually occurs within 1 to 6 mo after the completion of a RT course. The acute phase is characterized by congestion, edema, and cellular infiltration. Alveolar walls are infiltrated with cells and fibroblasts during the intermediate phase. Radiation toxicity may subside or progress to fibrosis in the chronic phase. A dose limit of 1,800 to 2,000 rads in 2 to 3 wk is recommended, and this dosage should be decreased if the patient is receiving concomitant chemotherapy.

A number of chemotherapeutic drugs have been implicated in causing drug-induced lung disease (DILD). The subacute pattern of DILD affects the interstitium, the alveolar wall, its lining cells, and occasionally the bronchiolar and arteriolar walls. Late in the course of the disease, a fibrotic process is evident. Factors that contribute to the risk of drug toxicity are: prior or concomitant RT, prior treatment with chemotherapy, the use of high fractions of inspired oxygen, preexisting lung disease, and high total dosage of antineoplastic agents. A dose-related risk has been identified for bleomycin and BCNU and has been suggested for busulfan and chlorambucil. Age, specific disease (e.g., lymphoma), and route of administration (e.g., IV vs. IM) of the drug are other factors that may predispose to DILD. With improvements in diagnosis and better description of the variables contributing to DILD, the incidence of lethal and nonlethal disease should decrease.

Respiratory failure may be caused by treatment- or disease-related factors. Pulmonary fibrosis secondary to RT or chemotherapy can lead to respiratory failure. Sepsis during neutropenia, intrapulmonary hemorrhage, pneumonitis, and fulminant pulmonary infection can also cause respiratory failure.

Nursing care for cancer patients with pulmonary problems focuses on symptom relief and prevention of common respiratory problems. An understanding of the complications arising from lung tumors and treatment permits the identification of nursing care problems encountered with cancer patients. **Airflow obstruction** may be acute or chronic and results from tumor or pneumonia. Symptoms of dyspnea and breathlessness and a laboratory pattern of restrictive lung disease are present in patients with **hypoxia and hypoventilation**. **Secretion clearance** is an important aspect of nursing care, whether caused by a tumor impeding airway clearance or by alterations in normal defense mechanisms. The prevention and early detection of **respiratory failure** must be an important consideration in the care of cancer patients. Table 13–2 illustrates the correlation between these nursing care problems and the medical diagnoses and may be used as a problem-identification tool when designing care for the cancer patient.

TABLE 13–2

Problem Identification for Nursing Care

Problem	Airflow obstruction	Hypoxia and hypoventilation	Inadequate secretion clearance	Respiratory failure
Cancer of the lung	Secondary to tumor obstruction of airflow.	Secondary to gas exchange impairment.	Secondary to obstruction of airflow.	Secondary to gas exchange impairment.
Neoplasms of the pleura, chest wall, diaphragm, and mediastinum	Secondary to bronchial obstruction or mediastinal shift.	Secondary to decreased chest wall or diaphragm motion.	Secondary to loss of adequate cough or gag reflex.	Secondary to gas exchange impairment.
Tracheal obstruction secondary to tumor or metastasis	Secondary to tumor.	Secondary to decreased ventilation from obstruction or pulmonary infiltrates.	Secondary to loss of adequate cough and/or altered defense mechanisms.	Secondary to obstruction of airflow and gas exchange impairment.
Pleural effusions	Secondary to fluid impeding chest expansion.	Secondary to restriction of lung expansion and ventilation-perfusion mismatch.	Secondary to postobstructive pneumonia.	Secondary to gas exchange impairment.

Pulmonary infections and infiltrates	Secondary to consolidation or secretions.	Secondary to decreased lung volumes; decreased surface area for O_2 diffusion.	Secondary to obstruction or increased secretions.	Secondary to gas exchange impairment.
Drug-induced lung disease	Secondary to impaired cough; increased secretions.	Secondary to fibrosis.	Secondary to altered defense mechanisms.	Secondary to fibrosis and gas exchange impairment.
Radiation fibrosis	Secondary to bronchial epithelial injury (cough, bronchospasm [asthmatic reaction]).	Secondary to radiation pneumonitis (in 4–11 wk, hypoxemia, and restrictive pattern on PFTs).	Secondary to altered defense mechanisms.	Secondary to fibrosis and gas exchange impairment.

PFTs, pulmonary function tests.

Assessment

Evaluation of lung function is dependent on a history, physical examination, and laboratory data. Table 13–3 lists the clinical findings of these three assessment areas for the patient with airflow obstruction, hypoxia/hypoventilation, inadequate secretion clearance, and respiratory failure. Although a complete history and physical examination are necessary for evaluating these patients, Table 13–3 is intended to focus on the pulmonary data base and move the reader from a specific assessment to interpretation of the data based on the four common problem areas.

Management

Improving the quality of life is the aim of managing pulmonary problems in cancer patients. The overall goals of therapy are (1) optimum oxygenation and ventilation, (2) decreasing the work of breathing, and (3) preventing infection. Management protocols for three of the common problem areas are provided (Tables 13–4 through 13–6).

Airflow obstruction. Airflow obstruction may be characterized by its location along the tracheobronchial tree, and by whether it occurs acutely or chronically. Obstructions, which are central or peripheral, originate in the airway lumen itself, the airway wall, or outside the tracheobronchial tree. The more central the location, the more severe the disturbance to airflow. Examples of intraluminal obstruction include: secretions (mucus plug), pneumonia, neoplasms, and foreign bodies. Obstructions arising in the wall of the airway may be caused by tumor or by more diffuse processes such as chronic obstructive pulmonary disease (COPD), fibrosis, or asthma. Finally, obstructions outside the tracheobronchial tree are caused by tumors (e.g., head/neck region, thorax, abdomen) that impede air and secretion movement. The management of acute airflow obstruction differs from that of chronic airflow obstruction because the focus is immediate removal of the obstruction and/or provision of an artificial airway.

The nursing management of airflow obstruction is detailed in Table 13–4. Because cancer patients face a high risk for pneumonia, a preventive protocol is presented. Breathing exercises and relaxation techniques are aimed at increasing expiratory flow and decreasing anxiety. Physical conditioning should be geared toward achieving maximal tolerance for activities of daily living. The treatment of reversible bronchospasm could include the use of methylxanthines, sympathomimetics, anticholinergics, steroids, and mediator blockers. The concomitant use of oxygen and mechanical assistance devices improves exercise tolerance, decreases symptoms of hypoxia, and prevents the development of cor pulmonale. A tracheostomy tube may be necessary to relieve obstruction on a temporary or permanent basis. Tracheostomy tubes also facilitate secretion removal and, when necessary, provide a medium for administering positive pressure ventilation. Other non-nursing aspects of managing airflow obstruction include: surgical removal of a tumor, irradiation, and chemotherapy.

Hypoxia and hypoventilation. Adequate tissue oxygenation is dependent upon an intact cardiovascular-respiratory-hematopoietic transport system.

Hypoventilation is the inability of the respiratory apparatus to maintain alveolar ventilation adequate for the metabolic needs of the body. Cancer patients, because of functional or structural impairments, have a propensity to hypoventilate. Fatigue and malnutrition are the most common examples of **functional** limitations that cause a patient to hypoventilate. Tumors obstructing air movement, surgery involving the thorax or lungs, treatment effects such as radiation pneumonitis or DILD, and pneumonia are all examples of **structural** causes of hypoventilation. Hypoventilation places a patient at risk for hypoxia, hypercapnia, and pneumonia. If air movement is diminished, so, too, is the oxygen available for transport across the alveolar-capillary membrane.

Hypoxia, or a decrease in oxygen tension, can result from hypoventilation or can occur in isolation. Problems of oxygen transport occur: (1) at the alveolar-capillary membrane, as in interstitial fibrosis or lymphangitic metastases; (2) as a result of hemodynamic dysfunction, as in pericardial effusion or adriamycin cardiomyopathy; or (3) because of an alteration in the chemical composition of the blood, as in anemia.

Prevention of hypoxia and hypoventilation and optimizing oxygen transport in irreversible lung disease are essential aspects in the care of the cancer patient. Factors for the nurse to consider include the prevention of pneumonia, oxygen administration, patient positioning, physical conditioning, and bronchodilator administration (all of these factors are discussed in Table 13–4). In addition, breathing exercises are essential for the patient, particularly thoracic expansion exercises (e.g., periodic deep-breathing, segmental breathing); incentive inspiratory devices; and coughing exercises (Table 13–5). Other aspects of management include transfusions, drugs to improve cardiac output, drainage of effusions or pleurectomy, and the administration of steroids, chemotherapy, or RT.

Secretion clearance. Hypoventilation or airway obstruction hampers secretion removal and predisposes to pneumonia. Immunosuppression secondary to chemotherapy, RT, malnutrition, disease, or advanced age add to the risk of pneumonia. Prevention is the hallmark of patient care management (*see* Table 13–5). Other aspects of

TABLE 13-3

Clinical Findings According to Nursing Care Problems

Assessment	Airflow obstruction	Hypoxia and hypoventilation	Inadequate secretion clearance	Respiratory failure
History	Dyspnea and/or shortness of breath, cough, hemoptysis, recurrent upper respiratory infections.	Dyspnea, tachypnea, lethargy, fatigue, restlessness, headache, irritability, confusion.	Cough, with or without sputum; inadequate cough; sputum: change in color, odor, consistency, and amount; fever; dyspnea; tachypnea; postoperative patient; generalized weakness; postoperative patient; history of smoking and/or COPD.	Rapidly progressive air hunger; restlessness, confusion, diaphoresis, headache. Refer to history data under Airflow obstruction, Hypoxia and hypoventilation, Inadequate secretion clearance.
Physical examination	Cyanosis; tripod posture: ↑ RR ↓ chest excursion; prolonged expiration; accessory muscle use; pursed-lip breathing; ↑ A-P diameter (if COPD); retractions, stridor; tracheal shift, ↓ fremitus;	Coma; cyanosis; tachycardia, hypertension, and then hypotension; ↓ respiratory excursion, ↓ breath sounds, ↓ diaphragm excursion;	Cyanosis; increased work of breathing — ↑ RR, accessory muscle use; rhonchi, rales, wheezing; signs of consolidation; systemic signs of dehydration.	Tachycardia; hypotension; cyanosis; confusion, coma, tremors, asterixis, ↓ respiratory excursion, ↓ RR; papilledema.

	flat or hyperresonant percussion; rhonchi, rales, wheezing; signs of consolidation if acute obstruction: snoring — partial, complete, marked; inspiratory effort without air movement.	rhonchi, rales, wheezing; signs of consolidation.		
Laboratory data	ABGs: ↓ PO_2; may have ↑ or ↓ PCO_2.	ABGs: ↓ PO_2; may ↑ PCO_2.	ABGs: normal or ↓ PO_2; may have ↑ PCO_2.	ABGs: ↓ PO_2; may have ↑ or ↓ PCO_2.
	CXR: may show tumor, pneumonia, COPD pattern.	CXR: may show pulmonary edema, pulmonary fibrosis, tumor, pneumonia.	CXR: may show pneumonia, tumor, fibrosis.	CXR: may show fibrosis, pneumonia, tumor, pulmonary edema.
	PFTs: obstructive defect.	PFTs: obstructive or restrictive defect.	PFTs: obstructive or restrictive defect.	PFTs: obstructive or restrictive defect.

ABG, arterial blood gas; A-P diameter, anterior-posterior diameter; COPD, chronic obstructive pulmonary disease; CXR, chest radiograph; PCO_2, partial pressure of carbon dioxide; PO_2, partial pressure of oxygen; PFT, pulmonary function test; RR, respiratory rate.

TABLE 13-4

Nursing Protocol for the Management of Airflow Obstruction

Factor	Intervention
Prevention of pneumonia (*see* Chapter 9A)	Wash hands.
	Decrease exposure.
	Practice aseptic technique, e.g., during suctioning.
	Use laminar air flow when available.
	Obtain surveillance cultures.
	Provide adequate nutrition.
	Decrease hospital stay.
	Perform tuberculin screening prior to immunosuppression.
	Hydrate adequately, encourage deep breathing, ambulation and, if necessary, institute chest physical therapy.
	If risk of aspiration pneumonia, refer below to Management of a Tracheostomy Tube, complications.
Position needs	
Acute (short-term)	Turn head laterally with neck extended and inspect mouth for cause of obstruction.
	Prepare for insertion of an artificial airway to relieve the obstruction, protect the airway, provide a route for secretion removal, and provide a port for supporting ventilation.
Chronic (long-term)	Reposition q 2 hr.
	Get patient out of bed to maximize thoracic excursion and improve oxygenation and secretion removal.
	Position for best alveolar ventilation:
	Check ABGs and lung sounds after position change and after the patient is stable (allow approximately 30 min).
	Patient will likely report being most comfortable in position with best alveolar ventilation.
	Have patient use tripod position (leaning forward on elbows) while sitting.
	While in bed use the position that provides the least obstruction to airflow. The patient should be less symptomatic, the lung sounds clearer and ABGs improved in this position.
	Educate patient and family as to rationale for management and patient care.

Breathing exercises and relaxation techniques	To slow respiratory rate and prolong expiration: Place hands over the lateral basal thorax or place one hand on the epigastric area and apply increasing pressure on expiration. Use pursed-lip expiration: deep inspiration; inhale through nose and exhale slowly and steadily through pursed lips. Use diaphragmatic breathing: place one hand (yours or patient's) on abdomen and one on thorax; inhale deeply through nose and push abdominal wall out; exhale through pursed lips while pushing abdomen in and up. For retraining of chronic patients, pursed-lip and diaphragm exercises should progress from the supine position to walking and to walking upstairs. Mechanical or electrical assistance can be used to strengthen the diaphragm further. Allow patient and family adequate time to learn exercises, particularly those that will be continued at home.
Physical conditioning	Collaborate with physical therapy department in designing program. Proceed from starting point to maximum tolerance: range of motion, to sitting, to walking with assistance, to level walking, to treadmill exercise, to bicycling, to stair climbing. Assist in energy conservation. Teach patient to: lift, push, pull, and go up a step on exhalation; pace activities, rest, sit when possible, eliminate unnecessary steps; use assistive devices, e.g., oxygen, a chair in the shower, devices to help in putting on socks. Involve family in activities, because they will be continued at home. Refer patient to agencies that provide assistance at home.
Bronchodilators	Maximize effects: control secretions — hydration, nebulizer treatment, breathing exercises, and early treatment of infection; provide low-flow O_2, if necessary, for continuous use or use with activities; collaborate with patient and family on how to avoid allergens, dust, fumes, and cigarette smoking at home or at work. Administer according to individual patient needs: evaluate effects, side effects, and optimum timing, and sequencing of drugs and activities, e.g., oral bronchodilator before inhaled bronchodilator and administration based on duration of action; ensure proper administration of inhaled drugs and proper dosage; encourage use before strenuous activity, breathing exercises, coughing, and conditioning exercises; teach patient and family about bronchodilators.

Factor	Intervention
Oxygen and mechanical assistance devices	Assess factors determining mode of delivery: The presence of an artificial airway, e.g., T-piece, tracheostomy mask. The fraction of inspired oxygen required: Low-flow system (e.g., nasal cannulas are less sensitive to changes in ventilatory pattern). High-flow systems (e.g., Venturi) provide a specific FIO_2 and bag reservoirs provide higher FIO_2. Assess patient comfort and tolerance, particularly if home oxygen candidate. Provide home oxygen. Delivery options: compressed O_2; liquid systems; concentrators. Factors determining type of delivery: oxygen requirement (e.g., FIO_2 and number of daily hours needed); portability (patient's life-style); cost of oxygen and financial status of patient and family. Patient and family education: machinery operation; cleaning and assembly; signs and symptoms of hypoxia and hypercapnia. Provide other devices: Nebulizers: vaporizer — increases humidity; aerosol mask — to administer water vapor; atomizer — to administer medications. Incentive inspiratory devices to encourage maximal inspiration. IPPB to increase ventilation. Pneumo belt — for severe diaphragm weakness (corset cuff intermittently inflates and deflates at preset rate).
Management of tracheostomy tube	Maintain airway patency: Provide a humidification source because the normal warming and humidifying mechanism, the nose, is bypassed. Remove secretions: hydrate and provide humidity; institute deep breathing and huffing cough (see Table 13–5); suction as necessary; reposition patient and get out of bed. Provide tube care: Suction as necessary: wash hands and wear sterile gloves; hyperoxygenate and hyperventilate before suctioning; use 12 or 14 French catheter and 120 mmHg pressure; introduce catheter and apply suction for a maximum of 15 sec; then withdraw catheter; reoxygenate and hyperventilate.

Clean inner and outer cannula: prepare equipment and suction; release lock, remove inner cannula, and place in a solution of 1:1 NS and hydrogen peroxide; clean inner cannula; clean outer cannula; dry inner cannula; suction outer cannula if necessary.

Change tracheostomy dressing and ties: remove dressing and ties and clean tracheostomy stoma with 1:1 solution of NS and hydrogen peroxide; wash hydrogen peroxide solution off with NS and apply antimicrobial ointment; replace precut tracheostomy dressing; replace ties.

Change tube 1 or 2 times/wk.

Prevent complications:

Pneumonia and mucus plugging: humidify and hydrate; mobilize sections, suction, and maintain asepsis.

Aspiration pneumonia: inflate tracheostomy cuff, if appropriate, for duration of feeding and 1 hr afterward; allow rest for 1 hr before and after meals; place in semi-Fowler's position for duration of meals and for 1 hr afterward.

Inadvertent extubation: have an extra tube available.

Promote communication and comfort with:

Assistance devices: trach talk, artificial larynx, esophageal speech.

Short-term solutions: letter board, writing tablet.

Comfort measures: mouth care; involving patient and family in care and care decisions; explanation of all aspects of care.

Extubate.

Gradually decrease tube size and/or tracheostomy plugs.

Use fenestrated tracheostomy tube.

Use tracheal button.

ABG, arterial blood gas; FIO$_2$, fraction of inspired oxygen; IPPB, intermittent positive pressure breathing; NS, normal saline.

TABLE 13-5

Nursing Protocol for the Management of Secretion Clearance

Factor	Intervention
Prevention of pneumonia	*See Table 13-4.*
Positioning	Reposition q 2 hr.
	Get patient out of bed to maximize thoracic excursion and improve oxygenation and secretion removal.
	Ambulate, if possible.
Coughing exercises	Hydrate patient adequately.
	Liquefy secretions by nebulization treatment, if necessary.
	Administer bronchodilators first, if prescribed.
	Encourage inspiration, followed by either a single cough or a series of smaller coughs.
	Manually assist coughing for patients with extremely weak abdominal muscles; manual pressure is applied over the abdominal wall during coughing.
Chest physical therapy and drainage (Fig. 13-1)	Provide adequate pain relief.
	Liquefy secretions: maximize fluid intake; humidify and/or nebulize.
	Define affected lung regions and therapy positions.
	Auscultate lungs before, during, and after treatment.
	Provide O_2 if breathlessness during chest therapy.
	Position for drainage of first lobe(s). If possible use Trendelenburg's position for lower and middle lobes.
	Percuss defined area with cupped hands in a rhythmic fashion for a given time, e.g., 3–5 min.
	Follow with vibration and instruct patient to deep-breathe. Place flat hand over area and vibrate on exhalation.
	Follow with coughing exercises.
	Proceed to next position, frequently to opposite lateral decubitus position.
	Coughing exercises.
Suctioning (if unable to cough effectively)	If intubated, refer to Table 13-4, Management of a tracheostomy tube.
	If not intubated: Use aseptic technique; preoxygenate and ask patient to take a few deep breaths; lubricate 12 or 14 French catheter tip and insert through a naris to the back of the throat; ask the patient to cough and pass catheter into the tracheobronchial tree to the level of the carina; apply intermittent suction, no greater than 120 mmHg for a maximum of 15 sec; rotate the catheter while removing it; reoxygenate and have the patient take a few deep breaths.

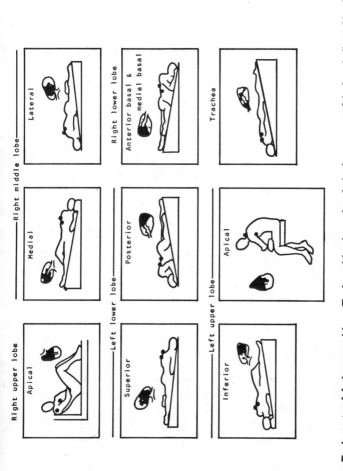

Figure 13–1.   Basic postural drainage positions. Each position is used to drain the segment of the lung indicated by the shaded areas. ● indicates the points where percussion and vibration are to be applied. *Adapted with permission from* Haas, A., H. Pineda, F. Haas, and K. Axen. Pulmonary Therapy and Rehabilitation Principles and Practice. Williams & Wilkins Co., Baltimore. 1979. p. 127.

management include antibiotics or antiviral drugs, judicious use of chemotherapy, granulocyte transfusion, bronchoscopy (e.g., for removal of mucus plugs), endotracheal intubation, and removal of airway obstruction.

Respiratory failure.   Respiratory failure is the inability of the respiratory system to maintain adequate oxygenation and carbon dioxide elimination. Identification of the oncology patient at risk and the early clinical manifestations of respiratory failure are the basis of decreasing patient morbidity and mortality. The critically ill cancer patients are those with sepsis, for example, or fulminant pneumonia, interstitial fibrosis, intrapulmonary hemorrhage, and large-airway obstruction. A more common cause of respiratory failure is narcotic suppression of respiration in an already compromised patient. Diagnosis and treatment of the cause of respiratory failure is of paramount importance. During the treatment phase, however, symptomatic management prevails (*see* Table 13–6). Additional treatment might include drugs to treat the cause of respiratory failure (e.g., antibiotics) bronchoscopy to aid in secretion removal, and chemotherapy or RT to treat tumor growth.

Bibliography

1. Carlon, G. C. Critical care of the cancer patient. *In* Burchenal, J. H., and H. F. Oettgen. Cancer Achievements, Challenges and Prospects for the 1980's (Volume 2). Grune & Stratton, Inc., New York. 1981.

   Discusses the care of the cancer patient with respiratory failure. Explains the possible causes, particularly infection and lung injury caused by chemotherapy and radiation therapy.

2. Dietz, J. H., Jr. Rehabilitation Oncology. John Wiley & Sons, Inc., New York. 1981.

   A short, practical text for health-care professionals that emphasizes the rehabilitation of patients from the time of hospital admission. Protocols for rehabilitation are based on patient goals and organized by anatomic region or organ system.

3. Fanta, C. H., and J. E. Pennington. Fever and new lung infiltrates in the immunocompromised host. *Clinics in Chest Medicine* (January 1981). 19–39.

   Presents a broad spectrum of diseases that present with fever and lung infiltrates in this patient group and describes possible etiologies. Emphasizes frequency and high mortality of the syndrome.

4. Ginsberg, S. J., and R. L. Comis. The pulmonary toxicity of antineoplastic agents. *Seminars in Oncology* (March 1982). 34–51.

TABLE 13-6

Nursing Protocol for the Management of Respiratory Failure

Factor	Intervention
Prevention of infection	Prevent pneumonia (*see* Table 13–4), remove secretions, and perform chest physical therapy and postural drainage (*see* Table 13–5). Change ventilator tubing q 24 hr. Secure the endotracheal tube. Use aseptic suctioning technique. Humidify inhaled air.
Oxygen and mechanical ventilation	Administer supplemental oxygen to bring PO_2 and PCO_2 to normal. Improve oxygen carrying capacity, e.g., Hb. Improve cardiac output. Decrease the work of breathing.
Positioning	*See* Table 13–4.
Hemodynamic and fluid balance	Hydrate adequately. Monitor cardiac output. Minimize the effects of positive pressure breathing: use intermittent mechanical ventilation; minimize peak airway pressure; restrict fluids if water retention secondary to vasopressin release; control pain, stress, and increases in CO_2; use diuretics.
Prevention of complications of mechanical ventilation	Maintain airway patency: humidify inhaled air and hydrate patient; remove secretions (*see* Table 13–5, Management of a tracheostomy tube, suctioning); secure endotracheal tube; sedate patient as necessary; have ambu bag and mask on hand. Prevent laryngeal and tracheal complications: secure endotracheal tube; use low-pressure cuffs; use minimal occluding volume in inflating cuff; measure cuff pressures. Prevent barotrauma: identify population at risk (patients with high peak airway pressures); minimize peak airway pressure: use intermittent mechanical ventilation; prolong expiratory time or decrease respiratory rate. Provide for mechanical emergencies: have ambu bag at bedside.
Communication and comfort	*See* Table 13–4, Management of tracheostomy tube.

PCO_2, partial pressure of carbon dioxide; PO_2, partial pressure of oxygen.

A sophisticated and comprehensive review of the pulmonary side effects of chemotherapy. Includes short- and long-term toxicity, the clinical course, and outcome.

5. Haas, A., H. Pineda, F. Haas, and K. Axen. Pulmonary Therapy and Rehabilitation Principles and Practice. Williams & Wilkins Co., Baltimore. 1979.
   The state of the art in pulmonary rehabilitation is presented in a most practical style. Good coverage of breathing exercises.

6. Jett, J. R., D. A. Cortese, and R. S. Fontana. Lung cancer: current concepts and prospects. *Ca-A Cancer Journal for Clinicians* (April 1983). 74–86.
   A clear, concise, and very readable review of the epidemiology, clinical manifestations, staging, detection, and treatment of lung cancer.

7. Johanson, B. C., C. U. Dungca, D. Hoffmeister, and S. J. Wells. Standards for Critical Care. C. V. Mosby Co., St. Louis. 1981.
   An excellent reference that presents protocols for the care of the critically ill patient. Organized according to organ system involved.

8. Lyons, R. J., and C. M. Yuska. Tracheostomy Care. Shiley, Inc., Surgical Products Division, Irvine, Calif.
   This detailed picture book was prepared for patients and their families and seems most useful for patient teaching and as an ongoing reference for at-home self-care. Copies are free.

9. Portlock, C. S., and D. Goffinet. Manual of Clinical Problems in Oncology. Little, Brown & Co., Boston. 1980.
   A short, practical manual that presents brief discussions of a broad range of clinical problems related to cancer and its treatment. Includes oncologic emergencies, diagnostic problems, and specific problems related to tumor types and metastases and provides annotated references.

10. Traver, G. A. Respiratory Nursing: the Science and the Art. John Wiley & Sons, Inc., New York. 1982.
    Excellent discussion of pulmonary physiology, pathophysiology, and nursing management. Highly recommended.

CHAPTER 14

OBSTRUCTIVE EMERGENCIES

A: INCREASED INTRACRANIAL PRESSURE

Karen K. Kane

A wide variety of cancer patients are at risk for the development of alterations in intracranial pressure (ICP) by virtue of their disease and treatments. Primary intracranial neoplasms, metastatic spread to the skull or brain tissue, metabolic encephalopathies, infections, vascular disorders, and side effects from chemotherapy and radiation therapy (RT) have the potential to increase ICP. The nursing implications include identifying patients at risk, assessing signs of neurologic dysfunction, and modifying nursing care activities to prevent further increasing ICP.

Pathophysiology

Intracranial volume consisting of brain tissue, blood, and CSF is essentially constant within the rigid skull. According to the Monro-Kellie doctrine, expansion of the volume of one of the three elements requires adjustment of the volumes of the other two in order to maintain ICP at a steady rate.

The body attempts to regulate ICP through compensatory mechanisms that allow an increase in the volume of intracranial components before ICP starts to rise. Once the limits of this regulation are reached and the volume is increased at a greater rate than the body can compensate for, an increase in ICP will occur.

Brain mass. Primary and metastatic tumors of the brain or skull, hematomas, hemorrhage, cerebral irritation, or infection with exudate will result in an increase in brain mass, because of the increased number of cells present within the cranium. Brain edema further expands the brain mass as fluid accumulates in the intracellular and/or extracellular spaces. Two major types of brain edema have been identified.

Vasogenic edema: Extracellular localized edema, the most common form of brain edema, is characterized by an increase in permeability of the blood-brain barrier (BBB). The increase in permeability allows larger molecules (plasma proteins) to leak through the capillary walls into the brain, drawing fluid from the capillaries into the surrounding tissue.

Vasogenic edema can be precipitated by primary and metastatic tumors, hemorrhage, brain necrosis, and infections. Regional swelling of tissue secondary to transudation occurs because fluid passes through capillary membrane pores into the extracellular space. The compression effects of this edema on surrounding veins may obstruct their outflow and further increase regional swelling. CNS infections caused by bacterial, fungal, viral, and parasitic organisms occur infrequently in the general oncology population, but there is a higher incidence in patients with lymphoma, leukemia, and CNS tumors. In addition, shunts, such as the Ommaya Reservoir, create a potential source for infection. The resulting inflammatory response and exudation will increase brain mass and may result in increased ICP.

Vasogenic edema can also occur as a result of acute cerebral irritation, caused directly by RT and indirectly by tumor-cell breakdown products. This irritation is an anticipated side effect of RT and is often treated with prophylactic steroids to minimize edema for the duration of therapy. Tissue necrosis and related edema may result as a delayed side effect of therapy in up to 25% of those individuals who receive 6,000 rads or more whole-brain irradiation. More frequently, necrosis is observed in individuals who have received CNS irradiation in conjunction with intrathecal (IT) and/or systemic use of the chemotherapeutic agent methotrexate. Irradiation is thought to produce thickening of capillary walls and progressive obliteration of small blood vessels, resulting in necrosis of tissue normally supplied by them. Characterized by diffuse destruction of normal brain tissue, this delayed reaction first manifests symptoms several months to 5 yr or more after therapy. The role of radiation in this delayed toxic syndrome may relate to its ability to perturb the BBB. Damage to the BBB may increase the neurotoxic effects of methotrexate by increasing its penetration into the CNS. Alterations of the BBB (secondary to radiation) may enhance CNS access of other drugs that otherwise would not have been able to permeate the BBB. This alteration in access may result in unsuspected neurotoxicities.

Cellular, or cytotoxic, edema: Intracellular localized edema is characterized by swelling of the brain cells, with a corresponding reduction in the extracellular fluid space. This increase in volume within the cells results in an increase in intracellular water and sodium content. Lactic acid accumulates within the cell, resulting in a dangerous state of lactic acidosis. Cell breakdown occurs, which increases intracellular osmolality and therefore increases cell swelling. As cells swell, the capillaries become compressed; the compressed flow of blood causes sludging, which results in depletion of oxygen and glucose and loss of consciousness. Increased resistance to arterial perfusion contributes to ischemia and necrosis. Edema is greatest where cell necrosis occurs but also develops in ischemic areas. Common causative factors include cerebral hypoxia, anoxia, syndrome of inappropriate antidiuretic hormone (SIADH), acute sodium depletion, or infections with exudates.

Blood volume. Alterations in blood volume can occur either through an increase in the overall cerebral blood flow or because of a decrease in the venous outflow. Normally, cerebral blood flow is maintained at a relatively constant level by a process known as autoregulation. Autoregulation allows the cerebral blood vessels to change their diameter in response to variations in systemic BP, thereby maintaining a constant flow of blood through the cerebral capillary bed. Severe hypotension, hypertension, hypoxemia, hypercapnia, trauma, or brain-tissue acidosis can impede or abolish autoregulation. The result of autoregulation loss is that cerebral blood flow and volume will be affected inappropriately by fluctuations in systemic BP. Increased intravascular pressure, caused by an increase in systemic BP, will push fluid out into the brain tissue, causing brain edema. The capillary bed may become overperfused. In cases of severe hypertension, hemorrhage could occur if the basement membrane of the capillary is weakened. Severe hypotension can cause underperfusion in peripheral areas and produce infarcts of brain tissue, resulting in edema.

Cerebral vasodilation will also increase blood flow. The most potent vasodilator is carbon dioxide. An increase in the partial pressure of arterial carbon dioxide ($PaCO_2$) in a person experiencing — or at risk for — increased ICP will further increase ICP. Likewise, a direct relationship exists between hypoxemia and increased ICP. As the partial pressure of arterial oxygen (PaO_2) falls below 50 mmHg, the ICP rises. Examples of situations producing increased $PaCO_2$ can be seen in patients with an accumulation of tracheobronchial secretions or those experiencing sustained labored breathing (*see* Chapter 13).

An interruption or decrease in venous return from the cranium will result in an increase in cerebral blood volume. The bilateral internal jugular veins (IJV) are considered the primary route of venous blood return from the cranium. Occlusion of the IJV causes increased ICP. Surgical resection in persons with head and neck cancers may involve excision of sections of the IJV. Partial or total mechanical compression of the IJV by adjacent cervical structures or tumors may be a factor in ICP changes.

Venous outflow is also hindered by increases in intra-abdominal or thoracic pressures. Activities that involve holding a breath after a deep inspiration, such as coughing and straining during defecation and urination, can increase ICP. Labored respirations and vomiting can also cause a rise in ICP in the patient at risk.

Compensatory mechanisms exist to protect against a rise in ICP because of an alteration in venous return. Not only will there be compression of the venous vessels, but collateral venous circulation will assume a greater role in cranial drainage.

CSF. Alterations in CSF account for the third mechanism of increased ICP. The major portion of CSF is produced in the choroid plexus, a highly vascularized structure, which projects into the lateral, third, and fourth ventricles. The CSF is circulated through the ventricles and leaves the fourth ventricle at the foramen of Magendie and the foramen of Luschka, exiting either downward into the spinal dural sac or upward over the surface of the brain to be reabsorbed. Normally, the volume of CSF in the intracranial cavity is 20 ml. The spinal sac holds 90 to 150 ml of CSF and may accommodate a larger volume should compensation for increased intracranial CSF be necessary.

The majority of factors that alter production, absorption, or flow of CSF are related to underlying pathology. Tumors of the choroid plexus can increase CSF production. Exudate caused by infections, hemorrhage, and products of cellular destruction can interfere with CSF resorption. Tumors, blood clots, tissue necrosis, and brain herniations can obstruct CSF pathways.

In summary, the following disorders place persons at risk for increased ICP:

1. Primary and metastatic brain or skull tumors.
2. Bleeding diatheses.
3. $\geq 6,000$ rads of whole-brain irradiation with or without methotrexate.
4. CNS infection.
5. Increased $PaCO_2$, decreased PaO_2.
6. SIADH or acute sodium depletion.
7. Alterations in IJV flow by head/neck tumor or by surgical resection.

Clinical manifestations

Early signs and symptoms of increased ICP are vague and indicate general impairment of cerebral function. They include altered mental status, headache, vomiting, dizziness, and seizures (Table 14A–1).

The **alterations in mental status** are characterized by undue irritability, emotional lability, a peculiar inertia, faulty insight, forgetfulness, reduced range of mental activity, indifference to common social practices, and lack of initiative and spontaneity.

TABLE 14A–1

Neurologic Alterations Associated with Specific Areas of Brain Involvement

Brain area involved	Associated impairments
Frontal lobe	Disturbed mental status. Personality/behavior alterations. Changes in emotional responsiveness. Speech disturbances. Impaired sphincter control. Contralateral paralysis.
Temporal lobe	Psychomotor seizures. Visual field changes. Memory impairment. Dominant hemisphere: aphasia, dysphasia. Nondominant hemisphere: nonverbal, auditory perceptual disturbances, musical impairment.
Parietal lobe	Focal seizures. Hypesthesia. Paresthesia. Dyslexia. Homonymous hemianopsia. Nondominant hemisphere: perceptual alterations, visual-spatial disturbances, body scheme disturbances, impaired cognitive processes, alteration in emotional sensitivities.
Occipital lobe	Visual disturbances. Hallucinations.
Cerebellum	Disturbed equilibrium. Impaired coordination.
Brainstem	Cranial nerve palsies (temporary or permanent).

Headache is an early symptom and varies in nature; the pain may be dull or sharp and range from mild to severe. Typically, the headaches are episodic, nocturnal, present upon awakening, and deep and nonpulsatile in quality. The mechanism of headache development is not completely understood. In the majority of cases, ICP is normal during the first few weeks of headache, and the pain can be attributed to local swelling of tissues or distortion of blood vessels. Later, the headache appears to be related to generalized rises in ICP. With elevated ICP, frontal and occipital headaches occur as a rule.

Vomiting usually accompanies headache and may be projectile, with or without preceding nausea. It is commonly unrelated to food ingestion and may occur upon awakening.

Patients frequently complain of **dizziness**. It is described as an unnatural sensation in the head, coupled with feelings of strangeness and insecurity when the position of the head is altered.

The occurrence of **focal or generalized seizures** is another major manifestation. A seizure might be an isolated event without associated symptoms or might occur with other symptoms suggestive of increased ICP.

Assessment

Ongoing assessment of the neurologic status of persons at risk is necessary for early diagnosis and treatment of increased ICP. Although the general signs and symptoms discussed are not routinely a part of a nursing assessment, their frequent occurrence as *initial* symptoms makes them important in the care of a person identified to be at risk. A standard assessment of signs and symptoms will assess level of consciousness, motor function, sensory perceptions, eye/pupil changes, and vital signs (*see* Chapter 10).

Level of consciousness. This most important indicator of cerebral functioning is maintained by the normal functioning of the frontal lobe, the reticular activating system (RAS), and the nerves connecting these two brain compartments. Increased ICP impairs cerebral blood flow and oxygenation, which affects the cells of the cerebral cortex and RAS. Consciousness is a continuum extending from full reaction to various amounts and kinds of stimulation to no reaction. The observation of subtle changes in a patient's level of consciousness can be the first indication of an alteration in neurologic status.

Motor capability and sensory perception. Normally, these functions are interdependent. Sensory and motor neurons are intimately connected at all levels of the nervous system, from the spinal cord to the cerebrum. Human activity depends on a constant influx of sensory impulses that are integral to motor adaptations. When disease occurs, however, motor and sensory functions may be affected independently. Alterations in motor function, muscle strength, equality of movements, and sensory perceptions can be signs and symptoms of increased ICP. Contralateral paresis and paralysis of voluntary movement may occur as a result of ICP changes in the motor areas located in the frontal lobe. An unsteady, ataxic gait may indicate cerebellar dysfunction. The general sensations of touch, pain, temperature, and proprioception are transmitted from the thalamus to the parietal lobes for sensory interpretation. Increased ICP may result in an absence or distortion of these perceptions.

Eye/pupil changes. The effect of increased ICP on the midbrain and therefore on the 3rd, 4th, and 6th cranial nerves is assessed by examining the eyes. These nerves are paired, with one nerve on each side of the brainstem. The pairs work together so that both eyes move simultaneously. Examination of the eye includes attention to pupil size, shape, equality, response to light, and eyeball movement. Pressure on the oculomotor nerve (3rd cranial nerve) is characterized by a dilated, nonreactive pupil, ptosis of the lid, and impairment of upward, downward, and inward eye movement. Weakness of downward and inward movement is characteristic of trochlear nerve (4th cranial nerve) involvement. Failure to rotate upward and outward indicates that the abducens nerve (6th cranial nerve) is affected. Damage to the sympathetic fibers that arise in the hypothalamus will result in pinpoint, nonreactive pupils.

Increasing ICP around the optic nerve can be detected with an ophthalmoscope. ICP increase will cause the retinal veins to dilate. The result is known as papilledema, or choked disk. The persistence of papilledema may permanently damage the optic nerve.

Vital signs. Frequent assessment of vital signs provides an important indicator of ICP changes. The vasomotor center in the brainstem controls the degree of vascular constriction and regulates heart activity. As ICP increases, the brainstem is compressed, causing ischemia in the vasomotor center. This excites the sympathetic vasoconstrictor fibers and raises the systolic BP. If ICP continues to rise, the vasomotor center loses its ability to excite the vasoconstrictor fibers and BP falls. Likewise, increased ICP on the vasomotor center transmits impulses through the parasympathetic fibers of the vagus nerve to the heart to decrease the heart rate. Further increases in ICP block parasympathetic impulses and cause heart rate to increase. Therefore, assessment of early increasing ICP may reveal increasing systolic BP, widening pulse pressure, and slowing pulse. Later changes include a sharp drop in BP and a rise in pulse.

The respiratory center's medullary rhythmicity area establishes respiratory rhythm by regulating rate, rhythm, and the inspiration: expiration ratio. As ICP increases, respirations become shallow, irregular, and slower, with periods of apnea. indicating increased pressure on — or an interruption of — the descending motor tracts at the midbrain level. Characteristically, a long hyperpneic phase is followed by a shorter phase of apnea. As $PaCO_2$ rises, cerebral vessels dilate, resulting in higher ICP and worsening of symptoms.

When observing and documenting respiratory rate, rhythm, and ratio, labeling the type of respiration accurately is often difficult. Therefore, descriptions of the duration of inspiration, of any periods of apnea, and of the expiratory phase will assist in evaluation of the respiratory pattern.

Involvement or compression of the hypothalamus may result in loss of the normal temperature-regulating mechanisms. The temperature may rise as high as 41 to 42°C, then fall to 33 to 34°C. In general, fever is not preceded by chills and the skin feels warm and dry.

Medical management

In the past, surgical intervention was the only option for the management of increased ICP. Today, a variety of medical approaches preclude the need for acute surgical measures. The management plan selected will be determined in part by the severity of the condition and the status of the patient.

Corticosteroids, such as dexamethasone (Decadron) and methylprednisolone (Medrol), may be given IV in large doses. Dexamethasone is more often the drug of choice. These drugs act as anti-inflammatory agents, preventing increased capillary permeability, and as diuretics. The initial dose of dexamethasone is 8 to 10 mg IV followed by 4 mg q 6 hr. Maximum effect is normally noted after 12 hr of therapy. Side effects include all those common to steroid administration:

1. Alteration in mental state (mood changes, anxiety, depression).
2. GI disturbances.
3. Immunosuppression (decrease of eosinophils and lymphocytes); increased susceptibility to infection; masking of signs and symptoms of infection; reactivation of tuberculosis.
4. Osteoporosis.
5. Thromboembolic phenomena.
6. Aggravation of preexisting hypertension or diabetes.
7. Impotence.
8. Increased appetite.

9. Increased protein metabolism.
10. Weight gain, salt and water retention.
11. Abnormal fat distribution around the pelvis.
12. Rounding of the facies, facial rubor, acne, hirsutism.
13. Insomnia, headache, fatigue.

Fluid restriction is an essential concomitant measure. IV administration of fluids must be restricted and strictly monitored. To properly monitor urinary output, a Foley catheter is inserted. In addition, the use of an anticonvulsant such as phenytoin (Dilantin) is an early measure.

More vigorous dehydrating agents may be used. The osmotic diuretics, such as mannitol (Osmitrol), are only a short-term treatment choice. A rebound effect may occur wherein mannitol causes a fluid shift into the brain tissue, creating a further increase in ICP. Given IV, as a drip or a bolus, mannitol is effective for only 3 to 10 hr. It produces its effect in 15 to 30 min. The usual adult dosage of mannitol is 50 to 100 g/day, either in a bolus or as a 20% solution. Side effects of osmotic diuretics include **dehydration, electrolyte imbalance** (decreased serum sodium and chloride), **increased circulating blood volume** that could cause pulmonary edema, periodic **BP elevations** secondary to increased circulating blood volume, and local **thrombophlebitis.**

In many cases of increased ICP resulting from intracranial tumors, the primary treatment is RT, particularly when the increased ICP is caused by a diffuse infiltration process such as leukemic meningitis or multiple metastatic lesions. RT is also used in instances in which surgery is contraindicated because of the patient's condition, treatment desire, or tumor location.

There are patients who present with increased ICP who require rapid surgical treatment. The basic surgical techniques are: needle drainage of ventricles by way of frontal or occipital burr holes, ventriculo-peritoneal (VP) shunting procedures, bony decompression, removing either the frontal or temporal bone, and tumor resection.

Nursing management

Certain routine nursing care activities have been associated with transient or sustained increases in ICP. Modifying these activities for patients at risk for or experiencing increased ICP may help to limit damage caused by a potential ICP increase (Table 14A–2).

Increases in cerebral blood volume resulting from vasodilation can be caused by both hypoxemia (PaO_2 <50 mmHg) and hypercapnia

TABLE 14A–2

Nursing Protocol for the Management of Increased Intracranial Pressure

Factor	Intervention
Airway/adequate ventilation maintenance	Auscultate chest sounds q 4–8 hr. Monitor the administration of oxygen. Use suctioning if necessary *only* after preoxygenating. Suction should be intermittent and *brief* (<15 sec). Use narcotics cautiously because they depress respirations. Monitor blood gases.
Body positioning	Maintain bed rest. Make use of pressure-distributing mattresses (eggcrate or alternating-pressure mattress), footboards, sheepskin paddings. Offer gentle body massage. Encourage patient to keep head in neutral position. Avoid rotated head positions, flexion or extension of the neck, and extreme hip flexion. Keep head of bed elevated 30 degrees to promote venous drainage. Side lying position will decrease risk of aspiration in patients with an altered level of consciousness. Avoid prone position.
Physical stressors Isometric muscle contractions	Encourage patient to allow passive movement. Use pull sheet to turn and move patient. Avoid stimulations that elicit decorticate or decerebrate posturing in the patient with brain damage to the internal capsule and corticospinal tract or to the midbrain, respectively. If the patient must actively move, encourage him to do so on exhalation. Avoid using restraints.
Cough	Determine etiology of the cough. A cough suppressant may be indicated.
Vomiting	Assess etiology of vomiting. Administer antiemetics.
Constipation	Discourage straining. Maintain bowel regimen to prevent constipation. Avoid the

Emotional stressors	Explore potential causes of emotional stress. Counsel family to maintain a calm atmosphere. Avoid disturbing conversations at the patient's bedside. Help to maintain open channels of communication between patient, family, and interdisciplinary team.
Environmental factors Excess stimulation	Explain the unavoidable hallway and equipment noises. Make attempts to minimize excess stimulation. Provide a quiet, darkened room. Discourage the use of television or radio. Restrict visitors to close family and friends. Make other hospital personnel (i.e., housekeeping, venipuncture team) aware of the need to avoid excess stimulation. Place sign in doorway.
Stability of surroundings	Provide consistent nursing personnel. Develop a predictable daily care routine. Provide periods of uninterrupted rest.
Treatment factors Steroids	Establish base-line mental status and monitor for changes. Minimize risk of GI disturbances. Steroids should be taken with meals, antacids, or milk. Avoid aspirin. Check for guaiac stools. Minimize risk of infection. Avoid invasive procedures. Encourage all persons who come in contact with patient to wash hands. Maintain nutritional status. High-protein, high-calcium diet. Monitor for hyperglycemia and glucosuria. Monitor electrolytes, especially sodium and potassium. Weigh patient daily. Teach patient and family about visible changes (acne, abnormal fat distribution, facial changes, hirsutism). Advise them that these changes are reversible and will subside when steroid therapy is discontinued.
Diuretics	Monitor serum electrolytes and chemistries. Keep an accurate record of intake and output.

($PaCO_2$ >42 mmHg). Therefore, the maintenance of a clean airway and the monitoring of gas exchange are important nursing concerns (*see* Chapter 13).

Outflow of venous blood and/or CSF may be impeded by certain head and neck positions. Head position deserves careful attention during all care activities. The patient's bed should remain elevated to 30 degrees to promote increased cerebral drainage by gravity. This elevation should be maintained whenever possible, even when transporting the patient. If the bed is elevated >30 degrees, neck flexion can result. A negative pressure caused by flexion may force intracranial contents downward toward the foramen magnum. Head rotation can also have an effect on the patency of the IJV, and obstruction of this venous channel will affect cranial outflow. For this reason, the patient should be encouraged to maintain a neutral head position. The patient need not remain supine; however, the prone position should be avoided. Lying prone combines the problems of head rotation with increased intrathoracic and intra-abdominal pressure. Side lying is an alternative to the supine position and will decrease the risk of aspiration in patients who have an altered level of consciousness. Pressure-distributing devices (eggcrate mattresses, alternating-pressure pads, footboards, sheepskin paddings) for the bedfast patient may help to prevent alterations in skin integrity.

Increases in BP can occur because of emotional and physical stressors, such as isometric muscle contractions, coughing, vomiting, and constipation. Isometric muscle contractions can be minimized or eliminated by encouraging the patient to allow passive movement. If the patient must actively move, thus using his upper trunk muscles, have him exhale during the movement. This prevents the use of the Valsalva maneuver, which increases intrathoracic pressure as the patient holds a breath, immobilizing the upper thorax and forcing the breath up against the glottis. This increase in pressure is transmitted to the CNS and decreases venous outflow and increases ICP.

Emotional stimulation has been reported to cause an increase in ICP. Nurses need to explore with each patient and family the actual and potential causes of emotional stress in this situation. Efforts should be made to keep the patient involved and informed about his care while maintaining a calm, caring, and confident atmosphere. An alteration in level of consciousness can be a frightening event for the patient and family. If an alteration does exist, attempts should be made to stabilize the patient's surroundings. Orientation is reinforced by providing meaningful stimuli. The family should be encouraged to bring familiar objects to the bedside from home. The nurse should provide consistent assignments of nursing personnel and develop a predictable daily care routine to alleviate the stress of seeing a new face and coping with a different plan of organization each day.

Excess environmental stimulation is often stressful for the hospitalized patient. Periods of uninterrupted rest should be provided (*see* Chapter 7B). Other hospital personnel (such as housekeeping, venipuncture team) need to be made aware that the patient is resting; a sign can be placed at the patient's doorway. Meaningless noise (hallway and equipment sounds) should be minimized and explained to the patient. Restricting visitors to immediate family and significant others may be necessary. The nurse must also coordinate care schedules to ensure that the patient is not overstimulated. The interdisciplinary care team must determine which activities have priority and how to schedule them.

Bibliography

1. Adams, R. D., and M. Victor. Principles of Neurology. McGraw-Hill Book Co., New York. 1977. Second edition.

    The emphasis in this text is on categories and clinical manifestations of neurologic disease.

2. Burgess, K. E. Neurological disturbance in the patient with an intra-cranial neoplasm: sources and implications for nursing care. *Journal of Neurosurgical Nursing* (August 1983). 237–242.

    An exploration of factors that might precipitate or exacerbate neurologic dysfunction in a person with an intracranial neoplasm.

3. Kornblith, P. L. Increased intracranial pressure. *In* DeVita, V. T., S. Hellman, S. A. Rosenberg, editors. Cancer: Principles and Practice of Oncology. J. B. Lippincott Co., Philadelphia. 1982.

    Diagnosis, medical evaluation, and management are described.

4. Ladyshewsky, A. Increased intracranial pressure: when assessment counts. *The Canadian Nurse* (October 1980). 34–37.

    The etiology of ICP is briefly described. The focus is on nursing assessment.

5. Lipe, H. P., and P. H. Mitchell. Positioning the patient with intracranial hypertension: how turning and head rotation affect the internal jugular vein. *Heart and Lung* (November-December 1980). 1031–1037.

    A description of two experiments designed to measure if body position changes and head rotation affected IJV flow velocity and its cross-sectional lumen size.

6. Mitchell, P. H. Intracranial hypertension: implications of research for nursing care. *Journal of Neurosurgical Nursing* (September 1980). 145–153.

    Questions concerning potential adverse effects of common nursing care activities on ICP are reviewed. The discussion is based on pathophysiology and ICP dynamics.

7. Pizzo, P. A., D. G. Poplack, and W. A. Bleyer. Neurotoxicities of current leukemia therapy. *The American Journal of Pediatric Hematology/Oncology* (Summer 1979). 127–140.

    Clinical, physiologic, and pharmacologic aspects of neurotoxicities associated with irradiation and chemotherapy are reviewed.

8. Taylor, J. W., and S. Ballenger. Neurological Dysfunctions and Nursing Interventions. McGraw-Hill Book Co., New York. 1980.

    The anatomy and physiology of the nervous system and related dysfunctions are discussed in detail. Nursing management of persons with neurologic dysfunction is systematically examined and is a significant portion of the text.

9. Zegeer, L. J. Nursing care of the patient with brain edema. *Journal of Neurosurgical Nursing* (October 1982). 268–275.

    Brain edema is classified, and selective nursing measures that may prevent and/or ameliorate edema are discussed.

B: SPINAL CORD COMPRESSION

Donna L. Couillard-Getreuer

Spinal cord compresssion (SCC) secondary to malignant disease may develop from metastatic tumors (including leukemic infiltration) (which account for ~95% of the total incidence of SCC) and primary spinal cord tumors (which account for ~5%). According to a study by Bruckman and Bloomer, patients with solid tumors have the highest overall incidence of metastatic SCC, accounting for 52% of the total. Cancers of the lung (16%), breast (12%), and prostate (7%) carry the highest relative risk. Hematologic malignancies that may cause SCC are lymphomas (12%) and multiple myeloma (9%). This section will focus on the metastatic process resulting in SCC. Permanent neurologic damage will result unless prompt and effective emergency care measures are instituted.

Numerous classification methods are used for SCC: **Level** of cord involvement (cervical, thoracic, lumbar, sacral, cauda equina) and **location** (extradural, intradural) are the most frequently employed. The thoracic spine is most often affected by malignant tumors. Extradural tumors are located within the spinal canal but outside the dura, and they usually result from metastatic tumors (Fig. 14B–1). Intradural involvement may be extramedullary (outside the spinal cord and within the meninges) or intramedullary (within the spinal cord).

Pathophysiology

A working knowledge of the normal components and function of the CNS is necessary for an understanding of metastatic impairment. [*See* Chapter 10 for a discussion of normal spinal cord function; particularly as it relates to sensation and mobility.]

The spinal cord contains motor and sensory fibers. Complete transection of the spinal cord at any point will result in paralysis below the level of the lesion. Partial spinal cord transection may result in unequal patterns of motor/sensory loss.

Disruption of reflexes and motor function arises from tumor impairment of neurons, the functional units of the nervous system. Tumors affecting the corticospinal (pyramidal) tract, or the upper motor neuron (UMN), can result in spastic paralysis below the level of the lesion. Lower motor neurons (LMNs) originate in the anterior horn of the spinal cord segments and form the peripheral nerves to voluntary

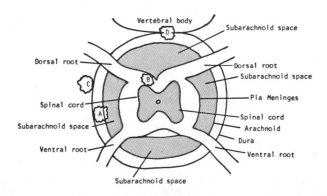

Figure 14B–1. The spinal cord, meninges, and location of various tumor types. A, Extramedullary tumor; B, intramedullary tumor; C, extradural tumor within the spinal canal; and D, bony metastasis to a vertebra outside of the spinal canal.

muscle. LMN damage causes interruption of motor and/or sensory nerve fibers, resulting in flaccid paralysis and/or sensory disturbance below the level of the lesion.

Damage to the spinal cord is caused by compressive and/or invasive growth of the tumor. The severity is dependent on the degree of tumor malignancy and tumor location within the spinal cord. Extradural involvement is the most frequent sequela of metastatic tumors. Most tumors invade the vertebral body and progress to the epidural space anterior to the spinal cord. This produces symptoms from the destruction of vertebrae, blockage of CSF, and pressure on the spinal cord (Fig. 14B–2). Intradural tumors mainly result from primary spinal cord tumors (e.g., gliomas, angiomas). Occasionally, metastatic growth may reach the intradural space through direct extension from vertebral metastases.

Clinical manifestations

The typical history of the patient with acute SCC is one of progressive back pain that occurs ≤6 mo before diagnosis. This **prodromal phase** is frequently accelerated, with up to 1 wk or more of local radicular thoracic pain. The pain may be aggravated by lying down, coughing, or motion, and may be relieved by sitting upright. Severe, agonizing pain may indicate sudden vertebral collapse, with paralysis developing over several hours. Spinal tenderness and local kyphosis may be found on physical examination.

The prodromal phase may be extended over a longer period of time, resulting in chronic compression. In most instances, the pain pattern is characterized by diffused or referred pain. As the tumor size increases — with the resultant pressure or irritation of the spinothalamic tract or

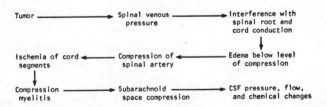

Figure 14B–2. Effects of direct pressure caused by a tumor on the spinal cord. *Adapted with permission from* Stockton, V., editor. Core Curriculum for Neurosurgical Nurses. American Association of Neurosurgical Nurses, Chicago. 1977. p. 129.

impingement on the nerves of the pia mater— pain intensity, character, radiation, and location patterns may change.

The emergency nature of acute SCC derives from the next — **compressive** — phase. The resultant sensory and motor impairment depends on the speed with which the diagnosis is made and the treatment is initiated.

Early in the disease process, sensory dysfunction occurs in ~75% of all SCC patients. Extremity paresthesia, numbness, tingling, and coolness may be present. These symptoms tend to ascend the body as time passes and as the lesion becomes more complete. Motor dysfunction may occur after or concomitant with sensory dysfunction. Common effects with either complete or incomplete UMN or LMN lesions include foot drop, weakness, balance disturbances, and locomotion impairment.

Combined motor and sensory dysfunction includes saddle anesthesia and paralysis. Saddle anesthesia most often results with metastases to the conus medullaris or cauda equina (frequently seen with prostatic carcinomas). Impaired micturition control (including hesitancy, precipitancy, retention, and overflow incontinence) is a hallmark of saddle anesthesia. Five major types of paralysis may occur with acute SCC (Table 14B-1). UMN flaccid paralysis is most often seen in early SCC (spinal shock), followed by UMN spastic in flexion (complete lesions) or in extension (incomplete lesion) in late stages. LMN flaccid paralysis may be found with cauda equina lesions, and mixed paralysis is usually found with conus medullaris lesions.

Later in the disease process, respiratory embarrassment secondary to metastatic involvement with lesions at cervical level 5 (C-5) or above may result from progressive paresis of diaphragmatic and intercostal muscles. In addition, wasting of the small muscle groups of the hands, forearms, and arms occurs with cervical involvement. Tendon reflexes are often absent at the level of the lesion, with exaggeration below the level of the lesion. Weakness and wasting of the extremities are viewed as late signs of SCC at any level.

Late signs and symptoms with metastatic compression at the cauda equina or conus medullaris level include saddle anesthesia (sensory impairment of the lumbar and sacral dermatomes; loss of urethral, vaginal, and/or rectal sensations; and loss of sphincter control).

Papilledema may be seen in patients with long-standing metastatic impairment at the thoracic and lumbar levels. This results from increased intracranial pressure secondary to increased protein in the CSF or from partial obstruction of the CSF, causing increased volume and pressure.

TABLE 14B-1

Types of Paralysis in Acute Spinal Cord Compression

Type	Tone	Bladder	Sensory	Reflexes	Comments
UMN flaccid (Total loss of sensory, motor, reflex, and autonomic function below lesion.)	Flaccid, toneless.	Painless retention, overflow incontinence.	Impaired.	All absent.	Absent sweating below lesion, and profuse compensatory sweating above. Abdominal distension due to ileus. Metastatic lesions with or without vertebral collapse.
UMN spastic in flexion (Loss of sensation and voluntary function below lesion level.)	Increased, flexion spasms.	Mass reflex, involuntary evacuation with spasms. Painless retention with overflow dribbling. Incontinence. Spontaneous filling and emptying.	Impaired.	Exaggerated tendon, extensor plantar present.	May follow UMN flaccid or with slowly progressive comprehensive lesions of spinal cord.

UMN spastic in extension (Weakness or paraplegia of lower limbs.)	Increased tone of extensors, spasms of extensors, spasticity.	Variable. Ranges from normal function, hesitancy, precipitancy, to complete loss of voluntary control with retention and overflow.	Variable impairment.	Exaggerated tendon, extensor plantar present.	Brown-Séquard syndrome with incomplete lesions. Incomplete lesions. Early SCC. Progresses to UMN flaccid or flexion.
LMN flaccid (Loss of tone of lower limbs and saddle anesthesia.)	Flaccidity, muscle wasting.	Retention, impaired micturition control.	Saddle anesthesia, absent rectal, vaginal, urethral.	Decreased or absent tendon, extensor plantar absent.	Acute or chronic lesions of cauda equina.
Mixed UMN and LMN (May have symptoms normally attributed to both UMN and LMN paraplegias; combinations of symptoms.)	Flaccid, wasting of upper extremities.	Retention.	Saddle anesthesia, impaired.	Absent, extensor plantar present.	Conus medullaris lesions. Cervical cord lesions. With respiratory failure.

LMN, lower motor neuron; SCC, spinal cord compression; UMN, upper motor neuron.
Adapted from Harries, B. Spinal cord compression. Part I. *British Medical Journal* (March 7, 1980). 611–614.

Assessment

Awareness of a high risk for the development of SCC in certain patients has resulted in earlier detection. Medical diagnosis is based on the patient's history, clinical signs and symptoms, laboratory values, and diagnostic tests. The laboratory values of the patient's erythrocyte sedimentation rate, electrophoresis, and CBC with differential should be used to determine the type of malignancy and to rule out inflammatory or other causes. The following diagnostic tests may be used to determine the type, size, location, and duration of the tumor: spinal x-rays, myelogram, CSF analysis (cytology, odor, protein, pressure, cell count, and glucose), angiography, CAT scan, and electromyelography. Clinical findings are determined by the following factors: (1) location of the tumor within the spinal column, and the functional role of that level, (2) vertical and horizontal dimensions of the tumor and compression, (3) duration of compression, (4) rate of onset of compression, (5) local blood supply to the area of compression, and (6) the patient's functional status and general overall state.

Nursing assessment of the patient with SCC should focus on the life-sustaining systems, which may be compromised. Nine major areas must be evaluated, with documentation of impairment or normal function. For each system, the patient's health history should focus on any recent changes in status and any prior impairments.

Vital signs. Interruption of sympathetic innervation from a spinal cord tumor may result in poor vasomotor tone. This manifests as hypotension, occurring most often with acute SCC. Bradycardia may indicate parasympathetic and sympathetic involvement. Involvement of the CNS may cause generalized hypothermia. The patient should be assessed for BP, pulse, apical heart rate, respiratory rate, temperature (core and extremities), and sweating patterns.

Motor status/body alignment. Muscle integrity and function, dermatome(s) marking, and the patient's ambulation status need to be appraised. This information can be used to help delineate the level of compression and the total extent of impairment. The stability of the spinal column and motor status will determine the patient's plan of care. The patient should be assessed for muscle strength (on a 0 to 5 scale) and tone, muscle wasting, atrophy, coordination (gross and fine motor), reflexes (deep tendon and plantar), ambulatory status (gait, assistive devices), spontaneous movements (spasticity, flaccidity), spinal condition (gross defects, stability), and movement of upper and lower extremities and digits. (*See* Chapter 10 for further discussion.)

Sensory status/pain. A complete assessment needs to be performed initially (*see* Chapter 10), with the patient's sensory status continually monitored. The extent of spinal cord involvement may be demonstrated by assessment of spinal tracts controlling temperature, touch, position, and vibration senses. The patient should be assessed for sensations (tingling, numbness, etc.), loss of sensations, dermatome sensory level to light touch and pinprick, and landmarks for dermatome involvement (*see* Chapter 10).

The site of vertebral involvement determines the character and location of pain. Vertebral percussion may elicit pain within one or two vertebral bodies of the level of compression. The patient's pain status should be assessed in terms of patterns (localized, radicular, dermatome, referred, diffuse, remote), character, associated symptoms (immobility, rigidity, reluctance to move or cough), quality, intensity (on a 0 to 5 scale), onset and duration, areas of tenderness to palpation along the vertebral column, location (back, neck, sacrum), aggravating qualities (e.g., Valsalva maneuver), and alleviating qualities. (A detailed discussion of pain is provided in Chapter 7A.) Finally, the patient should be assessed for level of consciousness and mentation.

Skin. Inspection of the patient's skin often reveals areas of breakdown or discoloration from sensory impairment and immobility. Evaluation of the integument can also highlight the duration of compression, with impaired integrity more likely to occur in longstanding impairment. The patient's skin should be assessed for color (extremities, general, sacrum, joints), bruising, petechiae, integrity (pressure sores, excoriation, infections), turgor, and temperature.

Ventilation. Ventilatory function may be affected in patients with high cervical lesions. The adequacy of air exchange and the mechanical process of inspiration and expiration are of paramount importance. The patient should be assessed for character of respirations; respiratory rate, rhythm, and amplitude; auscultation of lung sounds; character of chest motion (symmetry, use of accessory muscles); clear airway; cough, sputum production/character, and suctioning needs; and associated signs and symptoms (restlessness, nasal flaring, confusion, and facial color). In addition, laboratory values should be obtained for pulmonary function tests, arterial blood gases, Hct, and Hb.

Bowel. Bowel sphincter control will give further indications of the limits of impairment. Prior normal patterns and recent changes in elimination patterns need to be discerned. The patient should be assessed for bowel sounds, time of last evacuation, laxative history, abdominal distension, constipation, impaction, diarrhea, nausea, and vomiting.

Bladder. Assessment of bladder control will help indicate the extent of impairment. Prior patterns and recent changes should be discerned. On examination, the following factors should be assessed: urine output in the past 24 hr, time and amount of last voiding, and the presence of bladder distension, overflow, retention, dribbling, stress incontinence, frequency, urgency, and nocturia.

Sexual function. Evaluation of sexual impairment will help indicate the extent of motor and sensory impairment of the boundaries involved. The patient should be assessed for patterns of sexual function and recent changes, previous impairments, sexual dysfunction, and any associated signs and symptoms.

Rehabilitation needs. Finally, assessment must be made in light of current and planned medical therapy and the patient's rehabilitation potential. These areas and the total assessment of the patient will determine the patient management plan. The evaluation of a patient's rehabilitative potential should include a multidisciplinary approach with involvement including, but not limited to, physical therapy, occupational therapy, and home care nursing after the initial crisis has passed.

Medical management

The goal of medical management is to relieve the compression as rapidly as possible in order to prevent further damage to the spinal cord, thereby preserving maximum functional capabilities of the patient. The choice of medical treatment is dependent on the following factors: (1) the type of primary tumor; (2) the level, speed, onset, duration, and degree of the block; (3) the location of the lesion within the spinal cord (anterior, posterior, etc.); (4) the patient's functional level and prior therapy; and (5) the available treatment modalities and clinical experience/expertise.

The medical interventions of choice are being continually evaluated and revised. At present, the most common therapy for patients with acute SCC involves the concurrent use of radiation and glucocorticoids. This therapy has consistently demonstrated more frequent restoration of ambulation and sensation, and reduced pain. Radiotherapy should be instituted as soon as the diagnosis is made. Portals of treatment include the area of compression and one to two vertebral bodies above and below the site of the block. The goal is to administer 3,000 to 4,000 rads (the spinal cord tolerance level) over a period of 2 to 4 wk. According to a study by Greenberg et al., most radiation protocols follow the following schedule: 500 rads are administered daily for 3 days, followed by a 4-day rest, followed by 500 rads daily for 5 days (total dose: 4,000 rads). In addition, immediately after diagnosis, dexamethasone (100 mg IV) should be administered, followed by the administration of 24 mg IV q 6 hr for 3 days, at which point the drug dosage should be tapered off. The goals of dexamethasone administration are to decrease inflammation, improve neurologic function, and relieve pain.

Chemotherapy is not used for emergency treatment of SCC because it has not demonstrated the immediate effects desired in emergency situations; however, chemotherapy is used after radiation therapy if the underlying malignancy is known to be responsive to chemotherapy.

Surgical decompression of the obstruction site by laminectomy may be indicated when the need for prompt intervention exists. Indications for surgical decompression of SCC include (1) complete block with rapidly progressing neurologic defects, (2) no response or inadequate response to radiation and steroids, (3) palliation (pain control, maintainence of function), (4) high cervical lesions with risk of respiratory failure, (5) stabilization of spinal column, (6) unknown primary site, (7) uncertain diagnosis, and (8) prior radiotherapy to spine with spinal cord tolerance reached. In most cases, postoperative radiation is instituted to treat any residual tumor. Surgical treatment of SCC carries higher mortality and morbidity rates than other therapies. Several factors may help to explain this increased risk. Epidural tumors are usually located anterior to the spinal cord and do not lend themselves to ease of removal or spinal cord preservation by typical surgical posterior cord approaches. In addition, patients are often compromised because of their disease process.

Contraindications to surgical intervention center around the patient's physical status. Frequently, life expectancy at the time of diagnosis is short, and to prevent extended postoperative hospitalization is prudent.

Instability and pain ensue if the tumor destroys the vertebral bodies and the posterior body elements. In such a case, stabilization of the spinal column is indicated. External braces are often used with the cancer population for external stabilization. Internal stabilization is performed surgically by bone fusion or Harrington rod placement.

Regardless of treatment choice, evaluation of the efficacy of treatment is based on the patient's pre- vs. posttreatment ambulatory status, and the quantity and quality of pain, morbidity, and side effects. The prognosis for the recovery of motor and sensory function depends largely on the degree of disability at the time of diagnosis (Table 14B–2). The speed at which motor dysfunction occurs is more important than the duration of dysfunction. The best treatment results are obtained with patients who are ambulatory at the time of diagnosis. Conversely, those patients who are paraplegic or paretic will generally have residual paralysis or disability after treatment.

Nursing management

Nursing management is based on an individualized assessment, commonly recognized problems, and potential problems prevalent in acute SCC. Nursing management appropriately follows the nine areas of assessment (Table 14B–3).

TABLE 14B-2

Prognostic Indicators for Spinal Cord Compression

Indicator at diagnosis	Improved prognosis	Poor prognosis
Pretreatment motor status	Ambulatory	Paralysis
Rapidity/severity of motor dysfunction	Slow onset/less severe symptoms	Fast onset/more severe symptoms
Duration of motor dysfunction	<24 hr	>48 hr
Sphincter control	Present	Absent, bladder involvement
Tumor location within epidural space	Posterior	Anterior
Bony involvement of vertebral column	No structural loss, stable spine	Structural loss, unstable spine
General location of tumor	Lumbar, sacral	Cervical, thoracic

Adapted with permission from Bruckman, J. E., and W. D. Bloomer. Management of spinal cord compression. Seminars in Oncology (June 1978). 135–140.

Vital signs. Base-line measurement of temperature, pulse, apical heart rate, respiratory rate, and BP should be obtained at the time of admission or diagnosis. Ongoing monitoring by the nurse at hourly intervals until stability ensues is warranted.

Motor status/body alignment. Nursing actions center around the prevention of further damage to the spinal cord when suspected or documented vertebral instability is present. The nurse should consider the patient's spine unstable until proven otherwise.

Sensory status/pain. Pain control is an integral part of SCC management. Analgesics are usually required until the effects of treatment diminish the SCC pain stimulus. The nurse should explain the analgesic schedule to the patient and family. In addition, the nurse's ongoing assessment of patient needs is required for the titration of correct dosages as treatment commences (*see* Chapter 7A). If impairments in sensations of temperature and touch are present, the nursing care plan must include measures to ensure the patient's safety (e.g., avoid the use of hot water bottles if the patient is unable to discern between hot and cold).

Skin. Management of the potential for skin impairment needs to begin during the acute phase. A preventive approach is mandatory in order to prevent problems from occurring (*see* Chapter 9C). In addition, the rehabilitative phase after compression is easier without integument impairment.

Ventilation. The risk of respiratory impairment is present with cervical and high thoracic lesions. Acute respiratory insufficiency may result, and mechanical support of ventilation may be necessary. Pulmonary hygiene should be instituted to prevent pneumonia and atelectasis (*see* Chapter 13).

Bowel. Spinal cord impairment may result in loss of voluntary control over defecation. Although this is not an immediately life-threatening situation, measures should be instituted to assess impairment and prevent complications. Often, paralytic ileus and abdominal distension occur, followed by constipation and impaction. Patients will frequently present at the time of diagnosis of SCC with constipation or impaction. The immobility and analgesic use that are common with SCC patients compound the physiologic impairment. Patients should be started on a bowel maintenance program after relief of any preexisting impairment (*see* Chapter 11B).

Bladder. Loss of voluntary control of micturition may result in overdistension, retention, and urinary tract infection. Whereas severe distension may lead to vasomotor instability in patients with spinal shock secondary to trauma, this development is rare with malignant compressions. Ongoing observation to detect distension and prompt

TABLE 14B-3

Nursing Protocol for the Management of Acute Spinal Cord Compression

Factor	Intervention
Potential for vasomotor instability (from effects of CNS involvement)	Obtain base-line vital signs (apical heart rate, pulse, respiratory rate, core temperature, extremity temperature, BP).
	Perform ongoing assessments hourly until stabilized.
	Diagram base-line sweating patterns.
Potential for further injury to the spinal cord from unstable spinal column (increased risk with cervical and thoracic lesions)	Prevent rotation of the patient's head with cervical lesions (cervical collar, sandbags along either side of the head, no pillows on the bed, support head and neck at all times).
	Prevent further movement of the spine if there is suspected or documented vertebral instability.
	Evaluate the need for a Stryker wedge frame, CircOlectric bed, or Crutchfield tongs.
	Maintain spinal alignment during turning and positioning (log-roll to turn, pull sheet on bed for moving the patient in bed).
	Advocate bed rest until instability is disproven or treatment is completed.
	Determine if an external brace is indicated (consult with the physician).
	Position the patient with spine in proper alignment (supine with footboard, no pillows).
Potential alteration in comfort: pain related to tumor involvement of vertebral body and/or spinal cord	Provide ongoing pain assessment.
	Document methods used for pain control, and evaluate their effectiveness.
	Administer analgesics on a continuous schedule.
	Explore alternative methods of pain control.
	See Chapter 7A.

Actual or potential alteration in skin integrity related to motor and sensory impairment	Perform ongoing assessment of skin status q 2 hr. Provide skin care q 2 hr (turn and position q 2 hr, provide meticulous hygiene, massage bony prominences q 2 hr). Provide clean, dry, unironed, and unstarched bed linens. Provide an alternating air-pressure mattress on the bed. Provide nail and foot care. Provide a footboard on the bed to prevent foot drop.
Potential for ventilatory dysfunction related to impairment of intercostal and diaphragmatic muscles (increased risk with thoracic and cervical lesions)	Turn and position the patient q 2 hr. Perform pulmonary toilet q 2 hr (coughing, deep breathing, incentive spirometer [withhold percussion/vibration because of potentially unstable spine]). Suction as necessary. Provide ongoing assessment (need for ventilatory assistance [oxygen, IPPB, respirator, etc.], respiratory patterns and lung sounds, signs and symptoms of respiratory insufficiency). See Chapter 13.
Potential for alteration in bowel elimination related to loss of voluntary control, immobility, and sphincter dysfunction	Observe for signs and symptoms of paralytic ileus and impaction (check for abdominal distension, decreased or absent bowel sounds [hypotonic], nausea, and vomiting). Record and describe all stools. Perform digital examination on admission to determine if a stool is present in the rectal vault. Begin a bowel training program (see Chapter 11B). Obtain a physician's order for laxative. Encourage liberal fluid intake (~3,000 ml/day). Encourage a high-fiber diet (5–10 g/day) and the use of natural laxatives (prunes, juices, etc.).

Factor	Intervention
	Correct abdominal distension with antiflatulents, rectal tubes, and colon lavage.
	Provide ongoing assessment of bowel pattern with daily documentation of bowel sounds and stools.
Potential for alteration in urinary elimination related to overdistension of bladder and sphincter dysfunction from loss of voluntary control	Monitor urine output (check residual urine after each voiding, measure output q 1–2 hr, notify the physician if output is <60 ml/hr).
	Provide ongoing assessment (distension, retention, need for catheterization, signs and symptoms of urinary tract infection, laboratory values [BUN, creatinine, urinalysis]).
	Obtain daily urine culture.
	Begin program of intermittent catheterization (*see* Chapter 11C).
	Encourage liberal fluid intake (2–3 liter/day).

IPPB, intermittent positive-pressure breathing.

relief by catheterization are the best preventive methods (see Chapter 11C). All patients should be checked for residual urine after voiding. If impairment is present, the institution of a schedule of intermittent catheterization can be expedited during the acute treatment phase.

Sexual function. Sexual functioning in females with SCC is unimpaired, but genital sensation may be absent. Sexual function in male SCC patients is dependent on prior functioning, level and duration of compression, extent of damage to the spinal cord, and status of the sacral reflex pathways. In males and females with bowel or bladder sphincter impairment, concerns may include cleanliness. Pain may be an inhibitory factor as well. The nurse should help to direct the patient and spouse to appropriate sources for counseling and promote dialogues between the affected parties (i.e., patient, spouse, physician) (see Chapter 12).

Follow-up care

The acute phase of SCC ends when either the compression is relieved and function begins to return, or the compression is not relieved and paralysis becomes complete. Common nursing problems during this phase include respiratory impairment (pneumonia, atelectasis); nutritional disturbances (deficiencies, weight loss, anorexia); mobility impairment (immobility, thrombophlebitis, skin impairment, postural hypotension, foot drop, decalcification); sensory losses (safety); bladder and bowel dysfunction; pain control; concomitant cancer therapy; autonomic dysfunction; psychosocial coping; and sexual dysfunction. The reader should refer to the appropriate chapters in this text for detailed management of each of these impairments.

A thorough posttreatment assessment will delineate the extent of impairment and management priorities. The patient who has experienced SCC requires medical and nursing follow-up for an extended and indefinite period. The rationale for this close observation includes following residual debilities that may have remained from SCC (e.g., progression of paralysis, bowel or bladder dysfunction, contractures, pressure sores, mobility impairment); recurrence of the primary pathology; typical slow progressive recovery over many months; and common deformities or instability of the spinal column.

Nursing responsibilities during the follow-up phase include (1) referral to appropriate outpatient services; (2) referral for home-care nursing assessments and therapeutic management of residual debilities; (3) assessment of the need for occupational therapy, physical therapy, and psychosocial support, with appropriate referrals as indicated; and (4) assessment of any alterations in sexual function, with appropriate interventions and referral.

Bibliography

1. Arsenault, L. Primary spinal cord tumors: a review and case presentation of a patient with an intramedullary spinal cord neoplasm. *Journal of Neurosurgical Nursing* (April 1981). 53–58.

    Discusses clinical manifestations, diagnostic evaluation, and treatment of intramedullary tumors. Nursing assessment and care plan adaptable for extramedullary tumors.

2. Bell, M. A case study: astrocytoma of the cord. *Journal of Neurosurgical Nursing* (April 1981). 59–60.

    A case study with excellent background material. Outlines pattern of patient experiencing primary spinal cord tumor with compression.

3. Bruckman, J. E., and W. D. Bloomer. Management of spinal cord compression. *Seminars in Oncology* (June 1978). 135–140.

    Comprehensive medical discussion of metastatic epidural compression, including presenting symptoms, diagnostic evaluation, and treatment controversies. Prognostic determinants are highlighted by studies of primary malignancies and pretreatment status.

4. Carabell, S. C., and R. L. Goodman. Spinal cord compression. *In* DeVita, V. T., S. Hellman, and S. A. Rosenberg, editors. Cancer: Principles and Practice of Oncology. J. B. Lippincott Co., Philadelphia. 1982.

    The book is an authoritative reference on all forms of oncology. The chapter is an excellent, comprehensive overview of spinal cord compression and current status and includes summaries of current investigations and research.

5. Feustel, D. Alterations in neuron innervation associated with spinal cord lesions. *Journal of Neurosurgical Nursing* (April 1981). 48–52.

    Article deals with the effects of interruption to the spinal cord nerves from any cause; highlights the effects seen with lesions of motor neurons at cervical, thoracic, and lumbar regions. Helpful in understanding basis for symptoms at various levels.

6. Greenberg, H. S., J. H. Kim, and J. B. Posner. Epidural spinal cord compression from metastatic tumors: results with a new treatment protocol. *Annals of Neurology* (October 1980). 361–366.

    Study of 83 spinal cord compression patients treated with dexamethasone and radiation as outlined in this section. Early administration of dexamethasone substantially ameliorated pain in the majority of patients.

7. Harries, B. Spinal cord compression. Parts I and II. *British Medical Journal* (March 7 and March 14, 1980). 611–614 and 673–677.

    Deals with the significance of different types of paraplegia and early symptoms of spinal cord compression in part I. Part II discusses differential diagnosis and diagnostic testing.

8. Hodges, L. C. Human sexuality and the spinal cord injured: role of the clinical nurse specialist. *Journal of Neurosurgical Nursing* (September 1978). 125–129.

   Article outlines sexual dysfunction and nursing interventions for patients with spinal cord injuries. Adaptable to care of spinal cord compression patients; highlights expected dysfunction with lesions at various levels.

9. Wehrmaker, S. L., and J. R. Wintermute. Case Studies in Neurological Nursing. Little, Brown & Co., Boston. 1978. Chapter 16.

   Chapter 16 is devoted to spinal cord injury; however, many principles are common for spinal cord compression. Especially helpful are discussions of diagnostic evaluation, pathophysiologic basis for symptoms, and sexual functioning. Nursing management plan can be readily adapted to the management of the patient with spinal cord compression.

C: SUPERIOR VENA CAVA SYNDROME

Kristen Kreamer

Superior vena cava syndrome (SVCS) is a complex of symptoms and physical findings associated with obstruction of the superior vena cava (SVC). The SVC is the major venous channel returning blood from the head, neck, upper extremities, and upper thorax to the right side of the heart. Obstruction of the SVC interferes with venous drainage, resulting in increased venous pressure and dilation of superficial veins in these areas.

Pathophysiology

The SVC is particularly vulnerable to obstruction because of its physical properties, its location, and its relationship to surrounding structures. The vessel walls are thin and venous pressure low, so that it collapses easily. Tightly locked within the right anterior superior mediastinum, the SVC is bounded by rigid structures: sternum, vertebral bodies, right main bronchus, and trachea. It is encircled by the mediastinal and paratracheal lymph nodes at the junction with the azygos vein (Fig. 14C–1).

Malignant disease accounts for 95 to 97% of cases of SVCS; in a significant number of them it is the presenting condition that leads to a

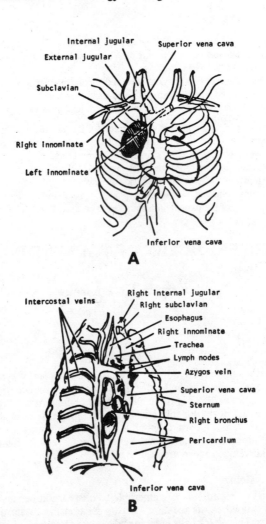

Figure 14C–1. Schematic representation of the frontal (A) and sagittal (B) sections of the thorax, showing the relationship of surrounding structures to the superior vena cava. Shaded area indicates classic site of obstruction. *Reprinted with permission from* Carabell, S. C., and R. L. Goodman. Superior vena caval syndrome. *In* DeVita, V. T., S. Hellman, and S. A. Rosenberg, editors. Cancer: Principles and Practice of Oncology. J. B. Lippincott Co., Philadelphia. 1982. p. 1583.

cancer diagnosis. Lung cancer is responsible for 70 to 85% of SVCS cases, 46% of those being cases of small cell carcinoma, 25% squamous cell carcinoma, 15% large cell anaplastic, 12% adenocarcinoma, and 2% other bronchogenic histologies. Lymphoma accounts for an additional 10 to 15% of cases. Other cancers that have metastasized to this anatomical site account for 3 to 7% of cases of malignant origin. Benign diseases (e.g., thyroid goiter, pericardial constriction, sclerosing mediastinitis, or aortic aneurysm) produce obstruction in the remaining 3% of all SVCS cases. SVCS is four times more prevalent among men than among women.

Partial or total occlusion of the SVC may result from extrinsic compression of the SVC and associated tributaries by malignant tumor itself or by metastatic disease in the mediastinal and paratracheal nodes; direct involvement of vessel walls by tumor; and/or thrombus formation within the vessels, secondary to inflammation, venous stasis, and platelet aggregation. Any of these factors, alone or in combination, can produce SVCS.

Clinical manifestations

Symptoms of <2 wk duration are reported by 20% of patients with SVCS, while 35% give a history of between 3 and 4 wk. Most frequently, patients complain of dyspnea and of facial and neck swelling experienced as a "tight collar" feeling; less often, the patient notes swelling of the trunk and upper extremities so that rings on fingers may become tight. Chest pain, cough, and dysphagia are not uncommon. CNS symptoms are relatively rare but may include headache, visual disturbance, anxiety, irritability, lethargy, or altered state of consciousness.

Physical findings on examination of the patient include thorax and neck vein distension, facial edema, and tachypnea of >30 breaths/min. The face may become ruddy and edematous and achieve an appearance likened to that of a "purple frog." Cyanosis and edema of the upper extremities may be apparent. Interference with the cervical sympathetic nerve supply may result in hoarseness, because of paralysis of the true vocal cord, and/or in Horner's syndrome, a condition in which there is unilateral ptosis with a small, regular pupil and loss of sweating on the same side of the forehead. Table 14C-1 presents an organized approach to the nursing assessment of patients at risk for SVCS.

The rapidity of onset of symptoms is the crucial factor in determining the patient's comfort and safety. More rapid onset, as in small cell lung cancer, prevents development of collateral circulation and leads to greater circulatory compromise. Small cell lung cancer is, however, more responsive to radiation therapy (RT) than squamous cell lung cancer, which is associated with a slower onset of SVCS.

TABLE 14C–1

*Nursing Assessment of Patients at Risk for
Superior Vena Cava Syndrome*

Factor	Assessment
Demographics	Gender
Base line	Vital signs Mental status Activity level Usual appearance
History	Malignant disease or its predisposing factors Duration of symptoms
Presenting symptoms*	Dyspnea Facial and neck swelling (tightness of collar) Swelling of trunk and upper extremities (rings tight on fingers) Chest pain Cough Dysphagia CNS symptoms: headache, visual disturbances, anxiety, irritability, lethargy, altered state of consciousness.
Physical findings*	Thorax and neck vein distension Facial edema Tachypnea (>30 breaths/min) Purple hue to face ("purple frog" look) Cyanosis and/or edema of upper extremities Hoarseness (caused by paralysis of true vocal cord) Horner's syndrome (unilateral ptosis with small, regular pupil and loss of sweating on same side of forehead)

*In order of most to least frequent.

Assessment

Identification of SVCS will be facilitated by a complete and accurate review of the patient's subjective symptoms, along with the nurse's objective findings. Because SVCS frequently indicates lung cancer, ascertaining whether there is a history of smoking or of exposure to environmental or occupational carcinogens is important. The diagnostic workup of a patient suspected of having SVCS will include a chest x-ray. Significant x-ray findings include evidence of a right superior mediastinal mass, mediastinal and paratracheal lympha-denopathy, and right-sided pleural effusion. If the chest x-ray is negative, a CAT scan with IV contrast may prove helpful. Procedures that may be undertaken to discover the histology of the lesion include bronchoscopy with biopsy; thoracotomy with biopsy; mediastinoscopy with biopsy; lymph node biopsy of scalene or supraclavicular nodes; and cytologic examination of sputum, of bronchial washings, or of fluid obtained by aspiration from a pleural effusion.

In some cases, when the patient is in acute distress and the complex of signs and symptoms is so dramatic as to be virtually diagnostic, emergency treatment of SVCS may be instituted without a tissue diagnosis of malignancy. The decision to treat without confirmation of the cause of obstruction may be made when it is determined that the delay for a diagnostic workup could be disastrous. In these cases, the diagnostic workup would be scheduled as soon as reasonably possible after the initiation of treatment.

Medical management

The primary goal of medical therapy of SVCS is to reduce the size of the tumor, thereby relieving the obstruction and restoring normal venous drainage. This goal is reached most commonly and most effectively through **RT**.

The determination of the total dose required is dependent on the type of tumor involved; e.g., lymphomas usually require a lower total dose than do lung tumors. Radiation may be given either on a high-dose or a conventional-dose schedule. High doses initially will result in more rapid shrinking of the tumor. On the high-dose schedule, the patient receives 3 to 4 daily doses of 300 to 400 rads/dose, followed by smaller daily doses of 180 to 200 rads until the total dose desired is reached. On the conventional-dose schedule, all daily doses are 180 to 200 rads throughout therapy.

Chemotherapy may be used in conjunction with RT in the treatment of SVCS; infrequently, it may be the only form of treatment. Specific drugs and dosage schedules are determined by the type of tumor involved.

Surgery is rarely used to treat these patients because it has been of limited benefit and carries a high morbidity; however, it may be tried if other methods fail.

Supportive medical management includes the prescription of oxygen for relief of dyspnea. Analgesics and tranquilizers may be ordered to decrease the patient's discomfort from chest pain and from the anxiety that often accompanies respiratory distress. Diuretics, particularly furosemide or ethacrynic acid, will be ordered to provide rapid — though temporary — relief of the symptoms associated with fluid retention. In addition, sodium and fluid restriction may be instituted. Steroids, although of questionable efficacy, may be ordered to reduce the inflammatory reactions associated with tumor and with RT. Anticoagulants, such as heparin and warfarin (Coumadin), and fibrinolytic drugs, such as streptokinase, may be employed if thrombus is present or suspected.

Symptomatic improvement is achieved for a majority of patients. Good to excellent symptomatic relief has been reported by 95% of lymphoma patients and 70% of lung cancer patients. The length of time from initiation of therapy to noticeable improvement varies; however, 77% report relief in 3 to 4 days, and an additional 14 to 15% note a decrease in symptoms in 7 days.

Overall survival for patients treated for SVCS is poor, with only 10 to 20% living longer than 2 yr. It must be kept in mind, however, that survival after SVCS depends on the type of malignancy involved and how responsive that malignancy is to current anticancer therapies (e.g., lymphoma patients, in general, live longer after developing SVCS than do lung cancer patients).

Nursing management

Institution of measures for symptomatic relief takes priority in the nursing care of patients experiencing SVCS. The nurse should proceed quickly to relieve hypoxia by adminstering oxygen, helping the patient to assume an orthopneic (e.g., Fowler's) position, limiting the patient's activity, and providing a calm, restful environment. A particularly distressing symptom for some patients may be the body-image change, or "purple frog" appearance. The nurse should reassure the patient that the purplish color and the edema will subside with successful therapy. The patient's objective response to medications, along with notable changes in physical findings, should be observed and documented.

The nurse must also monitor the patient for possible complications of diagnostic procedures. Because of venous engorgement in the area, excessive bleeding may occur after invasive procedures; the nurse should assess the patient for signs of blood loss. Other postoperative care should be instituted relative to the specific procedure employed (e.g., the postthoracotomy patient will have chest tubes and pleural drainage, whereas the postbronchoscopy patient needs to be evaluated for the return of the gag reflex).

The nurse should assess the patient for side effects of therapy and alleviate these when possible. The patient must receive adequate instruction to be able to participate by alerting the nurse to subjective symptoms.

Patients being treated with **RT** are likely to experience side effects, such as skin reaction, dysphagia, esophagitis, dry cough, fatigue, and nausea and/or emesis. Suggestions for relief of these side effects are provided in Table 14C–2.

Side effects experienced by patients receiving **chemotherapy** depend largely on the particular agents employed. In administering chemotherapy to these patients, it is usually necessary to avoid the right arm as a phlebotomy or IV site, because there is likely to be increased venous pressure on the right side of the body, increasing the risk of bleeding after venipuncture. Furthermore, when the right arm is used for chemotherapy, decreased circulation may result in accumulation of the drug locally, with poor absorption into the systemic circulation.

The nurse must also monitor the patient for the side effects of drugs instituted for symptomatic relief; in particular, the nurse should be aware of the implications of steroid, anticoagulant, fibrinolytic, and diuretic therapy (*see* Table 14C–2). Hyponatremia and hypokalemia are relatively common side effects of diuretic drugs; in lung cancer patients, maintaining electrolyte balance may be further complicated by the metabolic oncologic emergency known as syndrome of inappropriate antidiuretic hormone (SIADH) (*see* Chapter 15C).

The relatively rapid onset of symptoms and the atmosphere of emergency around the patient is particularly distressing for those who hitherto have had no idea that they had a malignant disease. Such patients and their families require additional support to deal not only with the immediacy of a medical emergency, but also with the diagnosis of cancer. When diagnostic procedures and therapy are being implemented without delay, time for thorough patient teaching may be inadequate. Nevertheless, the patient's need for information should be rapidly assessed and as much instruction provided as possible. Even a brief, simple explanation may alleviate the anxiety of the patient and family. More detailed information, along with continued reassurance and support, should be provided as part of the ongoing care of patients with SVCS.

Bibliography

1. Carabell, S. C., and R. L. Goodman. Superior vena caval syndrome. *In* DeVita, V. T., S. Hellman, and S. A. Rosenberg, editors. Cancer: Principles and Practice of Oncology. J. B. Lippincott Co., Philadelphia. 1982.

TABLE 14C–2

Nursing Protocol for the Management of Superior Vena Cava Syndrome

Factor	Intervention
Respiratory compromise with hypoxia Dyspnea, orthopnea, tachypnea	Administer oxygen. Vital signs q 4 hr till stable. Monitor for signs of increased respiratory distress (increased rate, increased use of accessory chest muscles, irritability, and restlessness). Position patient for maximal respiratory effort (probably orthopneic position, e.g., Fowler's). Limit activity by assisting with ADL.
Anxiety	Position call bell within reach and provide frequent reassurance of staff availability. Maintain a calm, restful environment.
Circulatory compromise Venous stasis	Remove rings and restrictive clothing. Avoid right arm for venipuncture and for administration of parenteral medications. Monitor for excessive bleeding after invasive procedures in areas of venous engorgement. Elevate upper extremities on pillows to promote venous return. Assess skin integrity in edematous areas.
Side effects of anticoagulants and fibrinolytics	Observe for spontaneous bleeding, i.e., petechiae, ecchymoses, bleeding gums, epistaxis, melena, hematuria.
Metabolic/electrolyte disturbance	Weigh daily. Record intake and output.
Steroid therapy	Check urines for steroid-induced glycosuria. Evaluate for weakness of voluntary muscles.

Diuretic therapy	Be vigilant for focal signs of infection in absence of systemic complaints. Monitor for euphoria, mood swings, or other signs of CNS stimulation. Monitor for signs and symptoms of: hyponatremia: listlessness, mental confusion, loss of skin turgor, postural hypotension; hypokalemia: muscle weakness, decreased bowel sounds, depression, cardiac arrhythmias, tetany.
SIADH	See Chapter 15C.
Emotional/psychologic concerns	Provide brief, simple explanations of planned procedures and treatments. Promote ventilation of concerns and feelings re: recent cancer diagnosis. Reassure that alterations in appearance will resolve with successful therapy.
Side effects of RT Skin reaction	Do not remove purple marks indicating radiation ports. Wash area within marks with lukewarm water only; pat dry with towel. Do not use soaps, creams, ointments, or deodorants within radiation marks.
Dysphagia and esophagitis	Monitor quality and quantity of nutritional intake. Provide soft diet — avoid irritants such as alcohol, spices, extremes of temperature. Encourage small, frequent meals. Suggest antacids for relief of burning on swallowing. Evaluate need for topical analgesia.
Dry cough	Increase humidity in room. Evaluate need for antitussives.
Fatigue	Assist patient in planning for periods of activity and rest.
Nausea and/or emesis	Evaluate need for antiemetic ½ hr before therapy.
Side effects of chemotherapy	See Chapter 2.

RT, radiation therapy; SIADH, syndrome of inappropriate of antidiuretic hormone

Medical text with details of pathophysiology, incidence, clinical implications, and treatment.

2. Donoghue, M. Superior vena caval syndrome. *In* Yasko, J. M., editor. Guidelines for Cancer Care: Symptom Management. Reston Publishing Co., Inc., Reston, Va. 1983.

Guidelines for nursing assessment and intervention, with outcome criteria.

3. Perez, C. A., C. A. Presant, and A. L. Van Amburg. Management of superior vena cava syndrome. *Seminars in Oncology* (June 1978). 123–133.

A review of 84 cases of SVCS, including presentation, incidence, diagnosis, and treatment.

4. Rubin, P., J. Green, G. Holzwasser, and R. Gerle. Superior vena caval syndrome. *Radiology* (September 1963). 388–401.

An early article comparing slow low-dose to rapid high-dose radiation treatment.

5. Spross, J., and R. Stern. Nursing management of oncology patients with superior vena cava obstruction syndrome. *Oncology Nursing Forum* (Summer 1979). 3–5.

Nursing considerations in caring for patients with SVCS.

D: TRACHEAL OBSTRUCTION

Lyn Sturdevant Davis

The trachea is a tubelike passageway through which air reaches the lungs. It is ~2.54 cm in diameter and 10.16 to 12.70 cm long and extends from the lower end of the larynx to the division of the right and left main bronchi.

Any reduction in tracheal lumen size (from tracheal stenosis, extrinsic compression, or a space-occupying luminal mass) compromises adequate gas exchange and respiratory functioning. Partial obstruction of the trachea impedes normal gas exchange, threatening life-sustaining respiratory and cardiovascular functioning. Complete obstruction of the trachea will rapidly lead to death unless there is emergency intervention.

Pathophysiology

Primary tumors of the trachea are exceedingly rare. The most common types are squamous cell and adenoid cystic carcinomas. These tumors affect males twice as often as females and are frequently diagnosed late in their course. Tracheal obstruction with primary tumors occurs as a result of intraluminal tumor growth.

Secondary tumors involving the trachea are much more common than primary tracheal tumors. The most frequently occurring types are carcinomas of the larynx, lung, esophagus, and thyroid. Metastatic carcinomas of the head and neck, breast, and lymphomas may also involve the trachea. Tracheal obstruction from secondary tumors can result from direct tumor growth into the lumen or from encroachment and extrinsic compression from adjacent masses.

Tracheal obstruction because of secondary malignancies is sometimes the result of tumor growth in the mediastinum. This obstruction occurs most often as a result of lesions developing in either the superior or posterior mediastinum (lymphomas and lung cancer). Lymphomas commonly cause impingement and collapse of the tracheal wall, whereas lung cancers within the mediastinum often directly invade the trachea. Mediastinal tumor involvement is often associated with the development of superior vena cava syndrome (SVCS) (*see* Chapter 14C).

Stenotic lesions resulting from **cuffed tracheostomy** or **endotracheal (ET) tube** use are the most common treatment-related cause of tracheal obstruction. A stenosis may develop at the tracheostomy site and/or at the inflatable cuff level. A *stomal stenosis* forms after the tracheostomy tube is removed and the margins unite by a fibrous scar. In a *cuff stenosis*, pressure that occurs between the inflated cuff and the tracheal wall leads to circumferential mucosal ulceration and tissue injury, with subsequent healing by concentric scar contracture. *Mechanical injury* resulting from movement of the tube and cuff within the trachea may also contribute to tracheal damage.

Because a tube will splint a cuff stenosis or potential stomal stenosis, obstruction appears after extubation in nearly all cases. Obstructive symptoms usually develop within 90 days after tube removal. In a small number of cases, however, obstructive signs have appeared as late as 1½ yr after extubation. Patients remain at risk for developing tracheal stenosis for at least 2 yr after extubation.

Stenotic lesions have been identified most frequently in patients who have received ventilatory assistance with cuffed tracheostomy or ET tubes; however, tracheal stenoses have also been seen in patients who have had cuffed tracheostomy tubes without ventilatory assistance. Cancer patients with a history of tracheostomy or ET intubation are at risk for developing tracheal stenoses. Patients undergoing head and neck surgery for malignant tumors are often managed with a cuffed tracheostomy tube. In addition, more aggressive management of cancer and its related complications has resulted in an increased incidence of intubation and assisted ventilation in the general oncology-patient population.

Radiation therapy (RT) is frequently employed to relieve malignant tracheal obstructions or to treat adjacent tumors before the appearance of symptoms of obstruction. Within the first few days of treatment of tumors in the tracheal region, there may be local tissue swelling, presumably due to intracellular and extracellular edema resulting from cell damage. Therefore, the risk of tracheal obstruction and subsequent respiratory compromise may be accentuated during the initial phase of RT.

Clinical manifestations

Reduction in tracheal lumen size, from whatever cause, impedes the normal flow of air to and from the lungs. Shortness of breath, especially with exertion, is an early sign of upper airway obstruction. Wheezing, stridor, and orthopnea appear with progressive narrowing of the trachea. Cough is common, and hemoptysis may be present with primary tracheal tumors. Episodes of difficulty in clearing secretions may occur as the airway narrows.

Assessment

Diagnostic studies undertaken to evaluate tracheal obstruction include lateral films of the neck; posteroanterior, lateral, and oblique views of the chest; tracheal fluoroscopy; and tomography. Pulmonary function studies will confirm a high degree of airway obstruction in patients with obstructing lesions of the trachea. Bronchoscopy is usually deferred until preparations have been made for definitive treatment of the lesion, because postbronchoscopy edema can precipitate complete obstruction.

When possible, the nurse obtains a history from the patient and/or family member regarding type, onset, and duration of symptoms, particularly shortness of breath, cough, wheezing. On physical assessment of the respiratory system, inspection of the thorax may reveal abnormal retraction of interspaces and the supraclavicular fossae during inspiration. Decreased breath sounds, rhonchi, and wheezes may be present on auscultation. Because patients with mediastinal malignancy are at risk for developing SVCS, the nurse should be alert for its associated signs and symptoms (*see* Chapter 14C).

Medical management

The most immediate concern in cases of tracheal obstruction is ensuring and maintaining a patent airway. Emergency or elective tracheostomy may be indicated before treatment of the cause is undertaken.

Primary tumors of trachea. At present, surgical resection is the only potentially curative treatment for obstruction arising from primary tracheal carcinoma. Tracheal resection with end-to-end anastomosis is the recommended surgical approach. RT has been employed as an adjunct to surgical resection, either preoperatively or postoperatively, with variable results. Repeated endoscopic resections and RT are used as palliative methods of treatment for obstructing primary tracheal tumors.

Secondary tumors. Secondary tumors involving the trachea are rarely amenable to tracheal resection, because in most cases the extent of disease precludes the potential for cure. Endoscopic resections are sometimes used to palliate obstructing tracheal lesions. A new technique of endoscopic intubation— involving permanent placement of a small metal tube in the lower trachea — has been performed in a small number of patients with malignant obstructing tracheal lesions. This technique can be used to relieve urgent respiratory obstructions and/or to provide long-term palliation.

Tracheal obstruction associated with mediastinal tumor involvement or extrinsic tumor compression is managed with RT. To reduce the potential for accentuating respiratory compromise during the initial phase of RT, oral prednisolone in dosages of 20 mg/day (1 day before and during the first 2 days of treatment) is recommended. In some cases, tracheostomy may be performed before RT is started to avoid accentuating respiratory compromise from edema during the initial phase of RT. Depending on the primary site, chemotherapy may also be included in the treatment plan.

Postintubation tracheal stenosis. The preferred treatment for significant postintubation tracheal stenosis is resection and end-to-end anastomosis of the trachea. In less severe stenoses, or in cases in which surgery is not feasible, repetitive bronchoscopic dilations or dilation with splinting (placement of an intraluminal tube, or stent, through stenosis) may be used to maintain a patent airway. Retrograde tracheal bougienage has been employed to provide urgent relief of airway obstruction caused by tracheal stenosis. This technique involves repeated passage of a small, cuffed ET tube past the stenotic segment and withdrawal with the cuff inflated. After this procedure, an ET or tracheostomy tube can be placed, in preparation for definitive surgical treatment of the stenosis.

Nursing management

Nursing interventions aimed at prevention and early detection of tracheal obstruction are outlined in Table 14D-1. The nurse should be alert to respiratory symptoms in patients with a history of tracheostomy or ET intubation. The early signs of airway obstruction (shortness of breath, cough) can easily be overlooked or mistakenly attributed to other factors, such as preexistent disease or smoking history.

Patients identified as being at risk for developing tracheal obstruction should be informed of respiratory symptoms requiring immediate medical attention. The nurse should educate patients who have obstructive tracheal tumors and are receiving pre-RT steroids as to the importance of taking the medication as prescribed and reporting signs of increasing respiratory difficulty.

Supportive nursing interventions for patients with tracheal obstruction are aimed at maintaining a patent airway and allaying anxiety. The nurse should closely monitor the patient's respiratory status and immediately report changes indicating hypoxia (such as restlessness and confusion) and increasing obstruction (e.g., wheezing, stridor, retraction of interspaces and supraclavicular fossae) to the physician. Because respiratory symptoms, such as dyspnea and difficulty clearing secretions, are often associated with high levels of anxiety, the nurse should direct interventions at reducing patient anxiety and promoting a calm, restful environment.

Bibliography

1. Cameron, S. J., I. W. B. Grant, J. G. Pearson, and C. Marques. Prednisolone and mustine in prevention of tumor swelling during pulmonary irradiation. *British Medical Journal* (February 26, 1972). 535–537.

   Reports results of a study examining the protective effect of preliminary treatment with prednisolone or mustine before irradiation in patients with partial obstruction of trachea, main, or lobar bronchus.

2. Clarke, D. B. Palliative intubation of the trachea and main bronchi. *Journal of Thoracic and Cardiovascular Surgery* (November 1980). 736–741.

   Presents new method of endoscopic intubation of malignant tumors of trachea and main bronchi with specially adapted esophageal tube.

3. Eliachar, I., K. Simon, J. H. Birkham, and H. Z. Joachims. Emergency management of tracheal stenosis. *Annals of Otology, Rhinology, and Laryngology* (January-February 1980). 46–48.

   Describes new technique, retrograde tracheal bougienage, for immediate temporary relief of airway obstruction due to tracheal stenosis.

4. Grillo, H. C. Surgery of the trachea. *Current Problems in Surgery* (July 1970). 3–59.

Provides thorough discussion of diseases of trachea amenable to surgical treatment (including postintubation stenosis and primary tracheal tumors) and operative techniques involved in tracheal resection and reconstruction.

5. Grillo, H. C. Obstructive lesions of the trachea. *Annals of Otology, Rhinology, and Laryngology* (November-December 1973). 770–777.

Describes the surgical management and outcome of 100 cases of obstructive lesions of trachea. Eighty-nine of the cases were benign tracheal stenoses; the remainder were primary tracheal neoplasms.

6. Guzman, L., and L. C. Norton. Minimizing cuff-related laryngeal-tracheal complications. *Focus on AACN* (February-March 1982). 23–25.

Reviews relevant research on cuff-related laryngeal-tracheal injuries. Includes valuable nursing protocol aimed at preventing laryngeal-tracheal complications in intubated patients.

7. Lokich, J. J. Pulmonary complications of malignancy. *In* Lokich, J. J., editor. Clinical Cancer Medicine: Treatment Tactics. G. K. Hall & Co., Boston. 1980.

Contains brief discussion of tracheal obstruction arising from mediastinal lesions and recommendations for management.

8. Portlock, C. S., and D. R. Goffinet. Tracheal obstruction. *In* Portlock, C. S., and D. R. Goffinet. Manual of Clinical Problems in Oncology. Little, Brown & Co., Boston. 1980.

Concise, up-to-date discussion of management of tracheal obstruction from benign or malignant causes.

9. Sise, J. G., and R. W. Crichlow. Obstruction due to malignant tumors. *Seminars in Oncology* (June 1978). 213–224.

Brief but valuable summary of tracheal obstruction secondary to malignant tumors. Clinical presentation and diagnostic workup are well discussed.

TABLE 14D–1

Nursing Protocol for Prevention and Early Detection of Tracheal Obstruction

Factor	Intervention
Malignancy Patients with metastatic/advanced cancers of lung, larynx, head and neck, esophagus, breast, and thyroid; lymphomas and mediastinal tumor involvement.	Assess respiratory system. Evaluate for obstructive symptoms: shortness of breath, wheezing, difficulty clearing secretions, cough. Monitor for signs of obstruction: retraction of interspaces and supraclavicular fossae, abnormal lung sounds: decreased breath sounds, rhonchi, and wheezes. Educate regarding signs and symptoms requiring medical attention: shortness of breath, persistent cough, wheezing, difficulty clearing secretions.
Current treatment Patients intubated with ET or tracheostomy tubes.	Monitor cuff pressures q 4 hr using three-way stopcock open simultaneously to cuff and manometer. Maintain at ≤30 mmHg. Use minimal-leak or minimal-occluding-volume technique whenever possible. Prevent excessive tube movement: stabilize head position; stabilize tube and tubing. Limit transient cuff pressure elevations by judicious use of bagging and vibration; sedation as indicated to prevent "fighting" the ventilator. Use upright body position when possible to promote venous drainage and reduce edema in tracheal tissue.

Patients undergoing RT to obstructing tracheal tumors.	Monitor respiratory status closely (*see* Malignancy *above*) during first 3 days of RT treatment. Observe for signs and symptoms of increasing obstruction. Educate regarding need to report to physician symptoms of increasing respiratory difficulty.
Patients with obstructing tracheal tumors receiving pre-RT steroid therapy.	Educate regarding need to report to physician symptoms of increasing respiratory difficulty. Reinforce importance of taking medication as prescribed.
Prior treatment Patients with prior history of ET or tracheostomy tube intubation, especially in conjunction with ventilatory assistance.	Assess respiratory system (*see* Malignancy *above*). Evaluate for obstructive symptoms. Monitor for signs of obstruction. Educate regarding signs and symptoms requiring medical attention (*see* Malignancy *above*), and importance of regular physician visits.
Patients with history of prior treatment (surgical resection, RT) for malignant obstruction.	Assess respiratory system (*see* Malignancy *above*). Evaluate for obstructive symptoms. Monitor for signs of obstruction. Educate regarding signs and symptoms requiring medical attention (*see* Malignancy *above*) and importance of medical follow-up.

ET, endotracheal; RT, radiation therapy.

E: BOWEL OBSTRUCTION

Lyn Sturdevant Davis

SMALL BOWEL

One of the primary functions of the small bowel, or intestine, is to absorb the products of digestion (*see* Fig. 8–1). During this process, there is an enormous exchange of fluids and electrolytes across the small-bowel mucosa. Saliva and gastric, pancreatic, biliary, and intestinal secretions deliver ~8 liters, or one-fifth of the total body water, to the small bowel in 24 hr. Most of this fluid is reabsorbed before it reaches the colon. Two unidirectional fluxes occur simultaneously in the small intestine. In **absorption**, fluids and electrolytes move from the intestinal lumen through the small-bowel mucosa to the interstitial fluid. Conversely, in **secretion**, fluids and electrolytes flow from the interstitial fluid to the intestinal lumen.

Pathophysiology

Mechanical bowel obstruction is the result of a physical block to the onward passage of intestinal contents. **Functional** bowel obstruction is caused by a loss of propulsive peristalsis (e.g., paralytic ileus occurring after surgery). This discussion is focused on mechanical causes of bowel obstruction, which can be subdivided into three types: intraluminal, mural, and extramural. **Intraluminal** obstructions are caused by obstructing matter in the bowel lumen, such as fecal impaction. **Mural** obstructions result from lesions of the bowel wall — such as colon carcinomas — that block the intestinal lumen. **Extramural** obstructions are caused by external compression of the bowel wall — e.g., by hernias or adhesive bands.

When the small intestine becomes obstructed, the block forces secretions from the stomach, pancreas, and biliary tree, along with swallowed air, to pool above the obstruction and distend the small bowel. The movement of fluid and electrolytes is disrupted. Once distension occurs, the functioning of the small bowel is altered, because distension impedes venous return and the absorptive process; the bowel wall becomes edematous and begins to secrete water, sodium, and potassium into the fluid pooled in the intestinal lumen. For reasons that are unclear, distension greatly stimulates the secretory activity of the gut but does not correspondingly increase the rate of absorption.

The distension process extends proximally, involving successive loops of bowel and further impeding absorption. The pooling of fluid in the intestinal lumen depletes the body's circulating fluid volume. Without treatment, profound hypovolemic shock will ensue.

Distension of the small intestine can lead to pressure necrosis of the bowel wall and result in strangulation. Strangulating obstruction occurs when the blood supply of the bowel wall is impeded, causing the wall to become necrotic and liable to perforate. The complications of septic shock are then added to the effects of obstruction. If corrective surgery for strangulating obstruction is delayed beyond 36 hr, the mortality rate is >25%.

Complete small-bowel obstruction is a life-threatening condition requiring immediate medical intervention. Fluid losses must be replaced to prevent hypovolemic shock, and close monitoring is necessary to permit early identification and treatment of strangulating obstruction.

Disease-related causes of small-bowel obstruction. **Primary tumors** of the small intestine are rare, comprising only 1 to 3% of all GI tumors. Carcinoid tumors, adenocarcinoma, leiomyosarcoma, and lymphoma constitute the great majority of primary small-bowel tumors. These malignancies can cause obstruction by progressive growth and occlusion of the lumen, kinking of the bowel, or intussusception. Carcinoid tumors are particularly prone to cause obstruction.

Secondary tumors involving the small intestine are the most common cause of small-bowel obstruction in cancer patients, occurring more than twice as frequently as obstruction caused by primary tumors. Small-bowel metastases may occur through direct extension of a primary tumor, by way of the lymphatics or blood vessels, or as the result of intra-abdominal carcinomatosis. Direct extension may occur from tumors originating in the pancreas, colon, or stomach. Small-intestinal metastases via the lymphatics and blood vessels may result from melanoma and cancers of the uterus, breast, and lung. Intra-abdominal carcinomatosis produces obstruction most frequently and is most commonly seen in ovarian, colonic, gastric, and pancreatic carcinomas. Metastases to the small bowel are often multiple. Obstruction results from the bulk of the growth, with angulation, fixation, and flattening of the bowel wall.

Treatment-related causes of small-bowel obstruction. **Bands of adhesions** or **scar tissue** from abdominal operations can constrict the lumen if they encircle a loop of bowel, thus resulting in small-intestinal obstruction. Adhesions constitute the most common cause of small-intestinal obstruction (60% of all cases). Cancer patients frequently undergo abdominal surgery during diagnosis and treatment of their disease and are consequently at risk for developing small-bowel obstruction.

Abdominal and **pelvic irradiation** may lead to late radiation injury to the small bowel. These late effects of radiation therapy (RT) can occur from months to 20 yr after completion of treatment. Small-bowel obstruction is the most common presentation of severe late radiation injury to the small intestine. Tissue changes that occur include mucosal and submucosal ulcerations, atrophy of glandular mucosa, collagen degeneration, and vascular damage. The wall of the small intestine is usually thickened secondary to submucosal fibrosis, and there may be segments of bowel with narrowed lumens and proximal dilation. The mesentery may also be thickened, resulting in shortening of the bowel.

The incidence of late radiation injury appears to be dependent on the radiation dose and the volume of bowel irradiated. The incidence of late effects increases with increasing total dose, although no formula has been developed that can predict damage based on dosage. The incidence of damage also increases when larger volumes of bowel are irradiated.

LARGE BOWEL

The major function of the large bowel (*see* Fig. 8–1) is absorption of water and electrolytes in the proximal half and storage of feces in the distal half until defecation occurs. Each day 1 to 2 liters of fluid is delivered to the large bowel from the small bowel. Of this fluid, all but 100 to 200 ml, which is excreted in the feces, is absorbed in the colon.

Pathophysiology

When the large bowel is obstructed, fluid and gas accumulation proximal to the obstruction occurs, but — in comparison with small-bowel obstruction — intraluminal fluid accumulation is slight and the metabolic results of fluid loss are generally not as severe. The urgent nature of large-bowel obstruction is related to the potential for rupture and perforation of the cecum, an event associated with a mortality rate of ~50%. If, in cases of complete bowel obstruction, the ileocecal valve remains competent — thus preventing reflux of colonic contents — the escape of fluid and gas proximally is prevented. A closed-loop obstruction results. This type of obstruction causes a rapid increase in intraluminal pressure as the colon distends. The cecum, with its large diameter and thin walls, is predisposed to rupture. Prompt treatment of large-bowel obstruction is required to avoid perforation.

In cases where the ileocecal valve permits reflux of colonic contents, small-bowel distension ensues, and the symptoms of small-bowel as well as large-bowel obstruction appear. An associated small-bowel distension is a frequent occurrence with large-bowel obstruction. High intraluminal cecal pressure may be present in cases in which reflux occurs, so that immediate intervention is urgent.

Disease-related causes of large-bowel obstruction. Obstruction in the colon and rectum occurs with about half the frequency of small-bowel obstruction, but >50% of large-bowel obstructions are caused by a primary malignancy of the colon and rectum. It is estimated that one in five patients with colon carcinoma will present with obstruction as a significant feature, and that in half of this number, an emergency operation will be required.

Right-sided colonic carcinomas may obstruct with luminal tumor growth, although this is usually a late development because of the relatively large diameter of the right side of the colon. Other mechanisms of obstruction include intussusception and swelling and edema of the bowel wall secondary to tumor.

Left-sided colonic carcinomas are a common cause of large-bowel obstruction. Of obstructing lesions in the colon, 75% occur distal to the splenic flexure. Left-sided lesions tend to grow annularly, producing a "napkin-ring" constriction. Severe stenosis and obstruction can be produced as the carcinoma encircles the bowel completely. A partial obstruction may be converted to a total one by swelling and edema secondary to tumor, or by the lodging of solid fecal material in the stenotic area.

Rectal carcinomas less commonly produce obstruction, because of the large diameter of the rectal ampulla, earlier recognition of symptoms, and the relative ease of diagnosis.

Occasionally, metastatic tumors may obstruct the colon or rectum by direct extension, usually from primary tumors arising in GU organs, such as the ovary and cervix. Metastases from distant primary tumors rarely obstruct the colon. When obstruction does occur, it usually arises from serosal deposits secondary to widespread metastatic carcinomas. The primary sites most often responsible are breast, stomach, pancreas, lung, ovary, and small bowel. Rarely, retroperitoneal tumors (such as leiomyosarcoma, liposarcoma, or lymphoma) will cause sufficient extrinsic pressure so that stenosis and obstruction result.

Treatment-related causes of large-bowel obstruction.   Late radiation injury to the large bowel, occuring months or years after treatment, is relatively uncommon. It generally presents as an obstruction or fistula of the rectosigmoid. Injury to the vascular and supporting tissues of the bowel is the presumed pathophysiologic cause.

The neurotoxicity of the vinca alkaloids, such as vincristine sulfate and vinblastine sulfate, places patients at risk for the development of constipation and paralytic ileus. Severe constipation, with resultant large-bowel obstruction, has required surgical intervention in rare instances. Elderly patients and those receiving vinca alkaloids for prolonged periods have an increased risk for developing vinca alkaloid neurotoxicity. Concomitant usage of other constipating drugs, such as narcotic analgesics and anticholinergics, further increases susceptibility to constipation (*see* Chapter 11B).

Many cancer patients are prescribed narcotic analgesics for pain management. Constipation is a frequent side effect of narcotics because these drugs inhibit peristaltic motility. Neglected constipation can lead to serious fecal impaction and bowel obstruction.

Clinical manifestations

Table 14E–1 presents a comparison of signs and symptoms for small- and large-bowel obstructions. Abdominal pain and vomiting are the most common symptoms in small-bowel obstruction. Episodes of crampy abdominal pain usually have a crescendo-decrescendo pattern, with a pain-free interval between attacks. Severe continuous pain may indicate strangulation. Vomiting occurs early and is profuse. Acid/base imbalances are common. Depending on the level of obstruction, vomiting may result in metabolic acidosis or alkalosis.

Characteristically, symptoms of large-bowel obstruction are insidious, developing over weeks or months. The most common complaint is abdominal pain or discomfort. The pain is usually crampy and generally milder than the pain associated with small-bowel obstruction. Abdominal distension is the most common physical finding and is frequently quite pronounced.

TABLE 14E–1

Comparison of Clinical Presentations of Small- and Large-Bowel Obstructions

Factor	Small-bowel obstruction	Large-bowel obstruction
Onset	Rapid	Insidious
Abdominal pain	Severe: crampy, intermittent attacks	Generally less severe; usually crampy
Vomiting	Occurs early; frequent and profuse	Occurs late; sometimes never
Bowel habits	Obstipation once distal tract emptied	Diarrhea, narrowing of stools, eventual obstipation
Abdominal distension	Often present	Pronounced
Dehydration	Early, life-threatening	Late
Electrolyte and acid/base imbalances	Common	Rare

Assessment

Diagnostic studies undertaken in cases of suspected bowel obstruction include three-way abdominal x-rays and laboratory studies. In instances of small-bowel obstruction, an abdominal flat plate classically demonstrates a ladderlike pattern of distended small-bowel loops, with air-fluid levels. In the case of large-bowel obstruction, abdominal x-rays display a distended colon, often with an associated picture of small-bowel distension. Evaluation of large-bowel obstruction also includes proctosigmoidoscopy, barium enema, and pelvic examination for women. If perforation is suspected, barium enema should be avoided or performed with a water-soluble contrast material.

Required laboratory tests include a CBC and electrolyte studies. An elevated WBC count (15,000 to 20,000 cells/mm³) suggests strangulation. Elevated Hct may reflect dehydration secondary to fluid shift. Hypochromic microcytic anemia may be seen in cases in which occult blood loss has occurred over the preceding weeks or months. Electrolyte imbalances — such as hypochloremia, hypokalemia, and hyponatremia — and acid/base disturbances are commonly present in small-bowel obstruction.

A GI history from the patient or family member may reveal such symptoms as anorexia, nausea, vomiting, abdominal distension, abdominal pain, change in bowel habits, constipation, obstipation, and GI bleeding.

On physical examination, gross distension is often observed with large-bowel obstruction. Distension may be great enough to raise the diaphragm and cause respiratory embarrassment. Waves of peristalsis in dilated loops of bowel are sometimes visible through the abdominal wall as the bowel attempts to propel its contents past the obstruction. High-pitched bowel sounds that occur in rushes during episodes of colic are frequently noted. If strangulation or long-standing obstruction is present, bowel sounds will be absent. Tympanitic percussion notes predominate because of gaseous distension. Localized tenderness on palpation suggests strangulation.

Medical management

Small-bowel obstruction is usually managed by surgery. The compelling reason for surgery is that strangulation, associated with high morbidity and mortality, cannot be excluded with certainty so long as obstruction persists. The operation may be preceded by a period of careful preparation and close observation. In selected cases, surgery may be delayed or avoided. Surgery is generally avoided in patients with a history of numerous operations for obstruction. Medical treatment may resolve some instances of partial small-bowel obstruction. During medical treatment, fluid and electrolyte imbalances are identified and corrected, and intubation with either a nasogastric or an intestinal tube for decompression is initiated. The patient is then closely monitored for signs of strangulation obstruction (elevated temperature, localized abdominal tenderness, elevated WBC count) which indicates the need for immediate surgery.

The management of obstruction arising from primary tumors of the small bowel is surgical resection. For cases of small-bowel obstruction secondary to metastatic tumor, surgery (consisting of side-to-side anastomosis) is usually indicated if there is no resolution of obstruction within a few days of medical management. Small-bowel obstruction secondary to RT injury is also treated surgically by side-to-side anastomosis if medical therapy is unsuccessful. Adhesive bands causing obstruction are lysed during laparotomy.

The management of **large-bowel obstruction** is also surgical. Immediate operation is required to avoid the life-threatening risk of cecal perforation. Surgery is delayed only long enough to correct any existing fluid and electrolyte imbalances. Preoperative intubation may be used to prevent vomiting and small-bowel distension, but it does not serve to decompress the large bowel.

The immediate goal of surgery for large-bowel obstruction is decompression of the obstructed segment. The secondary goal, when bowel obstruction is caused by primary carcinoma of the colon and rectum, is resection of tumor and the surrounding lymphatics. Tumor resection may be accomplished at the initial operation or planned as a second procedure 2 to 3 wk after decompression of the proximal bowel. Table 14E–2 outlines surgical approaches in obstructive colorectal carcinomas. One-staged procedures have recently been recommended for left-sided obstructive colonic carcinomas; however, these are generally considered unduly hazardous, because of the technical difficulties of left-sided-colon reanastomosis in an obstructed bowel, as well as the increased potential for postoperative septic complications.

For metastatic cancers resulting in large-bowel obstruction, diversion by colostomy or bypass procedures such as enterocolostomy are the operations most frequently used. Selected patients may be considered candidates for radical surgery, such as pelvic exenteration. Rectosigmoid RT injuries producing obstruction are usually managed by permanent end colostomy or low anterior resection (*see* Chapter 11A).

Nursing management

Nusing interventions should be aimed at **prevention** and **early detection** of bowel obstruction. The importance of regular rectal examination and sigmoidoscopy for persons >40 yr of age cannot be overemphasized. Digital-rectal examination can detect ~½ of all

TABLE 14E-2

Surgical Approaches in Malignant Large-Bowel Obstructions

Carcinoma	Surgical approaches
Right colon	One-stage procedure: Resection with primary anastomosis.
Transverse colon	One- or two-stage procedures.
Left colon	One-stage procedure: Decompression and resection.
	Two-stage procedures: Preliminary diversion (cecostomy or transverse colostomy); definitive cancer surgery 2–3 wk later.
Rectum	Two-stage procedures: Proximal diversion (sigmoid loop colostomy); definitive cancer surgery.

colonic cancers, and two out of three colorectal tumors can be visualized and biopsied with sigmoidoscopy. The nurse can play a valuable role in early detection by educating the public.

Patients at risk for developing bowel obstruction should be instructed to report symptoms such as vomiting, abdominal distension, and constipation. The nurse should be alert to GI complaints of patients with advanced malignancies and carefully evaluate symptoms that suggest possible bowel obstruction.

Supportive nursing interventions for patients with bowel obstruction are presented in Table 14E–3. Patients undergoing medical treatment for bowel obstruction must be closely monitored for signs of shock and strangulating obstruction. Careful attention to fluid and electrolyte status can help prevent dehydration or overhydration.

During both medical and surgical management of bowel obstruction, the digestive tract cannot be used for an extended period of time. Consideration must be given to how a patient's nutritional needs will be met. Cancer patients (especially those with advanced disease) are often depleted nutritionally, and the stress of surgery further increases nutritional requirements (*see* Chapter 8). Parenteral hyperalimentation may often be indicated until the enteral route is fully functional.

During the postoperative period, special attention should be given to wound healing. Poor nutritional status and immunosuppression places many cancer patients at risk for wound infection and impaired healing. Meticulous wound care and adequate nutritional support can help prevent these complications.

TABLE 14E–3

Nursing Protocol for the Management of Bowel Obstruction

Factor	Intervention
During medical treatment*	
Potential for hypovolemic or septic shock	Observe for signs of shock: cool, clammy skin, diaphoresis.
	Monitor vital signs frequently: report increased pulse, decreased BP; elevated temperature (sign of strangulation).
	Monitor urinary output; report output <40 ml/hr.
	Monitor central venous pressure as applicable.
	Report localized abdominal tenderness and elevated WBC count (signs of strangulation).
	Plasma, blood, and antibiotics may be administered.
Potential/actual fluid deficit and electrolyte imbalance	Monitor serum electrolyte values as obtained.
	Monitor urinary output; maintain accurate intake and output measurements.
	Check urine sp gr q 2 hr: high sp gr may indicate inadequate fluid replacement.
	Monitor IV fluid and electrolyte replacement.
Alteration in GI functioning	Assess GI system: abdominal pain; location, duration, character, abdominal distension; daily abdominal girths for prolonged medical treatment.
	Auscultate bowel sounds.
	Report abdominal tenderness.
	Check amount, consistency, guaiac of stools.
	Note volume, color, odor, of emesis or tube drainage.
	Nasogastric/intestinal decompression:
	Advance intestinal tube as prescribed.
	Maintain patency, irrigate as prescribed.
	Provide frequent mouth care, q 1–2 hr.
	Provide topical anesthetics for sore throat.

Nutritional deficit

Parenteral hyperalimentation often indicated (see Chapter 8).

Fear/anxiety

Provide clear, simple explanations of procedures, tests, treatments to patient and family members.

Provide emotional support.

Alteration in comfort

Use narcotics sparingly; may mask signs of obstruction and complications. Meperidine is preferred to morphine sulfate.

Provide comfort measures (see Chapter 7A).

During surgical treatment

Preoperative care
Potential/actual fluid and electrolyte imbalance

Goal: stabilize physiologically.
Monitor serum electrolyte values;
Administer fluid and electrolyte therapy as prescribed.

Potential anemia

Obtain CBC; blood transfusion may be indicated.

Potential infection/sepsis

Administer antibiotics as prescribed.

Need for information

Preoperative teaching for patient/family members when possible; give clear and simple explanations.

Fear/anxiety

Provide clear and simple explanations to patient and family members.

Provide emotional support.

Postoperative care
Potential infection

Administer antibiotics as prescribed.
Monitor respiratory status; check lung sounds; decreased breath sounds, abnormal lung sounds; assist with turning, coughing, deep-breathing q 1–2 hr.
Observe for signs and symptoms of urinary tract infection: dysuria, frequency, cloudy, strong-smelling urine; avoid prolonged catheterization.
Monitor for early signs of sepsis, especially hypotension.

Factor	Intervention
Decreased mobility	Check for calf tenderness ≥q 8 hr.
	Assist/instruct with leg exercises: flexion and extension, quadriceps setting, ankle turns q 2 hr.
	Promote self-care activities.
	Assist with progressive ambulation.
Alteration in GI functioning	Care for GI tube as above.
	Assess for abdominal distension; obtain daily abdominal girths as indicated; report increasing distension.
	Monitor return of GI functioning closely; check for return of bowel sounds and passage of flatus ≥q 8 hr.
	Monitor for nausea and vomiting as diet is advanced.
Alteration in comfort: incisional pain	Administer analgesics to provide adequate pain relief.
	Assist/instruct in splinting incision.
	Provide comfort measures.
Nutritional deficit	Parenteral hyperalimentation may be indicated.
	Consult with physician and dietician regarding need for oral supplements.
Wound healing	Monitor for signs of infection: redness, tenderness, warmth, drainage and impaired wound healing; poor approximation of wound edges.
	Provide meticulous wound care.
	Assess need for nutritional support as above.

sp gr, specific gravity.
*The medical management section applies primarily to patients with small-bowel obstruction who are receiving medical treatment. The majority of large-bowel obstructions require immediate surgical intervention.

Bibliography

1. Bizer, L. S., R. W. Liebling, H. M. Delany, and M. L. Gliedman. Small bowel obstruction. *Surgery* (April 1981). 407–413.

    Presents clinical material from 405 patients treated for mechanical small-bowel obstruction.

2. Greenlee, H. G., G. V. Aranha, and A. J. DeOrio. Neoplastic obstruction of the small and large intestine. *Current Problems in Cancer* (August 1979). 4–49.

    Lengthy but comprehensive discussion of malignant causes of small- and large-intestinal obstruction. Pathophysiology, clinical presentation, diagnostic evaluation, and alternative approaches in surgical management are presented.

3. Given, B. A., and S. J. Simmons. Gastroenterology in Clinical Nursing. C. V. Mosby Co., St. Louis. 1979.

    Chapter on intestinal obstruction includes discussion of pathophysiology, clinical presentation, and management of intestinal obstruction.

4. Ketcham, A. S., R. C. Hoye, Y. H. Pilch, and D. L. Morton. Delayed intestinal obstruction following treatment for cancer. *Cancer* (February 1970). 406–410.

    Presents results of study of 117 patients who had been treated for cancer and subsequently developed intestinal obstruction.

5. Kinsella, T. J., and W. D. Bloomer. Tolerance of the intestine to radiation therapy. *Surgery, Gynecology and Obstetrics* (August 1980). 273–284.

    Detailed description of acute and late effects of irradiation to bowel. Includes discussion of small- and large-intestinal obstruction.

6. Literte, J. W. Nursing care of patients with intestinal obstruction. *American Journal of Nursing* (June 1977). 1003–1006.

    Good overview of nursing management of patients with bowel obstruction. Includes helpful nursing interventions for patients undergoing intestinal decompression.

7. Osteen, R. T., S. Guyton, G. Steele, and R. E. Wilson. Malignant intestinal obstruction. *Surgery* (June 1980). 611–615.

    Reports clinical material from 66 patients treated for cancer who later developed intestinal obstruction. Suggested criteria for medical vs. surgical management are presented.

8. Sise, J. K., and R. W. Crichlow. Obstruction due to malignant tumors. *Seminars in Oncology* (June 1978). 213–224.

    Includes concise discussion of clinical presentation and management of small- and large-bowel obstruction caused by malignant tumors.

9. Spiro, H. M. Clinical Gastroenterology. Macmillan, Inc., New York. 1983. Third edition. 429–500, 661–662.

   Chapter on intestinal obstruction discusses pathophysiology, clinical features, diagnosis, and treatment of intestinal obstruction. Also contains a nice summary of small bowel metastases.

10. Wilson, R. E. Surgical emergencies. In DeVita, V. T., S. Hellman, and S. A. Rosenberg, editors. Principles and Practice of Oncology. J. B. Lippincott Co., Philadelphia. 1982.

    Includes brief discussion of clinical management of small- and large-bowel obstruction in cancer patients.

CHAPTER 15

METABOLIC EMERGENCIES

A: HYPERCALCEMIA
Joan Martin Moore

Hypercalcemia is a common and potentially fatal complication of malignancy. A rise in the serum calcium level may occur slowly and go unrecognized until severe symptomatology develops, or it may occur swiftly, causing a crisis within a short period of time. Hypercalcemia is considered an oncologic emergency because it can be quickly fatal. Fatal complications include: renal failure, coma, and cardiac arrest. Prompt, effective treatment will reverse hypercalcemia. The prognosis depends on the speed with which the condition is recognized and treated.

Although the exact incidence of hypercalcemia is unknown, it is estimated to occur in ~10% of cancer patients. For certain breast and lung tumors, however, the incidence may be 40 to 50%. While any tumor type can cause hypercalcemia, multiple myeloma, lymphomas, tumors of the breast, lung, kidneys, prostate, head, neck, and esophagus are the most frequently associated malignancies.

Pathophysiology

Care of the patient at risk for hypercalcemia requires an understanding of the mechanisms of normal calcium regulation as well as of the pathophysiology related to hypercalcemia in malignancy, the clinical manifestations, and the rationale for treatment.

Normal calcium regulation. Calcium concentration in the body is maintained within a narrow range of 9 to 11 mg/dl under normal conditions. Three organ sites are involved in this process: (1) bone, which contains 99% of the body's calcium; (2) the GI tract, which absorbs ingested calcium or eliminates it in feces; and (3) the kidney, which filters and reabsorbs ionized calcium (Ca^{++}).

Hormonal regulatory mechanisms.   Calcium homeostasis depends on sensitive regulatory mechanisms that are altered in response to the serum calcium level. These regulatory mechanisms include parathormone (PTH), vitamin D, and calcitonin.

PTH is a hormone, secreted by the parathyroid gland in response to low serum calcium levels, that stimulates osteoclasts, cells that act to break down bone tissue. Calcium is thus moved from bone into the extracellular fluid. PTH also stimulates gastric and kidney reabsorption of calcium. The net result of PTH secretion is therefore an increase in serum calcium. Vitamin D secretion also increases serum calcium by enhancing gastric absorption of calcium and release of calcium from bones.

Conversely, calcitonin, a hormone secreted by the thyroid gland in response to high serum calcium, decreases serum calcium levels by inhibiting osteoclast activity. This reduces bone destruction and release of calcium into the bloodstream.

When hypercalcemia occurs, the body's effort to maintain homeostasis should result in suppression of PTH and vitamin D secretion and enhancement of calcitonin secretion. If these measures are inadequate, normal regulatory mechanisms fail and the hypercalcemic condition worsens.

Mechanisms of hypercalcemia in malignancy.   Most frequently, hypercalcemia of malignancy is associated with bone disease. Of all hypercalcemic patients, ~85% have bone metastases. Therefore, patients with primary tumors that frequently metastasize to bone are at high risk for developing this complication (*see* Appendix B). Bony metastases accelerate bone resorption, causing destruction of the bone and release of calcium into the extracellular fluid. The resulting influx of calcium exceeds the capability of the body's calcium regulating mechanisms.

Hypercalcemia occurs in ~15% of cancer patients in the absence of bone metastasis. It has been found that some tumors, such as bronchogenic carcinoma and hypernephroma, secrete PTH-like substances. Recall that the net effect of PTH secretion is an increase in serum calcium. Therefore, any substance that mimics PTH will result in a rise in serum calcium.

Another cause of hypercalcemia in malignancy may be the release of prostaglandin (PG). Research has shown that tumors grown in culture produce a bone-resorbing substance identified as PG that results in increased serum calcium. At present, the source of the PG is unclear; it may arise from tumor, bone, or the renal medulla.

The fourth mechanism of hypercalcemia in malignancy is the existence of osteoclast-activating factors (OAF). Stimulation of the osteoclasts, with resulting bone demineralization, increases serum calcium. This mechanism is believed to be a factor in hypercalcemia associated with some lymphomas and multiple myeloma. The rationale for specific treatment used in hypercalcemia is interference with some of these mechanisms.

Role of calcium in metabolic functions. Calcium plays a vital role in many metabolic functions. In addition to its importance in maintaining bones, teeth, and normal clotting mechanisms, calcium is also crucial to muscle contraction and nerve impulse transmission. Cell membrane permeability is altered by changes in calcium levels. A decrease in extracellular Ca^{++} increases the excitability of nerve and muscle cells because it decreases the amount of depolarization needed to initiate changes in the cell membrane that produce action potentials and result in contractile activity. Conversely, an increase in extracellular Ca^{++} decreases excitability. Because calcium is involved in a wide variety of metabolic functions, abnormal calcium levels may be demonstrated in a wide variety of symptoms. This varied symptomatology may contribute to confusion over the initial diagnosis of hypercalcemia.

Assessment

Interpreting serum calcium levels. Circulating calcium amounts to 1% of the total serum calcium and occurs in three forms: 45% free ions, 45% bound to proteins (primarily albumin), and 10% complexed with a variety of anions. Only the ionized portion of calcium is biologically active and therefore of clinical significance. Because laboratories generally measure the *total* serum calcium level, it becomes necessary when interpreting calcium levels to estimate changes in the ionized, or active, calcium.

It is especially important to interpret calcium levels in relation to serum proteins. For example, when serum albumin is reduced, less calcium is protein-bound, creating an increase in ionized calcium. A normal calcium level associated with a marked reduction in serum albumin should be considered hypercalcemia. An abnormally high but asymptomatic calcium level may be found in a patient with hyperproteinemia, reflecting the increase in bound serum calcium. This relationship is especially significant in the hypercalcemia of malignancy, as many cancer patients have a low serum albumin. Recognition of the relationship between serum proteins and calcium is critical, particularly in a patient with suspicious symptoms despite a normal calcium level. If hypoalbuminemia exists, the measured calcium concentration should be increased by 0.8 mg/dl for each 1.0 g/dl of plasma albumin concentration below normal. Sample calculations to correct the calcium level in the presence of low albumin are included in Figure 15A–1.

Calcium level is correlated with the phosphate level; 85% of phosphate is combined with calcium in the skeleton. An inverse relationship exists between calcium and phosphate, so that factors that increase serum phosphate (PO_4^+) levels will decrease serum calcium levels.

Clinical manifestations of hypercalcemia. Because of the role calcium plays in a wide variety of metabolic functions, the variety of signs and symptoms that may occur complicate the diagnosis. The variation in onset and degree of severity of the presenting symptoms also make diagnosis difficult. Symptoms, such as anorexia, nausea, vomiting, constipation, and weakness, may be nonspecific and insidious in onset. Symptoms of dehydration, renal failure, and coma may develop swiftly, corresponding to a very rapid rise in calcium, and result in a life-threatening hypercalcemic crisis.

Table 15A–1 summarizes the clinical manifestations of hypercalcemia. Many of the early symptoms of hypercalcemia, such as anorexia, nausea, vomiting, constipation, and abdominal pain, are a result of the effect of hypercalcemia on smooth and skeletal muscle of

Calculate an additional 0.8 g/dl of Ca^{++} for every 1.0 g/dl of albumin below normal.

EXAMPLE: Laboratory reports calcium
         of 10.5 and albumin of 2.0.

1. Determine   3.5 normal albumin (low normal)
    albumin   -2.0 reported albumin
    value   ___
                     1.5 corrected (amount of albumin
                                    below normal)

2. Correct $\frac{0.8}{1.0} = \frac{x}{1.5}$
    for Ca^{++}
                     x = 1.2 g/dl Ca^{++}

3. Corrected   10.5 reported
    Ca^{++} + 1.2 correction
                    _____
                    11.7 corrected

Figure 15A–1. Rough calculation to correct calcium level with abnormal low albumin. *Adapted from* Doogan, R. A. Hypercalcemia of malignancy. *Cancer Nursing* (August 1981). p. 300.

TABLE 15A–1
Clinical Manifestations of Hypercalcemia

System	Signs and symptoms
GI	Anorexia, nausea, vomiting, constipation, abdominal pain, pancreatitis.
Neuromuscular	Apathy, fatigue, profound muscle weakness, lethargy, obtundation, coma, psychotic behavior (rarely).
Cardiac	Bradycardia, tachycardia, arrhythmias, increased P-R interval, shortened Q-T interval, widening of T wave.
Renal	Polyuria, polydipsia, nephrolithiasis, renal failure.
Miscellaneous	Metabolic alkalosis, bone pain, pruritus.

P-R, ECG interval between atrial and ventricular depolarization; Q-T, ECG ventricular depolarization and repolarization; T wave, ECG ventricular repolarization.

the GI tract. Obstipation and ileus may occur later in the course of the condition.

Neuromuscular and cardiac symptoms reflect interference with normal contractility of skeletal, smooth, and cardiac muscle, along with altered nerve impulse transmission. Initial ECG changes may be suggestive of hypercalcemia but are rarely diagnostic. A lengthening of the delay between atrial and ventricular depolarization (PR interval), shortening of the interval between ventricular depolarization and repolarization (Q-T interval), and widening of the T wave with a "covelike" appearance may be seen. Cardiac arrest may occur with high calcium levels.

The acute renal effects of hypercalcemia include polyuria and polydipsia. Polyuria is caused by a defect in renal tubular function that leads to an inability to conserve water. The resulting dehydration causes polydipsia. Chronic hypercalciuria resulting in nephrolithiasis may produce renal obstruction. These combined disorders lead to decreased renal function and potential failure. Metabolic alkalosis, often associated with the hypercalcemic state, is believed to result from renal hydrogen ion loss or excess buffer release from bone.

Hypercalcemic crisis.   A crisis exists when hypercalcemia results in severe nausea and vomiting, dehydration, confusion, coma, and renal failure. As the calcium level rises, the effect of hypercalcemia on the kidneys exacerbates the problem. Figure 15A-2 illustrates the dangerous cycles that develop.

The anorexia, nausea, vomiting, and polyuria caused by hypercalcemia result in dehydration. Dehydration accentuates the degree of hypercalcemia by compromising renal function. The body strives to correct the dehydration by decreasing the glomerular filtration rate (GFR) and increasing sodium reabsorption. Both mechanisms result in water conservation. However, a reduced GFR also results in decreased excretion of calcium, while increased sodium reabsorption enhances calcium reabsorption. Thus the volume-depleted patient cannot adequately excrete calcium.

Medical management

All measures to control the hypercalcemia of malignancy will be futile if effective tumor control is not achieved. Surgical removal of the tumor, effective radiation, chemotherapy, or hormonal manipulation is crucial.

Treatment of hypercalcemia related to malignancy is individualized according to the underlying disease, the degree of hypercalcemia, and the clinical presentation. If the patient is asymptomatic with a calcium

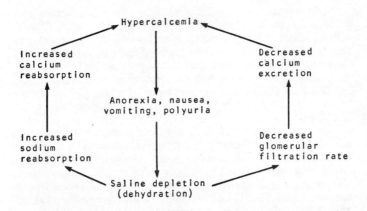

Figure 15A-2. Cycles in hypercalcemia. *Reprinted with permission from* Cunningham, S. E. Fluid and electrolyte disturbances associated with cancer and its treatment. *Nursing Clinics of North America* (December 1982). p. 586.

level of <13 mg/dl, tumor treatment may be the only therapy indicated.

For patients presenting with acute hypercalcemia, hydration with normal saline is the initial treatment. Not only is dehydration corrected, but the kidney's ability to excrete calcium is also enhanced as sodium reabsorption is reversed.

Diuretics, such as furosemide (Lasix) or ethacrynic acid, are often prescribed along with hydration. Furosemide promotes further diuresis of sodium by inhibiting the reabsorption of sodium in the proximal tubule of the kidney. Thiazide diuretics are contraindicated in this setting because they depress urinary excretion of calcium.

Patients with acute hypercalcemia refractory to these treatments or patients with impaired cardiac or renal function may be considered for hemodialysis if a rapid decrease in the calcium level is necessary to prevent heart block. In other cases, medications such as mithramycin and calcitonin may be added.

Mithramycin, an antibiotic with cytotoxic activity, has been shown to produce hypocalcemia, presumably by blocking PTH. It may also inhibit bone resorption. In doses of 25 μg/kg, its maximal effect is demonstrated in 2 to 4 days and lasts 4 to 6 days. No antitumor effect is seen with this dosage. Potential side effects of mithramycin include thrombocytopenia, hemorrhage, azotemia, and hepatocellular necrosis. Therefore, it is contraindicated for thrombocytopenic patients and not recommended for those patients with clotting, renal, and liver function abnormalities.

Calcitonin, a hormone that causes hypocalcemia by inhibiting osteoclast activity and thereby reducing bone depletion, is being utilized more frequently in the treatment of acute hypercalcemia because of its rapid onset of action and minimal toxicity. Dramatic decreases in calcium levels may be seen 2 to 3 hr after drug administration. Doses of 3 to 6 Medical Research Council (MRC) U/kg body weight are administered IM every 6 to 8 hr. When salmon calcitonin (Calcimar) is used, side effects are mild and infrequent, with ~10% of patients experiencing mild nausea and vomiting. Facial flushing, urticaria, and local dermatologic reactions may occur. Side effects may be minimized by administering injections at night.

Glucocorticoids, such as prednisone, have also been used in the treatment of hypercalcemia but are more appropriate for chronic than for acute conditions. The efficacy of these drugs may be attributable to an antitumor or to an anti-vitamin-D effect, or possibly to an inhibition of OAF. They have been most effective for hypercalcemia caused by multiple myeloma, non-Hodgkin's lymphoma, and breast carcinoma. Disadvantages of using glucocorticoids include the 7 to 10 days required for response and the many side effects that occur when they are used over extended periods of time.

Oral phosphates are frequently administered for chronic hypercalcemia. Doses of 30 to 60 ml/day inhibit bone resorption. Caution must be taken if the serum phosphate level is high, because of the danger of renal or soft-tissue calcification as a result of calcium precipitation. Diarrhea may be a bothersome side effect of these agents.

More recently, a new class of drugs called diphosphonates has been added to the treatment of hypercalcemia and is under further investigation. These agents stimulate osteoblast activity and thereby induce bone uptake of calcium. Indomethacin (Indocin), and aspirin, while once popular in treating hypercalcemia, are now rarely used because they cause variable and inconsistent decreases in serum calcium. More effective therapy is available.

Because immobilization enhances bone resorption, mobilization is critical to minimizing bone depletion. Calcium intake need not be restricted, because excess calcium arises from other mechanisms than dietary intake.

Nursing management

Although hypercalcemia may not be preventable, early recognition may prevent a crisis state with serious sequelae. Nurses need to recognize the population at risk, especially those with known or potential bone metastases. These patients and their families should be taught to recognize the signs and symptoms of hypercalcemia, such as anorexia, constipation, nausea, and lethargy. Visiting nurses must also be made aware of the risk so the patient can be monitored at home for signs and symptoms. Table 15A-2 outlines the nursing protocol for prevention/early detection of hypercalcemia.

The need and rationale for mobilization should be stressed. Pain and weakness often interfere with ambulation. Pain medication along with rest periods before and after ambulation may assist in meeting this goal. Those patients with multiple metastases to the bone are at risk for pathologic fracture. This risk must be considered in efforts to mobilize the patient. If a bony area is noted to be painful, x-ray evaluation is indicated and, if necessary, stabilization measures or radiation therapy (RT) undertaken before further attempts at mobilization are pursued (see Chapter 10). When mobilization can be achieved safely, it has the twofold benefit of minimizing bone destruction and helping to prevent constipation.

The importance of maintaining hydration cannot be overemphasized. Any condition leading to dehydration, such as nausea and vomiting, decreased fluid intake, or diarrhea is to be reported.

TABLE 15A–2
Nursing Protocol for the
Prevention/Early Detection of Hypercalcemia

Factor	Intervention
Tumor type	Recognize population at risk for hypercalcemia and those with bone metastasis.
	At each visit, check serum Ca^{++}, PO_4^+, and albumin.
	Evaluate for symptoms of anorexia, nausea, vomiting, constipation.
	Monitor pulse, BP, muscle strength, and mental status.
Immobility	Emphasize importance of mobility to patient/family.
	Ambulate patient tid, if possible.
	Evaluate for pathologic fracture if bone pain occurs.
Dehydration	Emphasize need to maintain hydration in high-risk patients.

Ca^{++}, ionized calcium; PO_4^+, phosphate ion.

Supportive management of hypercalcemia focuses on altered mental status, fluid and electrolyte balance, GI disturbances, effects of treatment, and potential cardiac and renal changes (Table 15A–3). The mental status of hypercalcemic patients ranges from confused and lethargic to fully comatose. The base-line mental status is recorded and carefully observed as treatment is undertaken. Attention is given to providing a protective environment until mental status returns to normal.

As normal saline is administered in large volume to correct dehydration, the patient is observed for signs of fluid overload or congestive heart failure. This is especially critical for patients with cardiac impairment. Caution is indicated for patients who have received doxorubicin and daunorubicin because of the possibility of cardiac damage. Strict intake and output records noting the response from diuretics are maintained. Renal function is monitored in this manner along with serum BUN and creatinine.

Serum calcium levels are monitored frequently to determine response to therapy. While being used to reduce hypercalcemia, potent drugs with rapid onset of action, such as calcitonin, may induce hypocalcemia. Patients should be observed for signs of hypocalcemia, including increased cardiac and neuromuscular irritability. Evidence of tetany may be demonstrated by positive Chvostek's and Trousseau's signs. Phosphate and albumin levels are monitored in conjunction with serum calcium for accurate interpretation.

TABLE 15A–3

Nursing Protocol for the Management of Hypercalcemia

Problem	Intervention
Altered mental status	Record base-line mental status and neurologic examination. Monitor for increasing fatigue, confusion, stupor, loss of consciousness. Provide protective environment.
Fluid imbalance	Correct dehydration by IV saline administration. Maintain accurate intake and output record. Observe for signs of fluid-overload: increased BP, shortness of breath. Administer diuretics and record response.
GI disturbance	Administer antiemetics to minimize nausea and vomiting. Correct constipation with laxatives as needed (*see* Chapter 11–B).
Electrolyte imbalance	Monitor electrolytes, especially K^+. Correct hypokalemia with IV KCl.
Effect of treatment for hypercalcemia	Evaluate response to hypercalcemia treatment by monitoring serum Ca^{++}, PO_4^+, albumin. Administer specified drugs to induce hypocalcemia and observe for side effects. Observe for symptoms of hypocalcemia (seizures, tetany).
Potential cardiac changes	Monitor for arrythmias: bradycardia, tachycardia, cardiac arrest. Observe ECG for increasing P-R intervals, and Q-T intervals, and widened T waves. Reduce doses of digoxin administered, monitor closely. Observe for signs of congestive heart failure.
Potential renal failure	Observe for oliguria, anuria. Monitor BUN, creatinine. Prepare for temporary hemodialysis.

Ca^{++}, ionized calcium; K^+, ionized potassium; KCl, potassium chloride; PO_4^+, phosphate ion; P-R, ECG atrial and ventricular depolarization; Q-T, ECG ventricular depolarization and repolarization; T, ECG ventricular repolarization.

Mithramycin is a potent irritant, causing local tissue necrosis if infiltration occurs. Therefore, the IV site must be observed carefully throughout the infusion for signs of infiltration. Clotting abnormalities and abnormal liver functions may result from mithramycin administration. Platelet status, clotting parameters, as indicated by prothrombin time and partial thromboplastin time, as well as liver function tests must be monitored for patients receiving mithramycin in the acute or chronic setting.

Because these patients are at risk for cardiac arrest when calcium levels are very high, monitoring for arrythmias and ECG changes is critical. The risk of tachyarrythmia is increased if the patient should become hypokalemic from hydration combined with furosemide diuresis. Because both hypercalcemia and hypokalemia increase cardiac irritability, monitoring electrolytes, including potassium, is essential. Hypercalcemia also potentiates the inotropic and toxic effects of cardiac glycosides, such as digoxin. When administering these drugs to the hypercalcemic patient, caution is indicated. Lowering the dose with careful monitoring is recommended.

Once the acute hypercalcemia has been brought under control, patients whose underlying disease is not well controlled may require continuous or intermittent medication to keep their calcium levels within a normal range.

Both patients and families must understand the dosage and the importance of taking medication prescribed for hypercalcemia and report inability to take the medication. If the medication, such as the oral phosphates, may cause diarrhea, patients and family need be aware of such side effects, along with measures to control it, so they will not discontinue the drug.

In the past, hypercalcemic patients were taught to avoid excessive calcium intake, but because the excess of calcium in the body comes from bone and not from dietary intake, calcium restrictions are unnecessary and may cause further eating difficulties for anorexic patients.

Bibliography

1. Chopra, D., and E. Clerkin. Hypercalcemia and malignant disease. *Medical Clinics of North America* (March 1975). 441–447.

   Provides a concise review of the pathogenesis, clinical manifestations, and treatment of hypercalcemia, including case studies.

2. Cunningham, S. E. Fluid and electrolyte disturbances associated with cancer and its treatment. *Nursing Clinics of North America* (December 1982). 579–593.

   Concise review of hypercalcemia with detailed explanation of the mechanism of dehydration complicating hypercalcemia.

3. Deftos, L. J., and B. P. First. Calcitonin as a drug. *Annals of Internal Medicine* (August 1981). 192–196.

   Reviews the use of calcitonin in hypercalcemic states. Side effects, dosage, and administration recommendations are included.

4. Doogan, R. A. Hypercalcemia of malignancy. *Cancer Nursing* (August 1981). 299–304.

Summarizes pathophysiology, clinical manifestations, and treatment of hypercalcemia. Detailed nursing management is described, including discharge planning and outpatient care.

5. Mazzaferri, E., T. O'Dorisio, and A. LoBuglio. Treatment of hypercalcemia associated with malignancy. *Seminars in Oncology* (June 1978). 141–153.

Provides comprehensive review of the clinical manifestation of hypercalcemia along with detailed descriptions of the drugs used in hypercalcemic treatment.

6. Myers, W. P. L. Differential diagnosis of hypercalcemia and cancer. *Ca—A Cancer Journal for Clinicians* (September/October 1977). 258–272.

Reviews normal calcium homeostasis and its disturbance in hypercalcemic states, using diagrams. Tables concisely display symptoms and treatment of hypercalcemia.

7. O'Dorisio, T. Hypercalcemic crisis. *Heart and Lung* (May/June 1978). 425–434.

Presents in detail the etiology of the hypercalcemic crisis state, including comprehensive medical care.

8. Zeluff, G. W., W. N. Suki, and D. Jackson. Hypercalcemia—etiology, manifestations and management. *Heart and Lung* (January/February 1980). 146–151.

Provides detailed summary of hypercalcemia in general. Descriptions of classification based on etiology, clinical manifestations, and management, using tables.

B: TUMOR LYSIS SYNDROME

Joan Martin Moore

Tumor lysis syndrome (TLS) is a disorder characterized by the development of specific metabolic and electrolyte abnormalities, which include: hyperphosphatemia, hyperkalemia, hyperuricemia, and hypocalcemia. TLS can be a very serious and potentially fatal complication for patients undergoing cytotoxic chemotherapy. The combination of electrolyte and metabolic disorders that exist create an emergency because they place the patient at high risk for renal failure and/or cardiac arrest. The syndrome occurs when rapidly growing tumors are treated with chemotherapy. As cells die and lyse after chemotherapy, large amounts of intracellular electrolytes and chemicals enter the bloodstream. The syndrome may also occur when malignancies characterized by rapid cell growth, such as leukemia and lymphomas, are accompanied by an increased breakdown of nucleic acids. Thus, both rapid cell lysis and rapid cell proliferation are etiologic factors in the development of TLS.

Pathophysiology

The mechanism of TLS is more easily understood when the physiology involved in rapid cell growth and rapid cell destruction is considered. A review of the electrolyte composition of cells will facilitate understanding of the specific metabolic and electrolyte abnormalities that result from TLS.

The electrolyte concentration within cells differs from extracellular fluid content in that sodium and chloride dominate the fluid outside of cells, whereas potassium and phosphorus dominate the fluid within the cell. Therefore, when cells lyse and release their contents, the result is increased serum potassium and phosphorus.

Another factor that contributes to hyperphosphatemia in TLS occurs when chemotherapy destroys circulating lymphoblasts. Because lymphoblasts contain more phosphorus than mature lymphocytes, destruction of these immature forms results in increased serum phosphorus. In the human body, an inverse relationship exists between phosphorus and calcium, so that an increase in serum phosphorus results in decreased serum calcium. This relationship accounts for the hypocalcemia that develops with TLS.

Cells undergoing rapid growth and division contain high concentrations of nucleic acids. When rapid growth is accompanied by increased catabolism of nucleic acids, the result is increased uric acid formation and hyperuricemia. Chemotherapy-induced cell destruction also causes hyperuricemia as a result of nucleic acid degradation. Because uric acid is relatively insoluble in body fluids, small increases can result in precipitation. Urate crystals then form in renal tubules and collecting ducts, causing renal insufficiency and failure.

The degree and duration of the metabolic disorders of TLS are related to tumor burden and renal function. Phagocytosis, hepatic metabolism, and renal excretion are all involved in clearing the products of tumor cell destruction. As the tumor burden is lessened through effective chemotherapy, the metabolic disorders of TLS are brought under control. If rapid tumor growth persists, the body cannot clear the products of tumor lysis, and the syndrome worsens.

Excretion of uric acid, potassium, and phosphate depend on adequate renal function. Patients with compromised renal function are at higher risk for developing TLS and experience more severe symptomatology.

Assessment

The clinical manifestations of TLS are listed in Table 15B-1. Signs and symptoms of TLS vary, depending on which metabolic imbalance predominates. If evidence for hyperphosphatemia (>2.6 mEq/liter), hyperkalemia (>5 mEq/liter), hyperuricemia (>8 mg/dl), and hypocalcemia (<9 mg/dl) are not sought together, confusion may arise over the etiology of a specific metabolic imbalance, obscuring the diagnosis.

The physical examination focuses on an evaluation of neurologic and mental status as well as on determination of muscle strength. Pulse and ECG are monitored for changes in rate and/or rhythm. Assessment of GI and renal function is also included.

Medical management

The primary treatment goals in the management of TLS are: (1) to prevent renal failure, and (2) to prevent severe electrolyte imbalance. Whenever cytotoxic treatment is being undertaken in patients with leukemia, lymphoma, or bulky disease, prophylactic treatment to prevent uric acid formation is essential.

Allopurinol is the drug most commonly used to decrease uric acid concentration and prevent acute renal failure. Allopurinol prevents the

TABLE 15B-1

Clinical Manifestations of Tumor Lysis Syndrome

Cause	Effect
Increased PO_4^+	Oliguria, anuria, azotemia.
Increased K^+	ECG changes, bradycardia, cardiac arrest, weakness, flaccid paralysis.
Increased uric acid	Nausea, vomiting, lethargy, oliguria, anuria, azotemia.
Decreased Ca^{++}	Cardiac: ECG changes, ventricular arrythmias, heart block. Neuromuscular: twitching, cramping, digital paresthesias, tetany, convulsions.

Ca^{++}, ionized calcium; K^+, ionized potassium; PO_4^+, phosphate ion(s).

formation of uric acid by inhibiting the enzyme xanthine oxidase, an enzyme essential for the conversion of nucleic acids to uric acid.

Renal failure may still occur in some patients despite allopurinol use. Patients with preexisting renal compromise are at high risk to develop renal failure. An alkaline diuresis may be added to their treatment. This is generally accomplished by administering 5% dextrose IV, plus sodium bicarbonate, 50 to 100 mEq/liter. Urine pH is then maintained ≥ 7. As the urine becomes more alkaline, uric acid becomes more soluble, thus minimizing uric acid precipitation and stone formation. Aggressive hydration is undertaken to correct dehydration and prevent uric acid crystallization.

If all of the above measures fail to increase the urine output, hemodialysis may be used to reduce serum uric acid and improve azotemia. In cases of ureteral obstruction, cystoscopy with alkaline lavages of the ureters has been recommended.

In addition to efforts to enhance renal function, treatment is also aimed at preventing electrolyte imbalance. Diuretics, such as furosemide, while inducing diuresis also cause potassium excretion. For this reason, diuretics are especially useful when TLS has resulted in hyperkalemia; however, the use of diuretics along with vigorous hydration may cause further electrolyte imbalances such as hypokalemia. Therefore, frequent electrolyte monitoring, with correction of imbalances, is essential.

Nursing management

Of primary importance in preventing TLS is recognition of the population at risk, i.e., those patients with large, rapidly growing tumors, lymphomas, leukemias, and small cell carcinoma of the lung. A prescription may be obtained for allopurinol prior to and during chemotherapy for this high-risk group. Patients and families are taught the importance of allopurinol in preventing hyperuricemia.

The second population at high risk to develop TLS are those patients with preexisting renal insufficiency (creatinine ≥ 1.6 mg/dl and uric acid ≥ 8 mg/dl). Maintaining hydration for both groups of patients is critical; urine alkalinization may be considered.

Lastly, because of the combination of metabolic disorders that characterize the onset of TLS, patients at risk for TLS development and their families are taught to report signs of hyperphosphatemia, hyperuricemia, hyperkalemia, and hypocalcemia.

Supportive nursing management of acute TLS focuses on maintaining fluid balance, monitoring for electrolyte and metabolic imbalances, and observing for signs of renal insufficiency (Table 15B–2). While vigorous IV hydration is administered along with diuretics, the

TABLE 15B–2

Nursing Protocol for the Management of Tumor Lysis Syndrome

Problem	Intervention
Fluid balance	Administer IV hydration. Monitor weight, intake and output, response to diuretics.
	Observe for signs of fluid overload, especially patients with potential or preexisting cardiac damage.
Electrolyte balance	Monitor electrolytes q day or q 6–12 hr as indicated. Correct imbalances as prescribed.
	Observe for signs of hyperkalemia: weakness, flaccid paralysis, ECG changes, cardiac arrest.
Potential renal failure	Monitor Ca^{++}, PO_4^+, uric acid, BUN, and creatinine daily for the 5–7-day period of cytolysis.
	Maintain hydration, especially if preexisting renal insufficiency (creatinine $>$ 1.6 mg/dl, uric acid $\geq$ 8 mg/dl).
	Administer allopurinol 300–800 mg PO q day.
	Monitor urine pH: maintain $\geq$ 7 by administering IV $NaHCO_3$ as prescribed.
	Report decreased urine output, lethargy.
	Prepare to manage patient on temporary hemodialysis.
Potential effects of drug therapy	Observe for side effects from allopurinol: skin rashes, GI disturbances, fever (rarely), vasculitis, and blood dyscrasias.
	Decrease doses of 6-MP and azathioprine if given concurrently with allopurinol.
Potential cardiac irritability	Monitor lab values for increased K^+ and decreased Ca^{++}.
	Check pulse rate and rhythm frequently. Report irregularity.
	Observe for ECG changes, cardiac arrest.
Potential neuromuscular irritability	Monitor serum Ca^{++} level.
	Observe for symptoms of hypocalcemia: tetany, positive Chvostek's and Trousseau's signs.

Ca^{++}, ionized calcium; K^+, ionized potassium; 6-MP, 6-mercaptopurine; $NaHCO_3$, sodium bicarbonate; PO_4^+, phosphate ion(s).

patient's weight and intake and output are carefully monitored. Response to diuretics can be recorded in this manner. Observation for signs of fluid overload is critical, particularly with patients having preexisting or potential cardiac damage.

Because of the combined metabolic and electrolyte disorders found with TLS, electrolytes, calcium, and phosphorus are monitored daily. Patients are observed for signs of hyperkalemia: weakness, flaccid paralysis, ECG changes, and cardiac arrest. Symptoms related to hyperphosphatemia, such as oliguria, anuria, and renal insufficiency, are watched for. Patients are also observed for symptoms related to hypocalcemia, such as increased cardiac and neuromuscular irritability.

Hyperuricemia may be demonstrated only by an elevated uric acid level or may be accompanied by nausea, vomiting, lethargy, and signs of renal insufficiency. Hydration is maintained to enhance urine output.

Allopurinol is administered in doses of 300 to 800 mg PO daily, to prevent further uric acid formation. Skin rashes and GI upset are common side effects of allopurinol. Rarely, fever, vasculitis, and blood dyscrasias develop from use of this drug. Allopurinol may potentiate the action of 6-mercaptopurine and azathioprine; therefore, doses of these drugs are decreased when used in conjunction with allopurinol.

Observing patients for signs of renal insufficiency and failure is critical. Daily BUN and creatinine are monitored. Any decrease in urine output or anuria should be reported. Patients failing to respond to hydration and diuretics may have an obstructive problem caused by precipitation of calcium phosphate or uric acid crystals in the kidney. In either event, hemodialysis will be undertaken to rapidly correct the metabolic imbalances, which are potentially lethal if uncontrolled. Nursing management then centers on care of the patient undergoing temporary hemodialysis.

The constant monitoring of renal function as well as of electrolyte and metabolic imbalances is continued for a period of 5 to 7 days. Thus, the time of greatest cytolysis following chemotherapy administration, which is the time of greatest risk to the patient, will be monitored.

Bibliography

1. Cohen, L. F., J. E. Balow, I. T. Magrath, D. G. Poplack, and J. L. Ziegler. Acute tumor lysis syndrome, a review of 37 patients with Burkitt's lymphoma. *The American Journal of Medicine* (April 1980). 486–490.

   Describes renal and metabolic complications of tumor lysis and outlines approach to metabolic management of Burkitt's lymphoma.

2. Cunningham, S. G. Fluid and electrolyte disturbances associated with cancer and its treatment. *Nursing Clinics of North America* (December 1982). 579–593.

Concise summary of tumor lysis syndrome and the metabolic consequences. Prevention and treatment are discussed.

3. Kjellstrand, C. M., D. C. Campbell, B. von Hartitzsch, and T. J. Buselmeier. Hyperuricemic acute renal failure. *Archives of Internal Medicine* (March 1974). 349–359.

Describes successful use of hemodialysis to treat hyperuricemia. Prophylactic allopurinol and diuretic administration not always successful in preventing acute renal failure.

4. Sagel, D., A. A. Fields, and R. G. Josse. Metabolic emergencies in cancer. *In* DeVita, V. T., S. Hellman, and S. A. Rosenberg, editors. Cancer: Principles and Practice of Oncology. J. B. Lippincott Co., Philadelphia. 1982.

Complete description of hyperuricemia as a result of cell destruction after chemotherapy. Development of acute hyperuricemic nephropathy and treatment options discussed.

C: SYNDROME OF INAPPROPRIATE ANTIDIURETIC HORMONE SECRETION

Joan Martin Moore

The syndrome of inappropriate antidiuretic hormone secretion (SIADH) is a disorder characterized by continued secretion of antidiuretic hormone (ADH). For the individual afflicted with the syndrome, the result is fluid retention, inability to excrete dilute urine, and dilutional hyponatremia. Because the most common etiology of SIADH is malignancy, oncology nurses need be aware of the pathophysiology involved in SIADH, and of the clinical manifestations and available treatment options.

Pathophysiology

ADH. An understanding of SIADH is contingent upon an understanding of how the body regulates water and the role of ADH in that regulation. The body constantly regulates water by either conserving or excreting it. This water balance is controlled by ADH, which is released from the posterior pituitary gland. The distal renal tubules and collecting ducts of the kidneys are the target site for this hormone. When ADH is released, water is conserved, as the word antidiuresis suggests. Increased reabsorption of water from the kidney is the mechanism by which this water conservation is achieved.

The mechanisms by which the brain regulates ADH secretion are twofold. First, baroreceptors detect increases or decreases of the BP in the left atrium. Increased atrial pressure stimulates the baroreceptors, which send impulses to the hypothalamus and posterior pituitary to limit ADH secretion. Conversely, decreased atrial pressure results in less baroreceptor stimulation so that more ADH is secreted. In this way hypervolemic and hypovolemic states, or changes in extracellular volume, can be corrected appropriately by an increase or decrease in ADH secretion.

The other major control of ADH secretion is determined by extracellular osmolarity. Osmoreceptors, sensitive to extracellular osmolarity, are located in the hypothalamus, where an increase in serum osmolarity (i.e., a more concentrated serum) causes increased ADH secretion and water conservation to produce a more dilute serum and concentrated urine. If the serum osmolarity decreases, ADH secretion is inhibited, resulting in more dilute urine as excess water is excreted. Normal serum osmolarity is 280 to 295 mOsm/liter.

In SIADH, the normal osmolar response of the osmoreceptors malfunctions. As serum osmolarity decreases, urine osmolarity is concentrated — indicating hyperosmolarity — rather than being lowered to excrete excess water in dilute urine.

Many factors are known to stimulate ADH release. Besides changes in extracellular volume, i.e., hypovolemic states (fluid or blood loss), and serum osmolarity, stress is known to increase ADH secretion. As part of the body's stress response, mechanisms to conserve water are necessary in the event of hemorrhage or sweating. This phenomenon may explain why pain, surgery, and trauma also result in ADH secretion. Lastly, medications such as narcotics, barbiturates, anesthetics, and tricyclic antidepressants have been found to stimulate ADH release.

Disease-related causes of SIADH. Disease-related causes of SIADH tend to fall into three categories: malignancy, pulmonary disease, and CNS disorders. Tumors with ectopic production of ADH are by far the most common cause of SIADH. Of the malignancies, lung carcinoma, especially of the small or oat cell carcinoma type, has the highest incidence. Other tumor types associated with SIADH are duodenal and pancreatic carcinoma, thymoma, non-Hodgkin's lymphoma, Hodgkin's disease, and uterine carcinoma. Laboratory research has shown that the ADH produced by neoplasms is identical to that produced by the posterior pituitary. The malignant lung cells of patients with SIADH have the capacity to synthesize, store, and release ADH.

A common feature associated with many pulmonary disorders is hyponatremia and SIADH. SIADH has been found in conjunction with aspergillosis, tuberculosis, and both viral and bacterial pneumonias. It is believed that benign pulmonary tissue also has the capacity to synthesize and secrete ADH.

The third major group of disorders associated with SIADH are those of the CNS. Meningitis, encephalitis, brain tumors and abscess, cranial trauma, and subarachnoid hemorrhage may all be acompanied by SIADH. It has been hypothesized that the mechanism responsible for SIADH is stimulation of the hypothalamic and posterior pituitary systems.

Recently it has been established that drugs may also cause SIADH. Of particular importance in oncology is that two cancer chemotherapeutic agents, cyclophosphamide (Cytoxan) and vincristine (Oncovin), have been shown to induce SIADH by stimulating release of ADH from the posterior pituitary. The drug chlorpropamide stimulates ADH secretion and causes water retention in diabetic patients. Tricyclic antidepressants, general anesthetics, narcotics, and barbiturates used in conjunction with surgery are believed to cause increased ADH secretion. Lastly, diuretics, both thiazide and others, may induce hyponatremia and SIADH.

Assessment

The presenting signs and symptoms of SIADH include: weight gain, lethargy, weakness, irritability, and confusion. Anorexia, nausea, and vomiting may occur. Edema is rarely seen. If untreated, the serum sodium concentration continues to drop, neurologic abnormalities develop, and symptoms progress to convulsions and coma.

The history and physical examination include evaluation of neurologic and mental status. An assessment of GI function is made, because anorexia, nausea, and vomiting may occur.

Laboratory data is generally suggestive of water retention and hemodilution. Hyponatremia is the most striking of the electrolyte disorders. Normally the serum sodium (Na^+) is 140 mEq/liter. In SIADH, serum Na^+ levels may fall <120 mEq/liter. Edema does not usually occur, because the hypervolemia that results from the excess water stimulates volume receptors that cause an increase in urinary sodium excretion with sodium concentrations of >20 mg/liter.

The clinical manifestations of SIADH consist of hyponatremia, with corresponding hypo-osmolarity in the absence of clinical evidence of hypovolemia. Urine is less than maximally dilute and has >20 mEq/liter concentration of sodium. BUN, creatinine, and albumin levels tend to be low or within normal range. Serum osmolarity will be low.

In order to make the diagnosis of SIADH with confidence, adrenal insufficiency and hypothyroidism must be ruled out because both may increase ADH secretion. Pain and hypotension must be corrected, as both may result in further ADH secretion despite hypo-osmolality. Dilutional hyponatremia may exist with congestive heart failure, renal failure, and liver disease with ascites. Thus, the coexistence of these states may complicate the diagnosis.

Determining the individual's response to a water load has been useful to help establish the diagnosis of SIADH. A water load is administered PO over a 15- to 20-min period. The patient is then monitored for water excretion and urine osmolality. Normally, 80% of water is excreted in ≤5 hr and the urinary osmolality falls to <100 mOsm/kg. In the presence of SIADH, water excretion is <40% after 5 hr and urine is less than maximally dilute. This procedure can be very dangerous if the serum sodium is not corrected to ≥125 mEq/liter prior to the water load.

Medical management

Fluid restriction is the initial treatment in the management of SIADH. When symptoms are mild to moderate, restriction to ~800 to 1,000 ml of fluid daily is adequate. Response is determined by loss of weight along with increases in serum sodium and osmolarity.

When symptomatology is severe, more aggressive therapy is indicated. Hypertonic saline, usually 3%, is administered over several hours. The addition of large doses of furosemide helps to improve symptomatology rapidly. Patients are then carefully monitored for potential electrolyte imbalances. Hyponatremia, once corrected, will recur if fluid restriction is not maintained. Any drugs that may contribute to water retention are withheld.

Other drugs used in the management of SIADH include demethyl-chlortetracycline (demeclocycline), urea, furosemide, and lithium carbonate. Demeclocycline, an antibiotic that decreases the renal response to ADH, has been shown to improve diuresis and hyponatremia when doses of 900 to 1,200 mg/day are administered. The major side effects have been azotemia, which promptly reverses when the drug is withdrawn, and the risk of superinfection.

Urea, administered PO in doses of 30 g/day, has also been effective in treating SIADH. Adequate hydration is maintained within the specified fluid restriction. Urea is contraindicated in the presence of GI problems, such as ulcers.

Furosemide, at 40 mg/day PO, may be useful for patients tolerant to demeclocycline and for whom urea is contraindicated. Salt must be replaced in the diet of those on PO furosemide therapy. Monitoring is also required to prevent alkalosis from a hypokalemic-hypochloremic state.

Lithium carbonate, an established ADH inhibitor, has been used with some success in treating both acute and chronic forms of SIADH. The use of this agent is, however, limited by toxic side effects, manifested by sluggishness, drowsiness, tremors, or muscle twitching, GI disturbances, cardiac irritability, and thyroid dysfunction.

Once symptoms are brought under control, successful treatment of the disease process responsible for the syndrome must be initiated. Surgery, chemotherapy, radiation therapy, or a combination of these treatment modalities may be indicated. In the face of advanced disease, therapy may be palliative to reduce the need for fluid restriction, which may increase discomfort and reduce the quality of life for cancer patients with this syndrome.

Nursing management

While prevention of SIADH may not be possible, serious consequences may be prevented through early detection. Early detection of weight gain, low urine output, hyponatremia, and mental status changes is essential. Symptoms of lethargy, weakness, weight gain, nausea, and irritability may not coincide. Unless a high index of suspicion is maintained, especially with patients at high risk, the cause of these symptoms may be overlooked or attributed to the malignancy itself. Lung cancer patients, particularly those with the small cell type, should be monitored carefully for symptoms suggestive of SIADH. Patient and family teaching may include those signs and symptoms to report to their care-givers.

Once the diagnosis of SIADH has been established, supportive nursing care is focused initially on fluid management (Table 15C–1). Restricting fluids to specified limits is essential. Intake, output, and weight are carefully monitored. Water retention places the patient at risk for fluid overload and congestive heart failure. Patients with known cardiac disease, or those having received doxorubicin or daunorubicin, with their potentials for cardiac impairment, should be closely observed for shortness of breath, hypertension, and dependent edema.

Electrolytes are continually monitored for hyponatremia and hypokalemia. The patient's mental status may range from fully alert to comatose, depending on the degree of hyponatremia. Frequent evaluation of mental status is essential as cytotoxic therapy is initiated and in progress. Mental status changes, evidenced early by confusion,

TABLE 15C–1
Nursing Protocol for the Management of SIADH

Problem	Intervention
Fluid balance	Administer diuretics as prescribed and document response. Restrict fluids to specified limits. Monitor for congestive heart failure secondary to water retention and impaired cardiac function.
Electrolyte balance	Monitor electrolytes frequently, especially Na^+ and K^+. Seizure precautions if serum sodium <120 mEq/liter. Observe for symptoms of hypokalemia.
Altered mental status	History and physical examination to include neurologic examination with evaluation of mental status. Observe and report changes: confusion, lethargy, coma. Ensure protective environment for confused or comatose patient.
Potential cardiac irritability	Monitor pulse rate and rhythm frequently. Observe ECG for arrythmias. Monitor for hypokalemia. Administer KCl as prescribed.
Potential effects of drug therapy	Observe for side effects related to drug therapy. Document response to treatment: weight loss, increased serum Na^+, increased serum osmolarity.
Lack of response to therapy	Examine factors contributing to ADH release. Minimize pain and stress. Limit use of narcotics, barbiturates, tricyclic antidepressants.
Patient/family education	Teach to report early signs and symptoms: weight gain, lethargy, weakness, nausea, mental status changes. Teach the importance of fluid restriction, dose, side effects, and rationale for prescribed medications.

ADH, antidiuretic hormone; K^+, ionized potassium; KCl, potassium chloride; Na^+, ionized sodium; SIADH, syndrome of inappropriate antidiuretic hormone secretion.

are frequently seen as the serum sodium drops to ~125 mEq/liter. Seizure precautions are indicated if the serum sodium falls <120 mEq/liter. Hypokalemia often results when high doses of furosemide are being administered. Serum potassium is closely monitored and at the same time the patient is monitored for cardiac irritability.

Because pain and stress are known to increase ADH secretion, successful efforts to relieve pain and minimize stress should have a therapeutic effect. When possible, the use of narcotics, barbiturates, and tricyclic antidepressants should be minimized because they are also known to enhance ADH secretion.

When drugs such as demeclocycline, urea, and furosemide are being administered in SIADH management, patients should be evaluated for side effects, adverse effects, and response to the therapy. Patients responding favorably to drug therapy will demonstrate weight loss, a rising serum sodium, and increasing serum osmolarity.

SIADH can only be permanently controlled by effective antitumor therapy. If tumor control cannot be achieved, the patient and family must learn to manage chronic SIADH. Their ability to manage the syndrome and enhance the quality of life for the patient depends to a large extent on how carefully they are taught about SIADH and their ability to understand and accept the treatment. They are taught to report weight gain, weakness, lethargy, nausea, and confusion as well as possible drug side effects. The importance of fluid restriction is emphasized. Discussion includes adapting the fluid restriction to the individual's normal fluid intake schedule. Dietary consultation may be indicated if severe fluid restriction is required.

Bibliography

1. Barter, F., and W. B. Schwartz. The syndrome of inappropriate secretion of antidiuretic hormone. *American Journal of Medicine* (May 1967). 790–801.

    Provides detailed review of the clinical features, pathophysiology, differential diagnosis, and treatment of SIADH.

2. Cunningham, S. G. Fluid and electrolyte disturbances associated with cancer and its treatment. *Nursing Clinics of North America* (December 1982). 579–593.

    Concise review of body saline-and-water balance in reference to SIADH. Nursing implications included.

3. De Fronzo, R. A., H. Braine, M. Colvin, and P. J. Davis. Water intoxication in man after cyclophosphamide therapy. *Annals of Internal Medicine* (June 1973). 861–869.

    Describes study of 17 cancer patients who developed impairment of water excretion following cyclophosphamide therapy. The mechanism of impairment is discussed.

4. Harrington, J. T., and J. J. Cohen. Clinical disorders of urine concentration and dilution. *Archives of Internal Medicine* (June 1973). 810–822.

   Detailed description of the body's water regulating capacity. Discussion includes circumstances resulting in impaired diluting capacity, including SIADH.

5. Levin, M. L. Hyponatremic syndromes. *Medical Clinics of North America* (November 1978). 1257–1271.

   Provides thorough review of clinical states associated with hyponatremia. Classifies the causes of SIADH.

6. Moses, A. M., M. Miller, and D. H. P. Streeten. Pathophysiologic and pharmacologic alterations in the release and action of ADH. *Metabolism* (June 1976). 697–717.

   Reviews physiologic factors involved in ADH release. Differential diagnosis and treatment of SIADH described.

7. Robertson, G. L., N. Bhoopalam, and L. H. Zelkowitz. Vincristine neurotoxicity and abnormal secretion of antidiuretic hormone. *Archives of Internal Medicine* (November 1973). 717–720.

   Describes hormone assays of one patient who developed SIADH while receiving vincristine. Mechanism may be related to neurotoxicity causing altered osmoreceptor control of ADH.

D: HYPERVISCOSITY

Tish Knobf

Pathophysiology

Viscosity is the resistance to flow created by the interaction of components in a fluid, or its internal friction. Blood is a viscous fluid composed of cells and plasma. Its viscosity is determined by the form, flexibility, and number of cellular components and by similar characteristics of serum proteins.

An increased viscosity (hyperviscosity) represents an increased resistance to blood flow caused by some alteration in the cells or plasma proteins. An increase in number of cells, loss of flexibility of cells, or overproduction of serum proteins can produce abnormally high viscosity levels (Table 15D–1).

Increase in cell number. An increase in the number of cells is the most common cause of blood hyperviscosity. As the number of RBCs increases, more friction is created among the blood components, and

TABLE 15D–1
Hyperviscosity: Causes and Disease States

Cause	Disease	Characteristics
Increased number of cells	Polycythemia vera	Increased number of RBCs resulting in abnormally high Hct ($\geq$50%)
Loss of cell flexibility	Sickle cell disease	Inability of the RBC membrane to stretch and change shape, resulting in markedly increased resistance to flow and anemia.
Increased serum proteins	Waldenström's macro-globulinemia Multiple myeloma	Malignant transformation and proliferation of cells resulting in overproduction of serum proteins (immunoglobulins).

increased resistance to flow results. Circulation is impaired because of the reduced flow of blood through the vessels.

Loss of blood cell deformity. Sickle cell disease and several other RBC disorders may produce blood hyperviscosity as a result of the lack of flexibility of the cell membrane. If the RBC membrane cannot be stretched, the cell is unable to change its shape to pass through the narrow capillaries. Resistance to flow is thus markedly increased.

Increase in serum viscosity. The viscosity of a protein solution is a function of the concentration and of the intrinsic viscosity of the individual proteins in the solution. The intrinsic viscosity is most commonly influenced by the size and shape of protein molecules.

The overproduction of serum proteins in Waldenström's macroglobulinemia and multiple myeloma — both neoplastic diseases — is associated with potential life-threatening consequences and requires immediate intervention. Both the concentration and the type of serum protein (immunoglobulin) in these diseases can affect blood viscosity. Hyperviscosity usually occurs when the immunoglobulins are present in high concentrations, are very large molecules, or are shaped so that they tend to clump together. The term hyperviscosity syndrome (HVS) describes the clinical signs and symptoms associated with high serum-viscosity levels observed in patients with Waldenström's macroglobulinemia and multiple myeloma. The syndrome includes bleeding from mucous membranes, retinal vein enlargement, retinal hemorrhage, loss of vision, neurologic disorders, and renal and cardiac complications. HVS occurs in 30 to 70% of patients with Waldenström's macroglobulinemia and ≤10% of patients with multiple myeloma.

Assessment

Laboratory. The viscosity of a fluid is expressed as a ratio of the rate of flow of that fluid: the rate of flow of water, at a given temperature and pressure. A viscometer is the measuring instrument used, and the procedure is simple, fast, and inexpensive. Symptomatology varies with the serum viscosity level, with no symptoms at a normal viscosity of 1.4 to 1.8, rare incidence at ≤4.0, and high incidence at levels >6.0. Levels may also be ≥10.0, at which point nearly all patients experience symptoms. Symptoms also vary greatly from one individual to another. The occurrence of symptoms associated with a specific viscosity level is referred to as the symptomatic threshold.

Clinical. The signs and symptoms of HVS are not always dramatic and are, in fact, often subtle and attributed to the underlying disease. Careful assessment and early detection are major nursing goals to prevent serious consequences. Hyperviscosity results in stagnation of blood flow and affects major organ systems (Table 15D–2). Severity of symptoms induced can be greatly reduced by early recognition and intervention.

In the absence of thrombocytopenia, chronic oozing of blood or spontaneous bleeding from a variety of sites is a frequent manifestation. And for patients who are thrombocytopenic, such as those with multiple myeloma after chemotherapy, hyperviscosity may still be a contributing factor to bleeding complications.

TABLE 15D–2
Clinical Manifestations of HVS

System	Potential signs and symptoms
Hematologic	Spontaneous bleeding from the GI and urinary tracts, nose. Prolonged bleeding from puncture sites. Low Hct, pallor, and fatigue.
Ocular	Visual disturbances, retinal vein distension, retinal hemorrhage, papilledema.
Neurologic	Headache, dizziness, vertigo, nystagmus, postural hypotension, wide-based unsteady gait, dementia, ataxia, somnolence, coma, and seizures.
Cardiovascular	Weakness, shortness of breath, tachycardia, rales, wheezing, edema, distended neck veins.

HVS, hyperviscosity syndrome.

Visual disturbances include blurred vision, amblyopia (dimness of vision), progressive, painless loss of sight, and acute total loss of sight. Ophthalmoscopic examinations are indicated and are valuable in detecting retinal venous distension and/or hemorrhage. These changes often precede serious visual impairment.

Mental status changes and other neurologic symptoms may be subtle. Vague and slight changes, which can be significant, are often detected by the nurse. The nurse spends the most time with the patient and family and, therefore, has the advantage of a solid physical and psychologic base line from which to measure change. More severe symptoms of neurologic dysfunction are usually correlated with increasing viscosity levels.

Cardiac complications are less frequent and less well understood. Congestive heart failure has been observed, secondary to circulatory overload, hyperviscous blood, and decreased RBC concentration. Circulatory overload may result from vascular stasis, hypervolemia, and edema. Decreased or inefficient cardiac function, because of the increased demand on the heart, may also lead to failure.

Medical management

Symptoms can be ameliorated and/or totally resolved in a dramatically short period of time by means of plasmapheresis, a process by which unit(s) of whole blood are removed from the patient, centrifuged, and the RBCs returned to the patient. This procedure removes large amounts of immunoglobulins from the blood, thereby reducing the viscosity levels. As many as 6 to 8 U of plasma are often removed over 1 to 2 days for acute symptoms, followed by a maintenance schedule of 2 to 4 U every week or every other week. The measurement of success is resolution of symptoms, not the absolute serum viscosity level. It must be stressed that plasmapheresis is a temporary measure, particularly in the case of patients with multiple myeloma. The best hope for prevention and control of HVS is primary treatment of the underlying disease with cytotoxic therapy.

Nursing management

The focus of the nursing approach should be preventive, because prevention ensures the best outcome for the patient. Preventive management includes close monitoring and patient teaching (Table 15D-3). Implicit in the concept of careful monitoring is accurate, detailed, and consistent documentation of nursing observations. Although symptomatic response to increased serum viscosity varies greatly from individual to individual, the response remains relatively constant within an individual patient. The history of prior episodes of

TABLE 15D-3
Nursing Protocol for Preventive Management of HVS

Problem	Intervention
Hematologic dysfunction	Monitor blood values: Hb, Hct, platelet count, serum viscosity.
	Observe patients for signs of bleeding: oral cavity, skin, urine, stool.
	Avoid trauma (e.g., invasive procedures, IM injections).
	Maintain bowel regimen to prevent constipation and straining at stool.
	Patient/family education on signs/symptoms of bleeding.
Ocular dysfunction	Ophthalmoscopic eye examination.
	Evaluation of any visual changes.
Neurologic dysfunction	Assess mental status changes.
	Observe patients for any physical signs of neurologic dysfunction.
	Patient/family education on neurologic signs/symptoms.
	Seizure precautions.
Cardiovascular dysfunction	Observe patients for any signs of fluid overload and congestive heart failure: weakness, dyspnea, shortness of breath, rales, wheezing, dependent edema, tachycardia, distension of neck veins.
	Record intake and output.
	Weigh routinely and evaluate for weight gain.
	If transfusion is required, administer slowly to prevent circulatory overload.

HVS, hyperviscosity syndrome.

HVS provides valuable clinical data for predicting the risk of clinical manifestation based on the serum viscosity level for a given patient.

Patient education about signs and symptoms should be clear and concise, with simple, understandable terminology, preferably supplemented by written information. It is very important that a support person (family member or friend) be included in the instruction, because many of the signs and symptoms will be obscure to the patient.

The complication of HVS in patients with chronic neoplastic disease processes adds physical and psychologic stress. Supportive nursing care must address the effects of the underlying disease and treatment on the patient and family while attempting to minimize the physical symptoms and psychologic response to HVS (Table 15D–4). Patients may experience one or any number of symptoms from a single body system or present with symptoms from all potentially affected systems.

The severity of the signs and symptoms is generally associated with increasing viscosity levels. Careful monitoring of these levels is essential to alert the nurse to further complications, to direct nursing care, to establish a pattern for the individual patient, and to assess the effect of plasmapheresis or primary disease treatment. The patient and family both require emotional support and reassurance throughout the illness. Once HVS occurs, there is a great likelihood it will recur unless the neoplastic process is under control. Many of the symptoms, particularly the visual and neurologic disturbances, produce fear, anxiety, and loss of control. Nursing care must be tailored to the individual according to the incidence and severity of symptoms and the associated distress, as perceived by the patient.

Bibliography

1. Bloch, K. J., and D. G. Maki, Hyperviscosity syndromes associated with immunoglobulin abnormalities. *Seminars in Hematology* (April 1973). 113–124.
    Comprehensive review: signs and symptoms, diagnosis, and treatment.

2. Fahey, J. L., W. F. Barth, and A. Soloman. Serum hyperviscosity syndrome. *Journal of the American Medical Association* (May 10, 1965). 120–123.
    Classic article describing HVS, clearly written and easy to understand. Discusses serum hyperviscosity, measurement, clinical syndrome, symptomatic threshold, and plasmapheresis.

3. Krol, T. C., and W. S. Wood. Hyperviscosity syndrome in Waldenström's macroglobulinemia. *American Family Physician* (August 1981). 187–189.
    Effective use of a case study to illustrate multisystem clinical manifestation of HVS. Pictures illustrate retinal changes before and after therapy.

4. Megliola, B. Multiple myeloma. *Cancer Nursing* (June 1980). 209–218.
    Review of the disease, treatment, complications, and nursing care.

5. Pruzanski, W., and J. G. Watt. Serum viscosity and hyperviscosity syndrome in IgG multiple myeloma. *Annals of Internal Medicine* (December 1972). 853–860.
    Report on 10 patients highlighting the immunoglobulin abnormalities

TABLE 15D–4

Nursing Protocol for Supportive Management of HVS

Problem	Intervention
Hematologic dysfunction	Ensure adequate rest. Monitor outcome of plasmapheresis: improved symptoms, decreased viscosity level. Provide pressure to all puncture sites. Practice frequent oral hygiene, because bleeding from the oral cavity is very common. Assess nutritional needs.
Ocular dysfunction	Monitor outcome of plasmapheresis: improved symptoms, decreased viscosity level. Provide careful explanation of all planned activity. Depending on degree of visual impairment, help with ADL, repeated orientation to immediate surroundings; ensure safe environment. Provide discussion and realistic reassurance of potential resolution of visual impairment.
Neurologic dysfunction	Provide safe environment. Assess and, if needed, provide orientation to time and place. Depending on severity of symptoms, assist with ADL. Assist with active and passive exercises if immobile to maintain muscle tone and function.
Cardiovascular dysfunction	Ensure rest. Evaluate laboratory values, especially electrolytes, and monitor for imbalances. Monitor intake and output. Restrict sodium and fluid intake, as indicated. Monitor cardiac status, if indicated, for signs or symptoms of pending failure. Monitor for side effects and complications of medications. Assist with ADL as needed.

HVS, hyperviscosity syndrome.

and the complexity of differentiating between disease manifestations and HVS.

6. Soloman, A., and J. L. Fahey. Plasmapheresis therapy in macroglobulinemia. *Annals of Internal Medicine* (May 1963). 789–800.

Good discussion of plasmapheresis (indications, procedure, outcome) with 10 patient cases presented to illustrate the points.

E: ANAPHYLAXIS

Kristen Kreamer

The immune system is one of the human body's basic defenses against foreign substances. Normally, the immune system mounts a protective and beneficial response to antigen assault by inactivating the antigen and rendering it harmless. In the case of a hypersensitivity response, however, the immunologic system is excessively stimulated; in such cases, tissue damage to the host may result.

There are four classes of hypersensitivity response: types I, II, III, and IV. Types II, III, and IV, while not benign, develop only after time has elapsed. Examples of these reactions include hemolytic anemia (type II), serum sickness (type III), and contact dermatitis (type IV). Type I reactions, however, are immediate; they include urticaria, allergic rhinitis, allergic asthma, and anaphylaxis.

Pathophysiology

Type I hypersensitivity is a two-phase process, the first phase being sensitization and the second phase being the hypersensitivity response.

Sensitization.   The first contact of the host with antigen results in the formation of IgE, the class of immunoglobulin associated with allergic reactions. These IgE antibodies, which are specific for the particular antigen, then bond with mast cells in tissue and with basophils in the circulation. Once this initial antigen-antibody response process is complete, the individual host is said to be sensitized to that particular antigen.

Hypersensitivity response.   Subsequent exposure to the antigen results in the reaction of that antigen with the complementary IgE antibodies already formed. This interaction of antigen with the cell-fixed IgE antibodies results in an alteration in the production of the enzyme adenylate cyclase. Since adenylate cyclase is a key enzyme in the generation of cyclic adenosine monophosphate (cAMP), there is a resulting decrease in the amount of cAMP.

The decrease in cAMP triggers a process known as degranulation within the mast cells and basophils. These cells contain granules in which are stored substances known as vasoactive mediators. These vasoactive mediators are thought to be responsible for the symptoms associated with the type I reaction of anaphylaxis.

The mediators believed to be implicated in the anaphylactic mechanism are histamine (H), slow-reacting substance of anaphylaxis

(SRS-A), eosinophil chemotactic factor (ECF-A), platelet-activating factor (PAF), bradykinin and lysyl-bradykinin (kinins), and the prostaglandins (PG). These mediators cause specific physiologic responses, explained in detail in Table 15E–1. Figure 15E–1 illustrates the process by which these mediators are released.

Some of the mediators (H, SRS-A, PAF, PG, and kinins) are thought to be potentiators of the anaphylactic response, while ECF-A is thought to decrease the anaphylactic response. When the potentiating forces overcome the regulating force, the patient exhibits an acute systemic reaction within minutes of exposure to the antigen. Anaphylaxis is characterized by the following:

Subjective symptoms:
1. Pain or tightness in chest, dyspnea.
2. Inability to speak.
3. Generalized itching.
4. Complaints of uneasiness, agitation, warmth, dizziness.
5. Nausea, crampy abdominal pain.
6. Desire to urinate or defecate.

Objective signs:
1. Respiratory embarrassment with or without wheezing, stridor.
2. Sneezing, coughing.
3. Local or generalized urticaria and/or erythema.
4. Angioedema of face, eyelids, hands, feet.
5. Hypotension, tachycardia, arrhythmia.
6. Cyanosis.
7. Unconsciousness.
8. Emesis and/or diarrhea.

All of the signs and symptoms listed above need not be present in order to make a diagnosis of anaphylaxis. Furthermore, it is recommended that immediate treatment be instituted in the face of a reasonable suspicion because, in severe cases, death may ensue rapidly because of respiratory failure, cardiac arrthymia, or complete vascular collapse.

Anaphylaxis and the cancer patient. It is imperative to remember that the person with cancer is subject to the same risks of anaphylaxis as any other patient. For example, a cancer patient may experience a type I anaphylactic response to an antibiotic given for infection. One antifungal agent often used to treat opportunistic fungal infections is miconazole; when given IV, this drug has been known to cause anaphylaxis. There is no evidence, however, that immunotherapy, a systemic form of cancer treatment, has caused any episodes of type I hypersensitivity.

The greatest number of anaphylactic reactions in cancer patients are caused by antitumor chemotherapeutic agents. The two drugs most

TABLE 15E–1

Mediators of the Anaphylactic Response

Mediator	Response
Potentiates response	
Histamine (H)	Contraction of smooth muscle Increased vascular permeability Increased mucous secretion
Slow-reacting substance of anaphylaxis (SRS-A)	Prolonged spasm of visceral smooth muscle Increased vascular permeability
Platelet-activating factor (PAF)	Aggregation and degranulation of platelets
Bradykinin and lysyl-bradykinin (kinins)	Increased vascular permeability Decreased BP Contraction of smooth muscle
Prostaglandins (PG)	Contract or relax smooth muscle
Decreases response	
Eosinophil chemotactic factor (ECF-A)	Attracts eosinophils, which: release histaminase to inactivate H; release sulfatase B to inactivate SRS-A; release phospholipase D to inactivate PAF.

Adapted with permission from Kreamer, K. M., Anaphylaxis resulting from chemotherapy. *Oncology Nursing Forum* (Fall 1981). pp. 13–16.

frequently cited in this regard are asparaginase and cisplatin. Other chemotherapeutic agents have also been implicated, though with less frequency. These drugs are neocarzinostatin, VM-26, doxorubicin, daunorubicin, mechlorethamine, bleomycin, cyclophosphamide, melphalan, and methotrexate.

In general, certain factors may contribute to an increased risk of anaphylactic response. The IV route of administration is more likely to cause anaphylaxis than the PO or topical routes. Drugs derived from bacteria, such as asparaginase, are more likely to cause exaggerated immunologic reactions than are drugs from an inorganic source. Crude preparations of drug are more likely to be highly antigenic; such preparations are more common in the early stages of investigational use, before refinement and isolation techniques have been perfected. Finally, it is important to remember that although the risk of a

Presensitization   Sensitization   Mediator
response

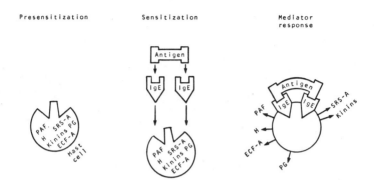

Figure 15E-1. Anaphylactic reaction and mediator response. ECF-A, eosinophil chemotactic factor; H, histamine; IgE, immunoglobulin E; PAF, platelet-activating factor; PG, prostaglandins; SRS-A, slow-reacting substance of anaphylaxis. *Reprinted with permission from* Kreamer, K. M. Anaphylaxis resulting from chemotherapy. *Oncology Nursing Forum* (Fall 1981). p. 16.

hypersensitivity response increases with successive doses of the drug, reactions have been seen in individuals with no known prior exposure to that particular drug (e.g., doxorubicin, cyclophosphamide). The explanation for this phenomenon may be that the individual had been exposed previously to contaminants or unrefined elements in the diluent.

Assessment

To identify those patients at increased risk, the nursing history should include a thorough review and documentation of prior allergic episodes, including the agent thought to be responsible and a precise description of the episode. Although there is no conclusive evidence that a prior allergic response predisposes to anaphylaxis, it is not unreasonable to identify persons with allergic histories as a possible high-risk group. Of particular interest is the patient who reports previous allergic reactions to antitumor drugs, because there is evidence of cross-reactivity within the classes of chemotherapeutic agents.

Medical management

Prevention. Preventive medical measures include administration of a test dose, a change in drug or route, and premedication with steroids and antihistamines. A small **test dose** of the drug may be given prior to full-dose therapy to assess for signs and symptoms of a hypersensitivity response. There is, however, little evidence to show

494 Handbook of Oncology Nursing

that such test doses are reliable predictors of an anaphylactic response. The physician may **change to another preparation** of drug, e.g., asparaginase derived from *Erwinia cartovora* may be substituted for asparaginase derived from *E. coli*, in hopes of averting a repeat of the anaphylactic episode. Also, the **route of administration** of a drug may be switched from IV to IM or PO. The physician may order **premedication** with hydrocortisone and diphenhydramine as a precaution against anaphylaxis. Although the value of this practice has not been well-documented, it is based on the clinical reasoning that these medications, proven useful in treating other hypersensitivity responses, may prophylactically decrease the severity of a type I reaction.

Support. Medical support measures may consist of maintenance of a patent airway, administration of epinephrine, correction of hypotension through fluid administration, and administration of antihistamines and steroids. **Maintenance of patent airway** may require simple repositioning, suction, or oropharyngeal intubation. In extreme cases, with glottic edema, tracheostomy may be performed. **Epinephrine** is the drug of choice for anaphylactic reactions and is administered for its bronchodilator and vasoconstrictive effects. A dose is given immediately and repeated in 10 min if required (Table 15E-2). A key physiologic change during anaphylaxis is altered vascular permeability, which results in fluid shift and hypotension. **Rapid fluid replacement** may be required to counter the drop in BP. **Antihistamines** are administered to control urticaria, and adrenocortical **steroids** to control abnormal vascular-wall permeability. These drugs do not contribute to the resolution of the life-threatening emergency but are instrumental in managing later symptoms.

Nursing management

Prevention. The nurse has two main responsibilities in preventive care of anaphylaxis: The first is the preparation of the setting, and the second the preparation of the patient. Preparation of the setting includes ensuring that emergency drugs and equipment are readily available. These preparations may vary, depending on whether the drug is being administered in a hospital, outpatient clinic, private physician's office, or in the home. In the latter case, the nurse should ensure that emergency services for the locale have been identified and relevant phone numbers have been obtained.

Base-line data on pulse, respiration, and BP should be obtained and recorded. When preparing the IV site, the nurse should ensure a view of the entire course of the vein along the extremity, unobstructed by clothing or tape. This area should be observed for localized urticaria or erythema. A critical aspect of patient preparation is that he be instructed in the subjective symptoms of anaphylaxis. While the nurse

TABLE 15E-2

Nursing Protocol for the Management of Anaphylactic Shock

Factor	Intervention
Prior to drug administration	Nursing history: Elicit specific information re previous allergic responses, especially to cancer chemotherapeutic agents.
	Educate patient in need to report subjective symptoms of allergic response.
	Ensure that emergency equipment is available.
	Secure base-line data: pulse, respiration, BP.
	Prepare IV site to expose complete course of vein.
Evidence of anaphylactic response	Stop flow of drug and keep line open with saline flush.
	Rapidly evaluate signs and symptoms.
	If anaphylaxis suspected, proceed to:
	Administer epinephrine (solution strength 1:1,000); repeat after 10 min if inadequate response.
	adults: 0.5–0.75 ml SC (smaller dose in elderly or those of slight build)
	children: 0.01 ml/kg SC (maximum single dose of 0.5 ml)
	Maintain patent airway: Suction and/or oropharyngeal intubation may be required.
	Place patient in supine position, with feet elevated, unless contraindicated by respiratory distress.
	Monitor pulse, respiration, BP.
	Reassure patient.
	Call for medical attention and/or emergency services.

Adapted with permission from Kreamer, K. M. Anaphylaxis resulting from chemotherapy. Oncology Nursing Forum (Fall 1981). p. 13–16.

should be careful not to alarm the patient, it is essential that he be aware that such symptoms, if experienced, need to be reported immediately.

Support. A nursing protocol for anaphylactic shock is presented in Table 15E–2. It is presented as a general guideline, which will need to be adjusted to the particular institution or chemotherapy-administration setting in which the nurse is practicing. There are two points that require further emphasis.

In the event that a physician is not immediately available in case of suspected anaphylaxis, the nurse should not delay in instituting supportive treatment for anaphylactic shock. As the protocol indicates, the nurse must stop the flow of drug, rapidly evaluate the patient's objective signs and subjective symptoms, and when indicated, administer epinephrine. Although other conditions can be mistaken for anaphylactic shock, the SC administration of epinephrine in correct dosage is not likely to be hazardous.

Finally, the nurse should be attuned to the patient's need for reassurance should a hypersensitivity reaction occur. The subjective symptoms experienced by the patient may be alarming. The situation requires a nurse who, while acting quickly, maintains an attitude of calm and provides support to the patient through verbal reassurance and physical contact. In the oncologic emergency of anaphylaxis, as in all other medical emergencies, the patient's need for psychologic safety must be a primary concern.

Bibliography

1. Dorr, R. T., and W. L. Fritz. Cancer Chemotherapy Handbook. Elsevier North-Holland Inc., New York. 1980.

   Contains a table of antitumor drugs thought to be responsible for allergic hypersensitivity.

2. Fruth, R. Anaphylaxis and drug reactions: guidelines for detection and care. *Heart and Lung* (July/August 1980). 662–664.

   A detailed discussion of the physiology of anaphylaxis and the clinical management of a type I response.

3. Groenwald, S. B. Physiology of the immune system. *Heart and Lung* (July/August 1980). 645–650.

   A nurse explains the components and function of the immune system.

4. Holt, D. Anaphylactic shock: a shock that's easy to see. *Nursing Mirror* (May 1979). 32–34.

   A general discussion of anaphylaxis and medical treatment.

5. Kreamer, K. M. Anaphylaxis resulting from chemotherapy. *Oncology Nursing Forum* (Fall 1981). 13–16.

   Mechanism of anaphylaxis and nursing implications.

6. Weiss, R. B., and S. Bruno. Hypersensitivity reactions to cancer chemotherapeutic agents. *Annals of Internal Medicine* (January 1981). 66–72.

A comprehensive review of the medical literature.

7. Young, P., editor. Anaphylaxis and the community nurse. *Nursing Mirror*
(September 1977). 41–42.

Guidelines for recognition and treatment of anaphylaxis by the home-
care nurse.

F: SEPTIC SHOCK
Jeanne M. Erickson

Infection is a life-threatening process and a leading cause of death in
cancer patients. Localized or systemic infection results from progression of the underlying disease or it develops as a complication of cancer
treatment. The clinical presentation of patients with systemic infections
can vary from a fever alone to extreme toxicity and shock. When shock
results from an overwhelming infection, the patient needs emergency
attention and treatment.

Cancer patients develop a variety of bacterial, fungal, parasitic, and
viral infections. Bacterial infections are the most common. Bacteremia
is the presence of bacteria in the blood, with or without clinical signs of
infection. Sepsis, or septicemia, refers to an infection in the blood with
clinical signs and symptoms of fever and chills. Septic shock implies
deterioration of the cardiovascular system, with inadequate tissue
perfusion and hypotension. The shock response to sepsis arises when
pathogenic endotoxins cause dilation of the vascular system and
pooling of blood in regional vascular beds, decreasing circulating blood
volume.

Pathophysiology

The sequence of events leading to septicemia begins when a
microorganism invades the body. Common portals of entry are skin,
nasopharynx, lungs, intestine, urethra, and perineum. The body's
immune system normally functions to recognize and destroy the
pathogens, either by phagocytosis or antigen-antibody reactions (*see*
Chapter 9A). If the immune system is deficient, however, or if the
pathogen is particularly virulent, the microorganisms adhere to the
cellular surface, multiply, and form a lesion. If uncontrolled, the lesion
spreads locally, causing regional symptoms of swelling, redness, and
tenderness, as well as a fever. Pathogens can then spread systemically
through the bloodstream by directly invading a blood vessel or by
entering the venous system through lymphatic channels. Specific signs

and symptoms may indicate that distant infectious lesions have formed, e.g., in the heart or lungs. Systemic symptoms of infection include fever, chills, and malaise. The infectious process can terminate in recovery or death at any stage, depending on the function of the host's defenses and on the pathogenicity of the invading microorganism.

Shock is the body's response to an overwhelming infection. While septic shock can be caused by a variety of pathogens, most cases involve infections by gram-negative bacteria. As bacteria undergo lysis and phagocytosis by leukocytes, endotoxins are released into the bloodstream. These endotoxins initiate antibody formation and complement interactions, which promote detoxification of the pathogens. Histamine, serotonin, and other cellular enzymes are products of these immune reactions. When these substances are produced in large quantities, as in an overwhelming infection, they cause general vasodilation and increased capillary permeability, allowing plasma volume to leak into interstitial tissue and pool in regional vascular beds. The progressive loss of intravascular volume results in hypotension and sets the shock response into motion.

The hemodynamics of septic shock are divided into an early and a late stage, separated by a transformation phase. Early septic shock is the vasodilative, high-output stage, or "warm shock." The patient usually has a fever and chills from the infectious process. The skin is warm and flushed as vessels dilate to dissipate heat. The endotoxic reactions producing histamine and serotonin cause blood to leak through capillaries and pool in peripheral tissues. Blood is shunted from arterioles into venules, which stagnates flow in the capillary bed. The result is a decreased circulating blood volume, which impairs tissue perfusion. In response, the heart rate and contractility increase to maintain adequate tissue perfusion. BP may be temporarily maintained but soon falls below the patient's normal range as vasodilation persists. The respiratory rate increases to provide more oxygen, but as hypoxemia develops, cells shift from aerobic to anaerobic metabolism. With this shift, lactic acid is produced, and its accumulation leads to metabolic acidosis and impaired energy production. Cells become incapable of maintaining an internal fluid-and-electrolyte balance, and chemical reactions are inhibited. A transient increase in urine output may develop as blood pools in the renal vessels.

The transformation stage varies in length and characterizes the body's response to progressive septic shock. Cool skin, peripheral edema, and pulmonary congestion result as more plasma volume without oxygen leaks into the tissues. As hypovolemia and hypoxemia progress, the body compensates by causing peripheral vasoconstriction. Though intended to increase venous return and BP, vasoconstriction precipitates classic "cold shock," or the late stage of septic shock.

The late stage of septic shock is the vasoconstrictive, low-output stage. Compensatory vasoconstriction traps blood in vascular beds and actually decreases venous return, cardiac output, and BP. Basic cellular reactions are inhibited because of inadequate oxygen supply and production of lactic acid, and tissues become ischemic. Excessive tissue damage and capillary leakage can force the clotting mechanisms into disseminated intravascular coagulation (DIC) (*see* Chapter 15G).

Eventually, hypovolemia and hypoxemia cause multisystem failure. As pulmonary perfusion declines, capillary leakage and edema lead to respiratory failure. Declining kidney perfusion leads to acute tubular necrosis, and poor cerebral perfusion leads to progressive somnolence and coma. Inadequate coronary perfusion causes arrhythmias and myocardial ischemia, and cardiac arrest is a likely cause of death.

Etiology.   A detailed discussion of the causes of infection in patients with cancer is included in Chapter 9. Numerous factors related to the disease process predispose the cancer patient to infections that could lead to septic shock. Because cancer is by definition an invasive disease, malignancies can erode through mechanical barriers, allowing pathogens to enter through skin and mucous membranes. Obstructive tumors allow overgrowth of normal, resident flora. A variety of malignancies affect host defense by interfering with bone marrow function. Severe granulocytopenia (granulocyte count <1000 cells/mm^3 of blood) often results from leukemia, while lymphoproliferative disorders, such as lymphoma, cause defects in cell-mediated and humoral immunity.

Cancer therapy is also responsible for increasing the patient's susceptibility to infection. Numerous chemotherapeutic agents cause profound bone marrow suppression, and administration of chemotherapy, as well as surgery and radiotherapy, can affect skin integrity. Other therapies that disrupt mechanical barriers include the placement of urinary catheters, IV catheters, and drainage devices. IV catheters, in particular, are significantly associated with septicemias, as they provide pathogens direct entry into the bloodstream for systemic dissemination. Impaired nutritional status, often associated with cancer and its treatment, causes immunologic deficiencies as well as delayed skin healing (*see* Chapter 8). Finally, the hospital environment introduces the patient to a variety of potentially more virulent and resistant microorganisms than would otherwise be encountered outside the hospital setting.

When a patient becomes granulocytopenic as a result of cancer and/or its treatment, the source of sepsis is commonly the patient's endogenous flora. *Escherichia coli, Pseudomonas* species, and *Klebsiella* species are gram-negative aerobic bacilli associated with a high incidence of sepsis in the granulocytopenic population. *Staphylococcus* species, gram-positive bacteria, and *Candida* species, opportunistic fungi, are also common causes of sepsis. Except for *Staphylococcus*, whose endotoxic reactions are less pathogenic, each of these organisms is frequently associated with septic shock.

In nongranulocytopenic patients, who primarily have solid tumors, septicemias are commonly caused by *Escherichia coli*, *Staphylococcus* species, *Bacteroides* species, *Klebsiella* species, and *Candida* species. These infections frequently occur in postoperative periods, arising from the GU tract, abdominal abscesses, peritonitis, wound infections, and pulmonary infiltrates. *E. coli*, *Klebsiella*, and *Candida* are likely to cause shock, while *Staphylococcus* and *Bacteroides* septicemias are less commonly associated with episodes of shock.

Regardless of the granulocyte count, the overall mortality rate of septicemias associated with shock approaches 70%. This astounding value compares with an overall mortality rate of 18% for septic patients who did not exhibit signs of shock.

Assessment

The patient can deteriorate unpredictably through the stages of septic shock over the course of days or in a matter of hours. Furthermore, the symptoms of septic shock may not always progress in an orderly fashion. Because the treatment of septic shock is most effective in the early stage, identification of patients at risk for sepsis and septic shock and prompt recognition of the early symptoms of shock are imperative for patient recovery.

Nursing measures to prevent septic shock begin with an assessment of the patient's susceptibility to infection, particularly septicemia (*see* Chapter 9). Patients should be educated about their risk of infection and taught to report early symptoms of infection. Granulocytopenic patients must be closely monitored, as the classic signs of inflammation may be absent or limited to only local tenderness and/or fever.

Mouth, nasopharynx, skin, lungs, perineum, and IV sites of susceptible patients should be inspected daily for signs of infection. Vital signs should be checked q 4 hr. Fever is defined as an oral temperature >38.5° C at a single reading or as 3 readings >38.0° C in a 24-hr period. For all granulocytopenic patients, patients with known or suspected septicemias or abdominal infection, and patients who have undergone pelvic or abdominal surgery, nurses should be alert for the signs and symptoms of early septic shock: tachycardia, tachypnea, vasodilation, and/or hypotension before, during, or following a febrile episode. The first sign of infection or septic shock should be immediately discussed with the physician and treatment initiated.

Assessment of the patient with signs of early septic shock should be increased to q 15 to 30 min and include monitoring of vital signs, mental status, and tissue perfusion. Mental status can be determined by noting the patient's level of awareness and consciousness and by asking the patient questions to check his orientation, memory, and cognitive functioning. Tissue perfusion is evaluated by checking the color of lips, nailbeds, and the temperature of the extremities. Blood cultures from two separate sites should be obtained at once, while other regional cultures and x-rays can be delayed.

Medical management

Early recognition and aggressive treatment of septic shock are imperative to increase a patient's chance for survival. The basic goal of medical therapy is to support the patient's cardiovascular system until the infectious process is controlled.

Antibiotic therapy must be prescribed to control the infection, but, at the time of shock, this treatment will not be sufficient to save the patient's life. A careful history and physical examination should be made to identify the source of infection, with particular attention to the nasopharynx, lungs, perineum, wounds, and sites of any invasive device. Urinalysis and chest x-ray, as well as routine bacterial and fungal cultures of throat, sputum, urine, stool, blood, and any drainage should be obtained to identify the organism and guide the choice of antibiotics. Any obviously infected device should be removed.

If the patient is granulocytopenic or unstable, antimicrobial therapy should be instituted immediately after blood cultures are obtained, without waiting for the completion of chest x-ray and regional cultures. A broad-spectrum antibiotic regimen, consisting of an amino-glycoside and a semisynthetic penicillin derivative, is usually ordered to cover the commonly infecting gram-negative bacilli. This regimen can be adjusted after culture results are known or if surveillance cultures have been done and indicate an unusual colonizing organism. If a patient remains febrile or has symptoms of shock while already on broad-spectrum antibiotics, antifungal therapy with amphotericin B is indicated for possible *Candida* sepsis, or candidiasis. Granulocyte transfusions may be prescribed for patients in shock who have prolonged granulocytopenia, gram-negative sepsis, and show poor response to antibiotic regimens.

For the patient with septic shock, fluid therapy to restore circulating blood volume is the most rapidly effective measure for improving tissue perfusion and vital signs. Because it is difficult to determine the status of myocardial functioning during an episode of shock, fluids are prescribed to be given incrementally with close monitoring. There is a tendency to give too little fluid in the early stage of shock, when the cardiovascular system is able to manage the volume, and too much fluid late in shock, when it is likely to cause cardiac and respiratory failure. Fluid boluses of 100 ml in 10 min are recommended and should be repeated until vital signs improve. If there is no initial response to fluid therapy, a central venous pressure (CVP) line and Swan-Ganz catheter are inserted to monitor cardiac and pulmonary function, respectively. Controversy exists about whether fluid replacement should be administered as a colloid or crystalloid solution. While less colloid solution is required for volume expansion, it carries a higher risk of pulmonary edema. Crystalloids require a larger volume of solution and can lead to systemic edema, which often makes the physician hesitant to administer the quantity necessary to restore an adequate circulating volume. Overall, crystalloid solutions of Ringer's lactate or normal saline are recommended during septic shock.

If the patient does not improve with fluid therapy, an inotropic agent is prescribed to improve tissue perfusion and cardiac output. Dopamine is frequently used in septic shock because of its flexibility. At low doses (3 μg/kg/min), dopamine improves splanchnic, mesenteric, and renal circulation, while at moderate doses (3 to 5 μg/kg/min), it increases cardiac output by increasing heart rate and stroke volume. Other inotropic drugs are generally not recommended because they increase myocardial oxygen demand at a time when tissues are hypoxic because of hypoperfusion.

All patients in septic shock have an increased oxygen demand because of increased metabolism and ensuing hypoperfusion. Oxygen therapy with arterial blood gas (ABG) monitoring is prescribed to maintain the arterial oxygen pressure (PO_2) >80 mmHg. If adequate blood gas values cannot be maintained or if respiratory distress persists, mechanical ventilatory assistance is indicated.

The hypoperfusion in septic shock leads to anaerobic metabolism and lactic acid production, resulting in metabolic acidosis. Sodium bicarbonate ($NaHCO_3$) is administered to keep blood pH in the normal range of 7.35 to 7.45. Serum electrolytes are also monitored and replaced as needed.

DIC can develop from excessive tissue damage and blood pooling. A continuous heparin infusion and fresh-frozen plasma may be prescribed if hemorrhage or other signs of DIC occur, although DIC secondary to sepsis is not readily reversed.

Renal damage and fluid overload may also complicate recovery from septic shock. If adequate BP and tissue perfusion has been attained but urine output remains low, a cautious trial of diuretics may be instituted.

Nursing management

Nursing measures to prevent and detect infection in susceptible cancer patients, as outlined in Chapter 9, may prevent overwhelming sepsis and septic shock. Once signs and symptoms of infection are documented in the patient, nurses become involved in controlling the infectious process. If the patient presents with shock related to sepsis, nursing interventions are directed toward reversing the shock response. Table 15F–1 outlines a protocol for the nursing care of patients in septic shock.

Because a patient in septic shock requires immediate medical and nursing interventions with careful monitoring, an intensive care setting may be indicated until the patient's condition has stabilized. Even after successful treatment, however, the patient remains at risk for septic shock and its complications and will continue to need frequent assessment. Because septic shock may develop in any patient with an infection, oncology nurses must be knowledgeable and skilled in monitoring and supporting the cardiovascular and respiratory systems during this emergency.

Bibliography

1. Cohen, S. Nursing care of patients in shock. *American Journal of Nursing* (June 1982). 943–964; (September 1982). 1401–1422; (November 1982). 1723–1746.

    This programmed instruction addresses the pathophysiology, pharmacology, and nursing care of patients in hypovolemic, cardiogenic, and septic shock.

2. Eskridge, R. Septic shock. *Critical Care Quarterly* (March 1980). 55–75.

    This article provides a detailed explanation of the pathophysiology of septic shock in addition to the clinical manifestations and medical treatment of septic shock.

3. Lamb, L. Think you know septic shock? *Nursing 82* (January 1982). 34–43.

    Two patients with septic shock are described and the goals of nursing care are highlighted.

4. Singer, C., M. Kaplan, and D. Armstrong. Bacteremia and fungemia complicating neoplastic disease. *American Journal of Medicine* (May 1977). 731–742.

    An analysis of 364 cases of infection in cancer patients with respect to causative organism, mortality, and prognostic factors, including shock.

5. Wilson, R. The diagnosis and management of severe sepsis and septic shock. *Heart and Lung* (May-June 1976). 422–429.

    An overview of the pathophysiology and medical treatment of septic shock.

TABLE 15F-1

Nursing Protocol for Management of Septic Shock

Problem	Intervention
Susceptibility to infection	Identify patients at risk for infection. Institute measures to prevent infection in susceptible patients. Inspect mouth, nasopharynx, skin, lungs, perineum, and IV sites of susceptible patients daily.
Septicemia	Obtain blood cultures at once, regional cultures, and chest x-ray. Institute prescribed antibiotic regimen at once and maintain on a strict schedule. Check patient's drug allergies. Know and monitor for side effects of antibiotics. Manage granulocyte transfusions if prescribed.
Inadequate circulating blood volume	Assure IV access with 1–2 large-gauge catheters. Infuse fluids as prescribed. Insert urinary catheter. Record hourly intake and output. Assess for effectiveness of fluid therapy: increased BP, urine output >20 ml/hr, improved mental status, and improved tissue perfusion. Anticipate insertion of CVP and Swan-Ganz catheters with continued fluid therapy. Manage dopamine infusion if prescribed for persistent hypotension: Administer via central or large vein on infusion pump; observe for signs of infiltration if given peripherally, as dopamine is an irritant. Record base-line BP, pulse, urine output, and tissue perfusion. Check BP and pulse q 2–3 min after each dose adjustment, then q 15–30 min until stable.

Inadequate oxygenation	Prescribe bed rest. Manage oxygen therapy per nasal cannula or mask at 2–4 liters/min. Monitor ABG results: Notify MD if pH <7.35 or PO$_2$ <80 mmHg. Assess rate, rhythm, ease of respirations, breath sounds, and tissue perfusion q 15–30 min until stable.
Abnormal body temperature	Monitor temperature q 30 min until stable. Administer antipyretics as prescribed. Use cooling blanket, ice packs to axillae and groin, or alcohol baths if temperature >39.0°C. Use warmed blankets during vasoconstrictive stage.
Acid-base, electrolyte abnormalities	Monitor ABG results and serum electrolyte values. Administer NaHCO$_3$ as prescribed to keep pH >7.35. Administer replacement of electrolytes as prescribed.
Potential for bleeding related to DIC	Monitor for signs of bleeding. Monitor results of coagulation profile. Be alert for elevated PT and PTT, decreased fibrinogen and platelet values. Apply pressure to sites of active bleeding. Manage heparin therapy as prescribed. Administer plasma and platelets as prescribed.
Potential for fluid overload	Assess for signs of fluid overload: pulmonary rales, dyspnea, wet cough, edema. Assess base-line BP, tissue perfusion, and electrolytes before administering diuretics. Administer diuretics as prescribed.

ABG, arterial blood gas; CVP, central venous pressure; MD, physician; NaHCO$_3$, sodium bicarbonate; PO$_2$, arterial oxygen pressure; PT, prothrombin time; PTT, partial thromboplastin time.

G: ALTERATIONS IN HEMOSTASIS

Anne R. Bavier

Normal hemostatic functioning is a delicate system that prevents either excessive hemorrhage or excessive clot(thrombus) formation. A change in the system, tipping the balance to either extreme, can cause diffuse venous thrombosis or the acute form of disseminated intravascular coagulation (DIC), either of which may be life-threatening. Nursing actions for the cancer patient at risk of developing an alteration in hemostasis are designed to promote normal coagulation and clot lysis.

NORMAL HEMOSTATIC MECHANISMS

To understand hemostasis, it is necessary to recognize the interrelationship among vasoconstriction, platelet plug formation, and clot formation (Fig. 15G–1). Vasoconstriction attempts to minimize blood loss and to decrease blood flow. Vascular spasm occurs immediately after a blood vessel is cut, thus reducing the blood loss from the wound. Nervous reflexes and local myogenic spasm initiate this vascular constriction. The degree of constriction is directly proportional to the extent of trauma to the vessel. The spasm lasts for up to one-half hour, during which time the other processes of hemostasis occur: platelet plug formation and blood coagulation leading to fibrin formation.

The platelet plug is a loose collection of platelets that acts as the base for the formation of a stable clot. Vessel-wall damage stimulates platelet aggregation by exposing the underlying collagen layer and releasing adenosine diphosphate (ADP). The platelets themselves release ADP, serotonin, and an enzyme that forms thromboxane A. Serotonin is a vasoactive substance that may enhance hemostasis by constricting small arteries and veins. Together, these chemicals attract additional platelets, which adhere to the mass and become the plug. The platelet plug is effective only in stopping blood loss through small rents in vessel walls, which are constantly occurring naturally. The absence of adequate platelet supplies to mend such small tears is noted in thrombocytopenic patients who develop petechiae.

While vasoconstriction and platelet plug formation contain the blood initially, blood coagulation begins to provide a stable clot and promote vascular healing. The general mechanism of blood coagulation has three parts: (1) formation of prothrombin activator; (2) conversion

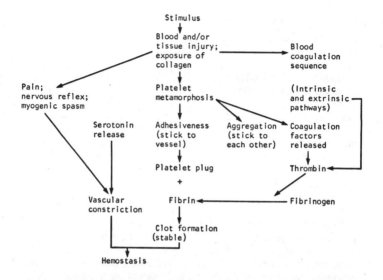

Figure 15G–1. Homeostatic mechanisms. *Reprinted with permission from* Bullock, B. L., and P. Rosendahl. Pathophysiology, Adaptations and Alterations in Function. Little, Brown & Co., Boston. 1984. p. 198.

of prothrombin to thrombin by the activator; and (3) conversion of fibrinogen to fibrin with thrombin as initiator and subsequent formation of solid fibrin strands.

There are two catalysts to the formation of prothrombin activator, the intrinsic and extrinsic pathways. The intrinsic pathway is initiated by trauma to the blood itself or contact by blood with a surface, such as collagen. An alteration of any blood component, such as the platelets, can initiate the intrinsic pathway. Tissue or vessel injury are the requirements for the extrinsic pathway initiation of coagulation. The extrinsic pathway begins with exposure of blood to tissue factor (tissue thromboplastin) released by traumatized tissues.

Within the blood are clotting factors that are utilized in sequence to reach the prothrombin activator stage. Clotting factors, which are referred to by Roman numeral (i.e., factor V, factor VIII), are inactive forms of proteolytic enzymes that become activated and, in turn, cause the next factor to be activated. The process requires nonenzyme cofactors to produce this cascading sequence. The vascular or tissue injury initiates tissue factor and tissue phospholipid formation and uses factor VII in the extrinsic pathway to prothrombin activation.

The intrinsic and extrinsic pathways converge at the formation of the prothrombin activator, and the remainder of coagulation follows a common pathway. These steps require adequate serum calcium levels to succeed.

The blood clot itself is composed of all blood-cell forms and plasma products caught in a mesh of fibrin threads, which holds the clot to the vessel walls. The action of factor XIII on the fibrin results in cross-links between the fibers, further stabilizing the clot.

Clot retraction is the next event. Its great importance is that it pulls the edges of the vessel closer together to promote healing. The fibrin strands contract, squeezing out the blood serum. Platelet secretion of fibrin-stabilizing factor is largely responsible for this vital phenomenon. Consequently, severely thrombocytopenic patients may be unable to mount this response; vessel healing is deterred and a less stable clot is formed.

It is important to note that the absence of any of the components of clot formation jeopardizes the patient. The danger is massive hemorrhage. Individuals may have a genetic condition, such as classic hemophilia A, in which factor VIII levels are inadequate, or an acquired condition. Massive trauma that has exhausted the supply of clotting factors or severe calcium depletion are examples of acquired states.

Balancing the clot formation process is clot lysis. Plasmin, or fibrinolysin, digests the fibrin strands and consumes coagulation factors. Fibrinogen degradation products result from fibrinolysis and act to prevent thrombin formation. Thus, the process of clot lysis also includes a mechanism that limits new clot formation. On the average, the relatively small quantities of these fibrinogen degradation products limit local expansion of the clot only, because the entire body's capability to form thrombin is not affected.

These two mechanisms of clot formation and lysis exist in a delicate balance that maintains blood flow through the vessels. Either or both mechanisms can become altered in cancer patients. Excessive clot formation, resulting in the blockage of vessels, occurs primarily as diffuse venous thrombosis. Chronic DIC is also associated with excessive clotting. Ineffective clotting, resulting in major hemorrhagic episodes, is the acute form of DIC, the oncologic emergency. Each condition is discussed separately below.

DIFFUSE VENOUS THROMBOSIS

Pathophysiology

Hypercoagulation results in the formation of a thrombus blocking a blood vessel. Two dangers exist: impairment of local/regional tissue perfusion, resulting in tissue death; and embolization of a portion of the clot to another body part, causing that tissue's death. If embolization to a vital organ, such as the lungs, occurs, then the patient's death may result. Knowledge about the cause of this condition is scant and the treatment is relatively ineffective.

One major difficulty is that it is hard to predict which patients are most likely to develop thrombosis. The cause as well as the incidence is unknown. The syndrome is associated with advanced cancer, however, and more often with solid tumors than hematologic ones. Mucin-secreting tumors of the pancreas, lung, and prostate are most commonly associated with thrombus formation.

Assessment

Typically, the thrombus develops in a large vein, often in the legs. Patients experience erythema and edema from blocked venous flow. In addition, severe pain associated with tissue death occurs. Once initial symptoms are observed, assessment of the originally affected limb as well as other body parts is prudent because the obstruction may gradually involve larger areas, expanding the affected region. For example, the edema of the lower leg may spread throughout the leg and lower abdomen. All body systems must be assessed for obstructive symptoms because of the propensity for embolus formation (Table 15G-1). A common cause of death is pulmonary embolism. Other similar complications are CNS infarcts, microangiopathic hemolytic anemia, and nonbacterial thrombotic endocarditis.

Medical management

Anticoagulants are given to control the syndrome (Table 15G-2). Withdrawal of the drugs frequently causes the return of symptoms, however. Successful treatment appears to be more directly related to control of the tumor than to anticoagulant therapy. Patients may require long-term SC heparin therapy while receiving antitumor treatments. Control of coagulation by drugs is delicate. Nurses should be alert for bleeding, which is indicative of excessive medication. Furthermore, the antidotes for both heparin and warfarin (Coumadin) should be available. Vitamin K (phytonadione) should be administered to counteract warfarin and protamine sulfate to counteract heparin.

Nursing management

All nursing care measures have the common goal of reducing the risk of embolization by maintaining a consistent venous pressure that is low (Table 15G-3). Low venous pressure encourages additional

TABLE 15G–1

Ongoing Assessments of Patients with Diffuse Venous Thrombosis

Body part	Nursing observations
Skin	Color changes, especially redness. Calf tenderness: Note any increase. Vascular filling: Check speed of return of normal color to nailbeds after compression. Vascular size/fullness: Look for localized abnormal areas of enlarged veins, e.g., over lower extremity.
Lungs	Breathing patterns: Note changes to more labored, shallow breathing and changes to more vertical posture, onset of coughing, symmetry of chest expansion, use of accessory muscles. Pain: Note sudden onset of shooting or stabbing pain and its location, especially if concurrent with temperature elevation. Quality of gaseous exchange in each lobe: Look for rales, wheezing, absence of breath sounds, etc.
Extremities	Measure girth at standardized point, noting gradual increase in size and differences between extremities. Pulses: Check for unequal, decreased, or absent pulses.
Neck	Check veins for distension.

TABLE 15G–2

Anticoagulant Therapy in Diffuse Venous Thrombosis

Drug	Administration/comments
Heparin	25–30 U/kg/hr Continuous IV infusion for 7–10 days Long-term SC administration often necessary
Warfarin (Coumadin)	5–10 mg/day PO Less effective than heparin

aggregation at a thrombus site. If there is a subsequent increase in pressure, the loosely attached elements can be swept away, becoming emboli.

TABLE 15G–3
Protocol for Nursing Management to Decrease Embolism Risk

Alteration in venous pressure	Bed rest initially; when ambulation allowed and sitting permitted, encourage frequent position change.
	Use elastic hose or extremity supports cautiously because excessive edema may cause device to actually constrict.
	No massages.
	Elevate affected extremities.
Alteration in fluid balance	Maintain accurate intake and output records.
	Encourage fluid intake to 2,000–3,000 ml/24 hr unless other physiologic conditions prevail, e.g., congestive heart failure.

Hydration poses a special challenge. Ideally, large-volume (2,000 to 3,000 ml/24 hr) intake is encouraged. The goal is to keep the blood diluted sufficiently so that the blood components are unlikely to contact each other or the existing thrombus, thus preventing expansion or creation of additional thrombi. Maintaining a consistent hydration level promotes a consistent venous pressure. These patients, however, who are often critically ill, may not be able to tolerate large fluid volumes because of other physiologic conditions, such as congestive heart failure. While maximum hydration may be impossible, nurses should be alert to prevent dehydration, which would promote contact among the blood's elements and alter venous pressure.

DIC

Pathophysiology
DIC is the common term used to describe an aberrant hemostatic mechanism. Other terms are acute intravascular coagulation and consumption-coagulopathy.

Unfortunately, the precise mechanism of alteration in hemostasis has eluded the understanding of researchers, so that no name provides an accurate description.

DIC may be either chronic or acute. In the chronic phase, DIC resembles the diffuse venous thrombosis described above. The chronic phase may culminate in the acute phase of active bleeding. It is believed that the chronic process eventually consumes all the clotting factors, making active bleeding inevitable. The precise mechanism of initiation of the problem is unknown.

Assessment

Although DIC in cancer patients is most often associated with acute promyelocytic leukemia and has an overall incidence of 10% in patients with cancer, any patient who develops unexplained or unexpected bleeding should be evaluated carefully (Table 15G–4). Nurses may detect subtle changes in patient status and thus greatly enhance early diagnosis and intervention. Particular attention should be given to cancer patients who experience other conditions associated with DIC development, specifically sepsis, volume deficits, and transfusion reactions.

While nurses may note early, subtle changes in patients, individuals often experience sudden dramatic changes that lead them to seek help. Patients may note decreasing ability to perform customary activities and petechiae (small changes) or may note frank bleeding (dramatic changes). The urinary and GI systems are frequent sites of acute blood loss.

Diagnosis is achieved through evaluation of laboratory values and clinical assessment. The most critical laboratory tests are prothrombin time, partial thromboplastin time, platelet count, thrombin time, and fibrinogen level. Consumption of platelets is reflected in markedly decreased platelet counts, <20,000 cells/mm³. As supplies of factor V and VII and prothrombin are exhausted, the prothrombin time and partial prothrombin times are prolonged. Fibrin-fibrinogen degradation products appear as fibrolysis proceeds. The Hct falls because of acute blood loss.

Medical management

As in diffuse venous thrombosis, treatment of DIC is aimed at the underlying tumor or other precipitating factor. Patients may receive coagulation factors through transfusion with cryoprecipitate and fresh-frozen plasma. RBC transfusions may be administered, as well as fluids to replace lost volume.

The use of heparin (300 to 600 U/kg/24 hr) is controversial, except in the case of leukemic patients. The theory is that heparin may interrupt the coagulation mechanism by its antithrombin effect. Heparin prevents the formation of prothrombin activator by factors V, activated X, Ca⁺⁺, and phospholipid via the intrinsic pathway when the concentration of these procoagulants is low. It may be used in situations where there is clinical evidence of severe bleeding while treatment of the precipitating cause or tumor is initiated. Heparin use is contraindicated in patients with open wounds, intracranial hemorrhage, or recent surgery. When heparin is administered, the patient's concurrent medications should be scrutinized for drug interactions

TABLE 15G–4

Ongoing Assessment of Blood Loss

Body site/system	Nursing observations
Renal system	Check urine for red color. Check for occult blood.
GI system	Check stool for occult blood (guaiac test). Observe for presence of bleeding hemorrhoids, which may respond to local measures. Check emesis for bright-red (fresh) blood or dark-brown (old) blood. Check emesis for consistency: stickiness and clots with red color or coffee-ground consistency with dark-brown color.
Skin/mucous membranes	Check blood loss around invasive devices: IV lines, venipuncture sites, surgical sites. Check blood loss on dressings. Measure loss by: removing dressing and weighing; marking saturated area of dressing and rechecking area hourly; removing dressing and estimating blood loss as extent of saturation, e.g., ½ saturation of a 4 × 4-in. gauze square. Check color (pale) and condition (oozing blood or irritation) of gingival tissue. Observe for ecchymosis. Observe for petechiae.
Cardiovascular	Observe for tachypnea. Observe for orthopnea. Observe for tachycardia. Observe for angina indicating deficit in myocardium.
Neurologic	Monitor mentation, especially for confusion or irritability. Observe for changes in consciousness: less conscious, more difficult to arouse, decreased awareness of light touch, changing responses to painful stimuli only. Check for headaches.
Eyes	Ask whether changes in vision, e.g., blurred, spots in visual field. Check for retinal hemorrhage by asking about pain in eyes, visual disturbances, and by use of ophthalmoscope to see vessels and bleeding.
Abdominal	Check for tenderness associated with palpation, indicating increasing fluid in abdomen or inadequate perfusion. Measure girth at consistent place, noting any gradual increase.

(e.g., digitalis, nicotine, tetracycline, and antihistamines deter heparin's effect, often requiring increased heparin doses). Insulin's effects may be promoted by heparin.

Nursing management

Nurses who care for patients with DIC must be aware of three major problems that patients experience: massive blood loss, altered fluid balance, and decreased oxygen-carrying capacity (Table 15G–5). The patient's inability to form a stable clot means that seemingly minor nursing acts can have major hemorrhagic consequences. Efforts to prevent blood loss should be initiated when DIC is suspected by such actions as using a small-gauge needle to obtain the blood samples. Awaiting confirmation of the diagnosis should not be allowed to delay precautionary measures.

Fluid volume may fluctuate between too much fluid or too little. Blood products as well as IV solution may be administered. Too much replacement volume can cause fluid overload, resulting in additional complications, such as congestive heart failure. With significant blood loss, however, hypovolemia can become a problem. Quantifying actual blood loss whenever possible and keeping accurate cumulative records of fluid intake that include all fluid types are important deterrents to the development of such problems.

Inadequate oxygenation may be manifested as tachycardia and dyspnea. These conditions represent the body's attempt to maximally oxygenate the blood volume remaining and move it throughout the system. RBC transfusions and supplemental oxygen are then indicated. Care-givers may help patients conserve energy expenditures and oxygen demands by doing whatever is necessary for them.

The great potential for alterations in hemostasis, whether bleeding or thrombus formation, requires nurses to monitor and report early subtle changes in patients. Moreover, patients and families need to recognize common symptoms for which they must seek professional help. In addition to the symptoms of bleeding caused by inadequate platelet production, a common side effect of many anticancer regimens, patients should be aware of the group of symptoms that indicate abnormal coagulation problems.

Bibliography

1. Brown, S. A. Venous thrombosis: another complication of cancer. *Oncology Nursing Forum* (Summer 1983). 41–47.

   Sophisticated presentation of complex material. Comprehensive description of nursing actions.

2. Bullock, B. L., and P. Rosendahl. Pathophysiology, Adaptations and Alterations in Function. Little, Brown & Co., Boston. 1984.

   Among the clearest pathophysiology texts available; content is well illustrated. Sections always include normal as well as altered functioning.

TABLE 15G–5

Nursing Protocol for the Management of DIC

Problem	Intervention
Potential for massive hemorrhage	Avoid medications that affect coagulation, e.g., aspirin-containing products.
	Avoid medications that interact with heparin (when it is used).
	Minimize trauma to patient: have patient wear slippers; pad side rails for restless, bedridden patient.
	Use smallest-gauge needles for fewest possible punctures of skin.
	Decrease trauma to gums by limiting toothbrushing to once a day.
	Apply direct pressure to any puncture site.
	Suction carefully.
	Minimize use of BP cuffs: do not inflate much above previous reading or release pressure quickly.
	Use existing infusion lines whenever safe.
	Avoid use of straight razors, IM and SC injection.
	Monitor for blood loss (*see* Table 15G–4).
	Count and weigh dressings saturated with blood. Calculate blood loss through suction devices.
Altered fluid balance	Use flow-control devices whenever possible, especially for heparin.
	Include volume of blood products in intake calculations.
Decreased oxygen-carrying capacity	Minimize requests for patients to move, do self-care, etc.
	Provide supplemental oxygen, when prescribed.
	Provide slow pace and rest periods for any patient activity.
Patient need for information	Provide patient and family with information on symptoms related to alterations in hemostasis caused by either excessive clotting or bleeding: swelling of arms, legs, abdomen or neck; change in the color of the skin anywhere; pain in swollen areas; change in the ability to perform customary activities, e.g., excessive fatigue or trouble breathing; frank bleeding from any injection site, nose, mouth, rectum, or urinary tract; development of petechiae.

3. Caplin, M. Disseminated intravascular coagulation: a multisystem problem. *Dimensions of Critical Care Nursing* (March-April 1984). 76–83.

   Thorough analysis of nursing interventions and their rationale. Presentation is systematic and detailed.

4. Franco, L. M. Acute disseminated intravascular coagulation. *Cardiovascular Nursing* (September-October 1979). 22–27.

   Emphasis is on a complex discussion of physiologic clotting mechanisms and their alterations in DIC. Only general nursing care information is provided.

5. Jennings, B. M. Improving your management of DIC. *Nursing 79* (May 1979). 60–67.

   Well-organized, thorough, and practical explanation of DIC using case examples well. Illustrations and descriptions of physiologic events are clear and concise, with emphasis on nursing care through all phases of the disease.

6. Kirchner, C. W., and C. E. Reheis. Two serious complications of neoplasia: sepsis and disseminated intravascular coagulation. *Nursing Clinics of North America* (December 1982). 595–606.

   Excellent review of these two conditions with good nursing care guidelines.

7. Minna, J. D., and P. A. Bunn. Paraneoplastic syndromes. *In* DeVita, V. T., S. Hellman, and S. A. Rosenberg, editors. Cancer: Principles and Practice of Oncology. J. B. Lippincott Co., Philadelphia. 1982.

   Comprehensive, sophisticated description of DIC medical management contained within this chapter focusing on several conditions. Controversies in management are clearly stated and suggestions for resolving issues outlined.

8. Portlock, C. S. Disseminated intravascular coagulation. *In* Portlock, C. S., and D. R. Goffinet, editors. Manual of Clinical Problems in Oncology. Little, Brown & Co., Boston. 1981.

   Concise description of medical phenomenona with good, annotated bibliography.

CHAPTER 16

INFILTRATIVE EMERGENCIES
Karen K. Kane

A: CAROTID ARTERY EROSION

Carotid artery erosion can be a devastating crisis for everyone involved in the care of the person with head/neck cancer. To recognize the cancer patients at risk, the nurse must be aware of the factors that influence tumor- and arterial-wall breakdown and wound healing. Identifying the patient at risk will allow the nurse to anticipate specific care needs.

Pathophysiology
There are three distinct layers to the artery: adventitial, medial, and intimal(Fig. 16A–1). The outermost(adventitial) layer is composed of connective tissue and carries 80% of the blood supply to the remaining walls of the artery. Although quite resistant to tumor invasion, this layer is most susceptible to drying and infection, and when it is exposed to the atmosphere, its tenous blood supply to the other layers is destroyed; soon the cellular elements disappear as well. Poor wound healing, exposure of the artery during surgery, tumor growth and invasion, previous treatment with radiation and/or chemotherapy, and infection are all mechanisms that can contribute to arterial erosion.

Once the artery is exposed to the atmosphere, destruction of its wall usually takes 6 to 10 days. It begins with the loss of the aventitial layer and the formation of an eschar. An eschar develops when a wound cannot be closed by epithelization. Instead, the open area becomes covered with dried plasma proteins and dead cells. The eschar eventually separates from the wound by a process known as sloughing. When this occurs, the underlying medial layer composed of circular smooth-muscle cells is exposed and undergoes the same process. The remaining fragile intimal layer, consisting of simple squamous epithe-

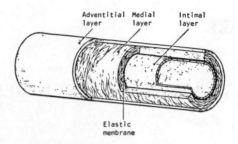

Figure 16A–1.   Cross-sectional view of an artery.

lial lining and loose connective tissue, is then the only tissue remaining between the bloodstream and the potential wound breakdown. This layer may become thinner or reach an aneurysmal state as a result of the exposure and drying process.

Wound healing is affected by many factors. Deficits in circulation, oxygen, and nutrients, as well as effects from certain therapeutic modalities will have adverse effects. Wound healing consists of a series of overlapping events. Initially, acute inflammation results in the elimination of clots, necrotic tissue, and bacterial contaminants from the wound. This cleaning within the wound is achieved through the release of vasoactive substances, such as histamine and serotonin, and through phagocytosis by leukocytes and macrophages. The release of vasoactive materials causes an increased perfusion of arterioles, capillaries, and venules. The phagocytosis results in the engulfment and destruction of microorganisms. This inflammatory process is essential in setting the stage for healing. The repair phase will begin as the inflammatory process abates. For healing to occur, a new vascular supply must be established to supply oxygen and nutrients to the injured tissue. This process of neovascularization occurs once the acute inflammatory reaction subsides. Fibroblast proliferation follows and functions primarily to synthesize collagen and other substances necessary to support the new vascular structure. Wound contraction decreases the surface area of the wound. Contractile myofibroblasts are responsible for the mobilization of adjacent wound edges. Concurrent epithelization functions to cover the wound with epithelium, preventing contamination and moisture loss.

A number of pathologic states and therapeutic modalities affect wound healing. Previous irradiation has been identified as the most common factor leading to carotid artery rupture because of the permanent changes that occur in all layers of the carotid arterial wall.

Therefore, it is important to know if the artery lies within the field of radiation treatment. Treatment with radiation affects the healing of tissue in neck wounds resulting from surgical procedures, from tumor growth that invades and causes breakdown, or from tumors that become necrotic themselves. The major effects of radiation on healing tissue are: impaired neovascularization; destruction of vascular supply because of inflammation of the intimal layer (endarteritis); impaired production of fibroblasts and myofibrils, resulting in impaired collagen synthesis and wound contraction; and impaired epithelization. Chemotherapeutic agents impair fibroblast replication, protein synthesis, and the necessary inflammatory response. Patients who are receiving anti-inflammatory steroids also have difficulty healing wounds because of impaired neovascularization, inflammation, contraction, and epithelization.

Slowly healing wounds are predisposed to infection, and wound infection further impedes healing. Infection can impede necessary collagen accumulation in the wound, disturb collagen deposition, and decrease the rate of epithelization. Depending on the physiologic state of both the patient and the wound, healing may not occur, and infection may cause continued deterioration of the wound. Further deterioration may result in invasion of the carotid arterial wall and exposure of the adventitial layer to the atmosphere, initiating the drying process and compromising the vessel wall's blood supply. The patient is then at risk for carotid erosion. A similar process occurs as tumor size increases and invades the arterial layers.

Assessment

Ongoing assessment of the neck wound, with documentation of any change, is necessary to detect evidence of progressive arterial erosion (Table 16A–1). A change in color from red to pale or black, a change of skin temperature from bilateral warmth to unilateral coolness, or the presence or increase of edema signifies impaired circulation. Progressive compromised blood supply to the vessel and surrounding area will result in continued deterioration. Normally, wounds will change in shape in response to skin tensions at the wound site. A change in turgor, as indicated by an increase in size and a change in the shape of the wound, will occur as tension at the site relaxes, resulting in wound deterioration. Changes in the type, amount, or odor of any drainage present will aid in the recognition of infection. Redness and tenderness may accompany infection. Obviously, evidence of bleeding, pulsations, or arterial exposure are important observations.

Only two warnings of carotid artery rupture are noted in the literature. Some patients will complain of sternal or high epigastric

TABLE 16A–1

Assessment of Wound and Surrounding Skin

Factor	Assessment
Color	Redness, pallor, black.
Temperature	Warm, cool, unilateral temperature changes.
Edema	Presence, absence, or changes.
Lesion	Location, size, shape, type.
Thickness	Inspect for level of repair or tumor invasion.
Turgor	Taut, mobile.
Moisture	Dry, sweating, drainage description.
Odor	Odorless, malodorous.
Tenderness	Presence, absence, or changes.
Vascularity	Evidence of bleeding and/or bruising, pulsations, arterial exposure.

Adapted from Bates, B. A Guide to Physical Assessment. J. B. Lippincott Co., Philadelphia. 1974. p. 10.

pain several hours before rupture. A small prodromal bleeding may be noted at the wound site 24 to 48 hr before a rupture. Because forewarnings are either lacking or inconsistent, ongoing assessment of the wound/tumor is the most accurate predictor of arterial erosion. Once the artery is exposed or invaded by tumor, the patient and family should be made aware of this change. An unexpected hemorrhage can be a horrifying event. Informing the patient and family that it might occur and what will be done to prevent and manage it might minimize anxiety. The staff should also be alerted.

Nursing management

Prevention.   It is an important role of the multidisciplinary team to facilitate the decision-making process by the patient and family in relation to the options of aggressive or supportive care measures. The nurse, as a member of that team, must know the patient's and family's understanding of the prognosis and their desires for treatment. The nursing care goals will differ, depending on the expectations for care.

A plan of preventive action should be developed once the patient is identified to be at risk (Table 16A–2). Preventive wound care requires strict aseptic technique. The dressing should support the wound,

TABLE 16A-2

Nursing Protocol for the Preventive Management of Carotid Artery Rupture

Factor	Intervention
Wound/incision care	Schedule dressing changes (based on amount of drainage and need for continuous nursing assessment of the area).
	Sample nursing orders: Change dressing q 8 hr (11 AM–7 PM–3 AM) or more frequently if excess drainage soils dressing. Initially document color, shape, mobility, skin temperature, presence or absence of edema, and odor of wound. Document changes as they occur.
Prevention of debridement	Remove dressing cautiously using normal saline applications to loosen dressing if necessary. Use a nonadherent dressing material (fine-mesh gauze).
Prevention of infection	Culture suspicious areas for infections and take appropriate isolation measures. Use nonocclusive dressing.
Wound stressors	
Respiratory efforts	Explore ways to minimize strenuous respiratory effects: reposition the patient; teach and encourage deep, sustained inhalations; consult the physician concerning the need for oxygen therapy or respiratory therapy treatments.
Coughing	Determine the etiology of the coughing. If pulmonary secretions are present, suction can be used. A cough suppressant may be indicated.
Vomiting	Assess the etiology of the vomiting. Administration of an antiemetic or nasogastric intubation may be necessary.
Constipation	Determine factors that cause constipation. Plan should be designed reflecting patient's ability/desire to eat and drink fluids, level of activity, and use of medications.
Emotional factors	Explore potential sources of emotional stress. Promote an atmosphere conducive to the expression of feelings, fears, and questions.

protect it from trauma and contamination, absorb drainage, and/or provide an aesthetic cover for what may be a necrotic, malodorous, and fungating neck mass. Wound healing may or may not be a realistic goal for this patient. The goal of wound care is to prevent drying and infection.

The optimal dressing material is fine-mesh gauze because it inhibits interweaving of granulation tissue into the dressing material. A nonadherent dressing soaked in normal saline or gauze impregnated with petroleum jelly may be used to ensure constant moisture, prevent debridement, and absorb wound drainage. A nonocclusive dressing will prevent growth of fungi, particularly yeast, which thrive in dark, moist, warm environments. Using porous tape to secure the dressing will allow circulation of air in the area. If tape cannot be used, an isolation mask tied around the neck may provide a snug bandage. Dressings should be changed frequently to reduce bacterial growth. If excessive drainage necessitates frequent dressing changes, remove only the external dressing and reinforce the inner layer of gauze. The dressing should be removed cautiously. Normal saline may be applied to loosen it without causing debridement, which could result in the unnecessary exposure of the underlying tissue layers to the atmosphere.

If normal wound healing does not occur, the risk for infection is great, because the normal skin barrier to bacterial invasion has been lost. All identifiable zones of necrosis, inflammation, and infection should be cultured. Depending on the microorganism, necessary wound and skin isolation precautions should be taken. Isolation procedures may differ slightly in each setting, but generally they include: disposal of contaminated linen and dressing materials in specified receptacles, always washing hands before entering and after leaving the patient's room, wearing gloves and gown when coming into contact with infected areas, and possibly wearing masks during dressing change procedures.

Any factor that increases physical stress on the wound may interfere with wound healing of the head and neck area. Strenuous respiratory efforts, coughing, vomiting, straining at defecation, and transient increases in BP are common stressors for the hospitalized cancer patient.

BP varies with emotional and physical activity because of changes in the blood-vessel diameter in response to the percentage of oxygen, carbon dioxide, electrolytes, hormones, and enzymes in the blood. Hemorrhage is an ever-present danger with an excessive BP. When the vessel is thinned and weakened, the BP may not need to be excessive to cause rupture.

Strenuous respiratory efforts call upon muscles not ordinarily used. Included in this group of accessory muscles are the sternomastoid and trapezius of the neck. The proximity of these contracting muscles to the wound and to the carotid arteries renders them a source of stress. Depending on the underlying disease and patient's condition, positioning the patient in a Fowler's or semi-Fowler's position, encouraging deep, sustained inhalations, and the administration of oxygen may be helpful to minimize strenuous efforts.

Vigorous **coughing** increases intrathoracic pressure, which may create cardiovascular and wound complications for the patient with a head/neck tumor. To reduce the excess pressure generated by coughing, nasotracheal, tracheal, or oropharyngeal suction may be the chosen treatment to remove pulmonary secretions. The stress that may be produced by intermittent suction may be lower and the treatment more satisfying than a continuous unproductive cough. Suctioning should be done with caution to prevent trauma and only after the presence of secretions has been documented.

The contraction of the diaphragm and abdominal muscles that accompanies **vomiting** raises intra-abdominal pressure, which in turn increases intrathoracic pressure, further stressing the wound site. Appropriate managment to prevent vomiting depends upon accurate determination of the etiology. Whether the treatment is the administration of an antiemetic or nasogastric intubation, there should be minimal delay. Prompt treatment is required to avoid contamination of the neck wound with gastric contents.

Many features of the hospitalized patient's condition predispose him to **constipation** (*see* Chapter 11). Patients with constipation strain excessively when trying to expel feces. The Valsalva maneuver, achieved by forced expiration against a closed glottis, causes maximum intrathoracic pressure. Management of this problem involves the patient's ability to eat, his level of activity, and the use of drugs. A fiber diet and/or appropriate fluid intake can assist in preventing this complication.

Emotional stress is also an important factor. The hospital setting itself, the location of the patient's room, visiting hour restrictions, fear of death, and fear of isolation are but a few of the identified emotional concerns common to patients. The nurse's recognition of emotional stress and its concurrent physical responses is an obvious and important aspect in the care of these patients.

Aggressive management. In many situations artery rupture and carotid hemorrhage may be treated successfully by ligation of the eroded arterial ends. This surgical procedure is not without associated morbidity and morality. The greatest morbidity is related to neurologic deficits, such as paresis or hemiplegia resulting from cerebral hypoxemia.

The goals of nursing intervention are: (1) to maintain an airway and prevent aspiration; (2) to minimize blood loss; and (3) to provide physical and emotional comfort to patient and family.

Anticipation of this emergency will allow for the maintenance of peripheral venous access with a large-bore needle. A central venous access might be preferred. Precautions should be taken to avoid delay in blood-product replacement. If an arterial rupture occurs, the normal blood volume must be restored before surgical ligation is attempted. Updated typing and cross matching and the availability of several units of blood products are important. Supplies at the bedside should include: vascular clamp, suction and resuscitation equipment, supplies needed for oxygen therapy, gloves, and absorptive dressing materials.

Placement of the patient at risk near the nurses' station ensures close observation. If a tracheostomy tube is in place, the cuff should remain inflated to prevent aspiration of blood from the wound. Cuff pressures should be monitored $\geq$ q 8 hr. This is also true if the patient has a stoma from a laryngectomy procedure. A cuffed laryngectomy or tracheostomy tube should be inserted and remain inflated.

When sudden hemorrhage occurs (Table 16A–3) the patient is placed in a head-down position. Pressure is applied to the bleeding area. This positioning should not increase blood loss if pressure is applied properly. If blood descends the oropharynx and no tracheostomy tube is in place, an oral airway should be inserted. Suctioning around the airway may help remove blood and secretions from the oro- and hypopharynx. Oxygen may be needed.

To prevent cardiovascular collapse, IV fluids should be continued, and blood product transfusions initiated. Vital signs should be monitored frequently to assess further changes in patient status. Providing support to the patient and family will be important during this crisis situation. Talking to the patient and family to reassure them and explain the procedure being done may help lessen anxiety.

Supportive management.   When aggressive treatment has failed, or is not possible or appropriate, easing suffering becomes the primary focus of patient care (Table 16A–4). The goals of nursing intervention are: (1) to maintain an airway and prevent aspiration; (2) to relieve discomfort and distress; and (3) to provide psychologic support to patient and family.

Supplies that will be needed for supportive care during a carotid rupture should be placed at the bedside prior to the occurrence. These include suction equipment, gloves, absorptive dressing materials, and a parenteral medication with an antianxiety/analgesic properties.

TABLE 16A–3

Nursing Protocol for the Aggressive Management of Carotid Artery Rupture

Factor	Intervention
Airway maintenance	Inflate cuff of tracheostomy or laryngectomy tube to prevent aspiration of blood.
	Insert oral airway if patient does not have a tracheostomy.
	Suction aspirated blood.
	Administer oxygen.
Minimizing blood loss	Position patient in Trendelenburg's position to minimize cerebral hypoxemia.
	Determine site of bleeding.
	Apply digital pressure with gauze or dressing material to the bleeding site.
	Notify other care-givers of the emergency situation.
Stabilization of cardiovascular status	Maintain rapid infusion of IV fluids.
	Initiate blood-product transfusion.
	Monitor vital signs.
Comfort	Reassure patient and family that everything is being done.
	Act in a calm, organized manner.
	Administer analgesics as prescribed.

TABLE 16A–4

*Nursing Protocol for the Supportive Management of
Carotid Artery Rupture*

Factor	Intervention
Airway maintenance	Tracheostomy tube cuff or laryngectomy tube cuff should be inflated.
	Position patient supine with head turned toward the affected side or laterally to facilitate drainage.
	Absorb bloody discharge with dressing materials.
	Suction to remove blood from oral cavity or tracheostomy/laryngectomy.
Comfort	Administer appropriate drugs to relieve anxiety and alter sensitivity to pain.
	Provide emotional support to patient and family. Allow family members the opportunity to leave the bedside.
	Do not leave the patient alone.

Maintenance of an airway may not be possible. If hemorrhage occurs externally, the patient can be positioned supine with the head turned to the affected side or laterally to facilitate drainage and prevent aspiration. Absorptive dressing materials may be used to suppress a pulsive discharge from the site, even though control of bleeding may not be achieved. If hemorrhage occurs internally, nothing can be done to prevent aspiration. Suction may be used in an attempt to remove blood that ascends into the oral cavity or through a tracheostomy to ease the patient's discomfort.

The nurse at the bedside remains aware of the family presence and their needs. Allowing the family members the opportunity to leave the bedside may lessen the shock of this sudden death. Treating the patient with gentle respect will have a calming effect on both the patient and family during the crisis of carotid artery rupture.

An important nursing role at this time is to give appropriate drugs to alleviate the patient's anxiety and alter the sensitivity to pain. Drugs that are effective against pain and anxiety must be parenteral, rapid acting, and available at the bedside for prompt administration. Morphine sulfate is often the drug of choice.

Many times the patient dies in the absence of family. The patient, realizing that death is near, may be apprehensive and should not be left alone. Reassuring the patient that he is not alone and explaining procedures may provide comfort.

Bibliography

1. Bruno, P. Nature of wound healing. *Nursing Clinics of North America* (December 1979). 667–682.

   The healing process is clearly defined. Indicators of normal healing and negative influences on wound repair are discussed.

2. Copper, D. M., and D. Schumann. Postsurgical nursing interventions as an adjunct to wound healing. *Nursing Clinics of North America* (December 1979). 713–726.

   The importance of nursing care on postoperative wound healing is presented, with emphasis on identification and management of wound stressors.

3. Kane, K. K. Carotid artery rupture in advanced head and neck cancer patients. *Oncology Nursing Forum* (Winter 1983). 14–18.

   Nursing interventions for the advanced head/neck cancer patient at risk for carotid erosion are derived from pathophysiology.

4. Keith, C. F. Wound management following head and neck surgery. *Nursing Clinics of North America* (December 1979). 761–778.

   A variety of concerns unique to the surgical head/neck cancer patient are presented, and nursing implications are highlighted.

B: LEUKOSTASIS

Leukostasis is intravascular or perivascular sludging that can occur in patients with acute or chronic leukemia when the leukocyte count is ≥100,000 cells/mm^3 and a high percentage of the cells are myeloblasts or lymphoblasts. The result is capillary obstruction, microinfarctions, and organ dysfunction. While any organ may be affected, symptoms are most life-threatening when the lungs or brain are involved. Emergency treatment is necessary to prevent fatal respiratory distress or pulmonary or intracranial hemorrhages. Nursing responsibilities include collaborating with physicians to recognize patients at risk for leukostasis, observation for early signs and symptoms of organ dysfunction, and monitoring the prescribed medical treatment.

Pathophysiology

The exact mechanism underlying the development of leukostasis is not clearly understood. It is known that myeloblast and lymphoblast cells, immature forms of granulocytes and lymphocytes, are larger, more rigid, and more internally viscous than normal mature leukocytes (Fig. 16B–1). These cells can cause an increase in blood viscosity, stagnation of blood flow, and mechanical obstruction of small

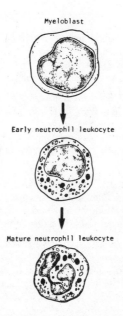

Figure 16B-1.   Three stages in the development of a myelogenous leukocyte.

capillaries when they are present in abnormally large numbers. The obstruction is caused as the cells adhere to the blood vessel endothelium and to each other. Release of toxic substances from these cells damages the vascular endothelium and further enhances cell stasis and aggregation.

The vascular endothelium is further compromised by hypoxemia secondary to several factors: (1) anemia; (2) impaired pulmonary gas exchange; (3) high oxygen consumption by myeloblast and lymphoblast cells; and (4) local vascular obstruction. The vessel wall is eventually weakened to the point of rupture, and bleeding occurs.

Circulatory compromise caused by leukostasis in the CNS results in increased intracranial pressure (*see* Chapter 14A). Pulmonary leukostasis causes fluid to fill the alveolar and/or pleural spaces, impeding oxygenation and ventilation (*see* Chapter 13).

Assessment

Persons with leukemia who are at risk for leukostasis are identified by laboratory examination of peripheral blood. A leukocyte count

$\geq$100,000 cells/mm³ with a high percentage of immature cells has been implicated as the factor responsible for the development of leukostasis.

Once these patients have been identified, the primary role of nursing is to observe for signs and symptoms of organ compromise. Patients who present with a high leukocyte count and percentage of immature cells remain at risk for hemorrhage or vessel occlusion during the early induction treatment period in spite of a lowered leukocyte count. This circumstance may be caused by preexisting endothelial damage or rapid cell lysis. Initial neurological and pulmonary assessments will establish a base line. Frequent follow-up assessment is indicated until it is determined that therapy has significantly reduced the risk of hemorrhage and/or vessel occlusion.

The neurological assessment for early signs of increased intracranial pressure is described in Chapter 14A. Abrupt onset of neurological dysfunction, e.g., decreased level of consciousness or pupil changes, may indicate intracranial hemorrhage.

Fever, dyspnea, and tachypnea accompany pulmonary leukostasis. Patients typically encounter problems with airflow obstruction, secretion clearance, hypoxemia, and hypoventilation. Pleural effusions result when leukostasis occurs in the pleural space. Chapter 13 provides a discussion of these problems in depth.

Medical management

Emergency treatment of a patient with a high and premature leukocyte count is necessary to prevent serious organ dysfunction and/or hemorrhage. Cytotoxic therapy is initiated immediately to lower the circulating myeloblast/lymphoblast count.

Hydroxyurea (Hydrea) inhibits DNA synthesis and causes a rapid fall in the leukocyte count within 24 to 48 hr. The drug is administered PO, often in one of two schedules: (1) 3 g/m² daily for 2 days, or (2) 50 to 100 mg/m² daily until the leukocyte count is <100,000 cells/mm³. IV single-dose cyclophosphamide (Cytoxan) is sometimes used in place of hydroxyurea (Hydrea) to rapidly lower the leukocyte count. This alkylating agent primarily causes a defect in DNA replication. A recommended dose range is 20 to 30 mg/kg. In patients with acute nonlymphocytic leukemia, the leukocyte count is often rapidly reduced using a combination of the anthracycline antibiotic daunorubicin (Daunomycin) and the antimetabolite cytarabine (ARA-C). Both of these drugs work by interfering with DNA and RNA synthesis.

Additional therapies can help to reduce the leukocyte count and the risk for fatal intracerebral and pulmonary hemorrhages and respiratory distress. The delivery of single dose (600 R) cranial irradiation will destroy intracerebral leukostatic aggregations. Leukapheresis and exchange transfusions are temporary measures that rapidly remove excess circulating leukocytes, but they have no effect on established foci of leukostasis.

Cytotoxic therapy or a combination of therapies will always result in cellular destruction. Uric acid is a normal end product of this breakdown. Normally, uric acid is excreted by the kidneys at a rate of 300 to 500 mg/day. In patients with leukemia, the serum concentration is abnormally high. If this condition is not treated, the renal clearance and urine concentration may increase to the point at which the urate precipitates in the renal tubules, causing renal failure. The antigout xanthine oxidase inhibitor, allopurinol (Zyloprim) is given to reduce serum uric acid concentrations. Allopurinol works by inhibiting the enzyme xanthine oxidase, which is needed to convert xanthine and hypoxanthine to uric acid. Absorption of allopurinol is excellent by the PO route. The usual adult dose is 300 mg daily, yet ≥800 mg/day may be prescribed for a patient at great risk of uric-acid nephropathy.

Nursing management

The major life-threatening complications of leukostasis are respiratory distress and pulmonary and intracranial hemorrhage. The goals of nursing intervention are: (1) to ease respiratory distress; (2) to minimize increases in intracranial pressure; and (3) to support patient and family during a life-threatening medical crisis (Table 16B-1).

Pulmonary complications are usually attributed to leukostasis only after other causes of respiratory distress are ruled out. When a hemorrhage does occur, the patient will experience increasing respiratory difficulty.

Dyspneic patients will naturally assume the posture that allows them to breathe with minimal difficulty and discomfort and with maximum efficiency. Upright or sitting positions are usually preferred. These positions help to prevent the abdominal organs from pressing upward on the diaphragm and lungs, and they allow for easier expansion of the lungs. If bleeding is occurring, turning the patient onto the affected side may help to prevent the blood from entering the unaffected lung. If a pleural effusion is causing distress, having the patient lie on the affected side will help aerate the unaffected lung.

To ensure optimal airflow, the airway must be kept clear of obstructing secretions and body fluids. Hemoptysis is a sign that hemorrhage may be occurring. The blood is coughed up and usually preceded by a tickling sensation in the throat. Ordinarily the blood is frothy and bright red in color.

Immediate medical treatment of hemorrhage may be to aspirate the blood from the pleural cavity by thoracentesis. If bleeding continues, a chest-tube drainage system may be instituted. Depending on the amount of blood lost and the patient's CBC, transfusions of red blood cells, fresh frozen plasma, and/or platelets may be indicated. Intubation and mechanical ventilation may be required, depending upon the goals of medical therapy and the desires of the patient and family.

Symptoms of an intracranial hemorrhage may be insidious in onset. Depending on the location of hemorrhage in the brain, the patient may experience alterations in the level of consciousness, visual disturbances, or loss in motor function (*see* Table 14A–1). Early signs and symptoms are general and vague. These include restlessness, irritability, confusion, headache, and nausea.

Modification of certain nursing care routines can provide comfort and lessen increases in an already increased intracranial pressure resulting from an obstruction or hemorrhage (*see* Table 14A–2).

Patients who are experiencing severe respiratory distress may appear apprehensive and withdrawn. Most of the patient's energy is directed toward trying to breathe. Alterations in the level of consciousness as a result of hypoxemia or intracranial hemorrhage can be frightening and frustrating for the patient and family. An important role of the nurse will be to help the patient and family identify and address these concerns.

Individuals who experience leukostasis are persons who have leukemia. In order to anticipate how the patient and family might respond to this crisis, it is imperative to know how long it has been since diagnosis, how the patient and family reacted to the diagnosis initially, and what they are feeling at the present time. At the time of crisis, the patient and family may be facing the need to define their hopes in relation to treatment response, quality of life, and survival. The nurse can be an invaluable resource at this time. The availability of empathic care-givers to reinforce information given by physicians, to explain nursing routines and procedures, and to offer the comfort of presence at the bedside will help to lessen the intensity of stress in this crisis situation.

Bibliography

1. Bloom, R., A. Taveira Da Silva, and A. Bracey. Reversible respiratory failure due to intravascular leukostasis in chronic myelogenous leukemia. Relationship of oxygen transfer to leukocyte count. *The American Journal of Medicine* (October 1979). 679–683.

TABLE 16B-1

Nursing Protocol for the Management of Leukostasis

Factor	Intervention
Pulmonary function	Monitor vital signs q 2–4 hr. Assess pulmonary status q 2–4 hr. Monitor blood gases. Monitor the administration of oxygen. Monitor intake and output.
Dyspnea	Provide extra pillows and elevate head of bed. Assist positioning of the patient to promote ease of respiration and gas exchange.
Cough	Assess tracheobronchial secretions. Encourage coughing, deep-breathing exercises, and maintenance of mobility. Offer respiratory treatments and medications as needed. Culture sputum if indicated. Intermittently suction for brief periods (<15 sec) after preoxygenating.
Hemoptysis	Assess amount and character of hemoptysis. Help patient to turn onto affected side of suspected pulmonary hemorrhage. Prevent aspiration. Administer blood products. Assist with thoracentesis or chest-tube insertion.
Neurological status Increased intracranial pressure*	Assess neurological status q 2–4 hr (*see* Table 14A-2).

Emotional factors Anxiety	Explain to patient and family the need for frequent nursing assessments. Explore with patient and family potential causes of anxiety (respiratory distress, pain, fear of sudden death). Administer appropriate drugs to relieve anxiety. In collaboration with the physician, support a realistic assessment.
Communication	Tell the family that persons experiencing respiratory distress tend to be silent, because talking requires a tremendous effort. Explore alternate means of communication and providing comfort (family should do most of the talking when at the bedside, not overstimulating the patient and allowing for periods of rest; sitting quietly at the bedside providing the comfort of presence, listening to music together).
Treatment complications Metabolic alterations (hyperuricemia, hyperkalemia, hypoglycemia, hyper-/ hypophosphatemia, hypocalcemia)	Know recent blood/plasma electrolyte and chemistry results. Administer medication to correct abnormality. Assess for side effects of imbalance.

*See also Table 14A–2 for specific guidelines for the care of the patient experiencing increased intracranial pressure.

Case presentation of a 49-year-old man, diagnosed with chronic myelogenous leukemia in blast crisis with leukocytosis, who experienced severe hypoxic respiratory failure. Correction of hypoxemia occurred after WBC reduction with hydroxyurea therapy.

2. Hug, V., M. Keating, K. McCredie, J. Hester, G. P. Bodey, and E. J. Freireich. Clinical course and response to treatment of patients with acute myelogenous leukemia presenting with a high leukocyte count. *Cancer* (September 1, 1983). 773–797.

The natural history of acute myelogenous leukemia and treatment response of patients with pretreatment leukocyte counts >100,000 cells/mm^3 was reviewed to identify clinical features and response characteristics.

3. Lichtman, M. A. Rheology of leukocytes, leukocyte suspensions, and blood in leukemia. Possible relationships to clinical manifestations. *Journal of Clinical Investigation* (February 1973). 350–358.

The effect of leukemic cells on blood flow and oxygenation by virtue of their structure is explored in detail.

4. Myers, T. J., S. R. Cole, A. U. Klatsky, and D. H. Hild. Respiratory failure due to pulmonary leukostasis following chemotherapy of acute nonlymphocytic leukemia. *Cancer* (May 15, 1983). 1808–1813.

Four patients with acute nonlymphocytic leukemia and at risk to develop pulmonary leukostasis, with leukocyte counts >200,000/mm^3, experienced respiratory distress within 10 to 48 hr after initiation of chemotherapy. The pathophysiologic basis of pulmonary leukostasis and potential treatment modalities are discussed.

5. Vernant, J. P., B. Brun, P. Mannoni, and B. Dreyfus. Respiratory distress of hyperleukocytic granulocytic leukemias. *Cancer* (July 1979). 264–268.

A description of the sudden appearance of acute respiratory distress in 25 patients with hyperleukocytic leukemias with rapid blood leukocyte doubling rates. The symptoms seemed related to leukostasis by mechanical obstruction of the pulmonary capillaries and responsible for a septal and alveolar edema.

CHAPTER 17

PARENTERAL CHEMOTHERAPY

Jean F. Jenkins

Chemotherapy is one of the major methods of treating cancer. There are many classes of chemotherapeutic agents that have proven effective in causing toxicity to cancer cells. Unfortunately, they are also toxic to normal cells, producing potentially serious problems, such as local tissue necrosis caused by extravasation of drug from the vein. Venous access lines, such as Hickman or central catheters, may be used to administer drugs and thereby decrease the risk of local irritation to veins. The toxicities associated with systemic therapy have led scientists and physicians to develop better ways to administer drugs. The desirability of delivering large concentrations of drug directly to the site of disease while sparing normal tissue is the rationale behind several of the access devices discussed in this chapter. Nurses need information about how to assess, prevent, and manage problems that may be encountered in care of patients receiving parenteral chemotherapy. The following guidelines address these issues for a variety of access routes in delivery of parenteral chemotherapy.

IRRITANT AND VESICANT DRUGS

Despite precautions taken by physicians, nurses, and other health professionals, there is always potential for local tissue reaction to antineoplastic drugs. This may be as a result of the properties of the drug, volume of diluent, site of drug injection, or technique of administration. Agents that have commonly produced local necrosis or irritation are dactinomycin, aclacinomycin, adriamycin, daunomycin, DTIC, mithramycin, mitomycin-C, nitrogen mustard, streptozotocin, vinblastine, vincristine, and vindesine.

Vesicants can cause tissue inflammation and pain when extravasated. Skin discoloration and loss of venous patency may follow erythema. Drugs that are true vesicants (e.g., doxorubicin [adriamycin], nitrogen mustard) can cause ulcers that require surgery, debridement, or skin grafting to repair extensive tissue damage. Irreversible changes in tendons and underlying tissue can result in loss of limb function. Other drugs labeled as vesicants may cause severe irritation but not result in blisters, ulceration, or skin burns (e.g., BCNU, etoposide, DTIC).

Management

Nursing management consists of preventive and supportive measures.

Prevention.   Awareness of which drugs are potential problem agents can allow the nurse to better prepare and evaluate the patient. Patient education regarding side effects of the chemotherapy should include information on signs and symptoms to be reported during drug administration. Complaints of pain, burning, swelling, or redness at the injection site might be a signal of extravasation. Hypersensitivity to the drug is often hard to distinguish from actual tissue seepage. Suggestions for monitoring chemotherapy instillation are given below.

Chemotherapy procedure: Take time to evaluate both arms for best vein selection. Proceed from the hand to the forearm. Avoid the side of a mastectomy. Lower extremities should not be used because they are more susceptible to emboli formation. Do not use the antecubital fossa, sites distal to recent venipuncture, or bruised, sore areas. Impaired venous circulation would also be a reason to avoid a site. Use heat to distend veins to aid in finding a site.

Procedure 1. Wash hands.

2. Apply the tourniquet after positioning the arm comfortably.

3. Cleanse the site with alcohol or povidone-iodine (Betadine) swab.

4. Insert the needle, observe for blood backflow, remove the tourniquet, and tape to allow observation of exit site as well as to stabilize the needle.

5. During administration of the drug, observe for signs of infiltration such as redness or swelling at injection site, decrease in IV flow rate, inability to obtain a blood return, or pain experienced by the patient.

6. Irrigate the line with solution of normal saline or sterile water between drugs and posttreatment.

Itching, inflammation, and rash may appear at the point of drug entry but usually disappear within seconds if the patient is only hypersensitive. If there is any doubt as to the patency of an existing IV line, this line should be removed. A new IV should be started either proximal to the previous insertion site or in the other areas.

Support. Management of vesicant extravasation is controversial. Several antidotes have been proposed in the literature, but little experimental data has been published to substantiate which is best. Further research is needed to evaluate the effectiveness of the agents listed in Table 17–1. Until then, each institution responsible for chemotherapy administration needs to formalize standard orders for treatment should vesicant seepage into tissue occur.

Supportive nursing management requires knowledge of possible treatments for drug infiltration. Use of isoproterenol HCl (Isuprel), dimethylsulfoxide (DMSO), corticosteroids, and sodium bicarbonate have been reported. Heat or ice may be indicated. The following management plan is one that may be used for suspected drug extravasation of anthracycline antibiotics (courtesy of A. Barlock and D. Howser, National Institutes of Health, Washington, D. C.).

TABLE 17–1
Extravasation Treatments

Antidote*	Agent
Sodium thiosulfate	Nitrogen mustard Dactinomycin Mithramycin Mitomycin-C
Sodium bicarbonate Dexamethasone	Daunorubicin Adriamycin Vinblastine Vincristine
Hydrocortisone	Adriamycin
Vitamin C	Dactinomycin Mitomycin-C
Hyaluronidase (Wydase)	Vinblastine Vincristine Vindesine
General antidotes: Lidocaine HCl (Xylocaine) Isoproterenol HCl (Isuprel) DMSO	EDTA

*May be injected through existing IV line or SC at extravasation site. *See* Oncology Nursing Society Guidelines for more information.

Extravasation treatment: If extravasation occurs, immediately (1) remove the IV needle and apply ice pack to the site; then (2) inform the patient's primary physician; (3) initiate appropriate treatment measures according to physician's order and/or standardized order sheet:

Procedure 1. Anesthetize the skin surface with ethyl chloride.
2. Inject hydrocortisone sodium succinate (Solu-Cortef) 100 mg/vial intradermally and SC into the site, using 25-gauge straight needles. Multiple injections are administered from the periphery inward, covering the entire erythematous area and along the borders of the infiltrate. The dose of hydrocortisone sodium succinate is from 50 to 200 mg, depending on the size of the infiltrate and the area of erythema.
3. Apply a film of 1% hydrocortisone cream to the area and cover with a sterile 4 $\times$ 4-in. gauze pad secured with paper tape.
4. Apply an ice pack to the area and instruct the patient to keep ice on as continuously as possible for 24 hr ($\geq$50 min q hr).
5. Instruct the patient to apply steroid cream bid — or more frequently if skin tension in the area occurs — until all the redness has disappeared.
6. Instruct the patient to exercise the affected extremity and not allow pain to restrict full range of motion. Pain medication may be necessary initially.
7. Fully document the incident in the patient's chart, including site of extravasation, treatment, and recommendations for follow-up.

The extravasation site should be observed carefully and status documented on a daily basis for 7 days. If the patient is to be at home, he should be instructed in care of the extravasation site (use of hydrocortisone cream, ice) and supplied with hydrocortisone cream, gauze, and paper tape. Instructions should be written and the nurse should assess his condition by telephone daily (for 7 days). The patient should also be instructed to report any prolonged pain or redness to the physician or nurse. It is important to provide emotional support while the extravasation site heals. On the next patient visit, the area of extravasation should be assessed and observations documented in the patient's record.

VENOUS ACCESS LINES

One way to avoid drug extravasation is to use a central line for administration of chemotherapy. This is only one of the indications for a central venous catheter placement. The patient with cancer often needs therapy over a long period of time and much of the treatment is administered IV, often with sclerosing agents. Large volumes of fluid are often necessary prior to administration of certain drugs. Blood studies are frequent. All these factors can create poor venous access, because of deterioration in peripheral veins, and can subject patients to an excessive number of venipunctures. Methods for improved venous access have been developed and are presented here.

There are several types of central or long-term venous access devices now available. These devices may be used in any patient with cancer, in all kinds of situations. The Hickman catheter is made of silicone rubber with a single, double, or triple lumen. This catheter requires surgical placement. It has a dacron cuff that anchors the catheter SC and provides a barrier to infection (Fig. 17–1).

The Centrasil and Intrasil catheters are silicone elastomer central venous access lines. The Centrasil is a 16-gauge, 9-inch-long catheter that is placed in the subclavian vein under local anesthesia (Fig. 17–2). The Intrasil is a 16-gauge, 20-inch-long catheter that is also placed under local anesthesia but in a peripheral vein (*see* Fig. 17–2). Both catheters are threaded into the central veins and used for long-term IV therapy.

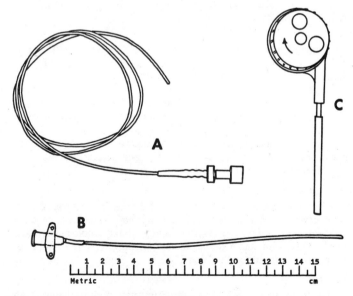

Figure 17–1. Venous access lines. (A) Hickman catheter; (B) Centrasil; (C) Intrasil.

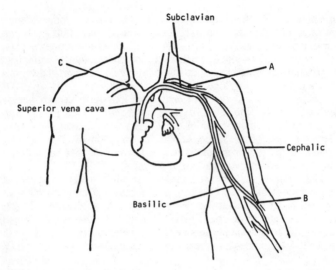

Figure 17–2.   Sites of catheter placements: (A) Centrasil; (B) Intrasil; (C) Hickman.

Other catheters, made of different materials, such as Teflon or polyvinyl, are used for central venous access and are cared for in a similar manner to the Centrasil.

There are several indications for use of these catheters. Total parenteral nutrition (TPN) benefits depend on the reliability of a central venous catheter for TPN delivery. Long-term antibiotic therapy, continuous drug infusions, provision of blood products, and bone-marrow transplantation are also reasons a reliable venous access site is needed. Cancer pain relieved by long-term drug administration may also require an indwelling catheter system.

Assessment

The nurse should have knowledge of the types of central or long-term access lines available and of the benefits and risks of each, enabling her to assess patient needs and potential problems preplacement, at insertion, and postplacement. Nursing interventions for these concerns are discussed in Table 17–2.

Management

The medical team is responsible for insertion of central lines. They may need to replace or reposition the catheter if complications occur.

They also need to make the decision as to whether to use streptokinase or urokinase to dissolve a clot in a catheter.

Nursing management of patients with a central line is threefold and consists of monitoring for complications; developing procedures for care of the catheter; and educating the patient about the care and risks involved. Each institution should set standards of care for the central line. These guidelines will be based on whether the hospital uses a Hickman, Intrasil, or another type of catheter. Patient education should also include a method for heparinization of the catheter between cycles. The dressing change procedure, the flushing procedure, and special precautions should be taught to the patient, because he will assume catheter care while at home. Frequency of dressing change, frequency of flushing, and volume of irrigation may vary, but a suggested care management plan follows (courtesy of Regina Carelli, National Institutes of Health, Washington, D. C.).

Hickman exit site dressing change: Sterile technique is not required when changing the exit site dressing of a Hickman catheter. Supplies (often available in a kit) include (1) 3 povidone-iodine (Betadine) swab sticks; (2) 1 small packet povidone-iodine (Betadine ointment; (3) E-Med strip; (4) Skin-Prep swabs; (5) alcohol swabs (optional); (6) 1-in. micropore tape (optional); (7) sterile 4 × 4-in. gauze (optional).

Procedure 1. Explain procedure to patient.
2. Wash hands with povidone-iodine scrub solution or a cleansing soap.
3. Remove old dressing.
4. Observe site for redness, irritation, or drainage around exit site.
5. Clean catheter with alcohol swabs prn.
6. Clean area with povidone-iodine swab sticks 3 times.
7. Squeeze povidone-iodine ointment on exit site.
8. Apply Skin-Prep to area where E-Med strip will be applied.
9. Apply E-Med strip according to package directions.
10. Loop catheter under flap of E-Med strip.
11. Coil remaining catheter, cover with 4 × 4-in. gauze and tape securely if desired.

Hickman flushing procedure: Supplies (often available as a kit) consist of (1) syringe of heparin (the usual heparin dose is 1.8 ml of 1,000 U heparin/ml normal saline but may vary according to physician's orders); (2) 1 3-ml/syringe with 25-gauge needle; (3) IV cannula clamp; (4) povidone-iodine swab.

Procedure 1. Explain procedure to patient.
2. Wash hands.
3. Clean infusion cap with povidone-iodine swab and allow to dry.

4. Attach syringe of heparin, which should contain an amount ≥catheter volume plus 0.2 ml.
5. Flush line gently.

Another benefit of having a Hickman catheter is that it can also be used for blood drawing. (It is also possible to draw blood through both the Centrasil and Intrasil catheters. Greater caution is required than with the Hickman, however, because the Centrasil and Intrasil are very flexible and break with too much pressure.)

Hickman blood drawing procedure: The supplies needed include (1) 1 12-ml syringe with 22-gauge needle for discard; (2) 1 3-ml syringe with 25-gauge needle with prescribed amount of heparin; (3) syringe(s) for amount of blood to be drawn, with 22-gauge needle(s); (4) povidone-iodine swabs; (5) labeled collection tubes for blood specimens; (6) sterile 3-way stopcock (optional); (7) 1 10-ml syringe with normal saline. The following special precautions must be observed during the blood drawing procedure: (1) To avoid air embolus or hemorrhage, the catheter is either clamped with a smooth-edged occlusion clamp or capped with an intermittent infusion cap. The clamp prevents air from entering the catheter and blood from leaking out when the catheter is unclamped. Clamps and caps are not used when IV solutions are being infused continuously or a syringe is attached directly to the catheter. (2) Hickman catheters are fragile and susceptible to breaks and leaks; therefore, *only* smooth-edged occlusion clamps (cannula clamps) are used; a cannula clamp must be on the patient's person at *all* times; wetproof tape *must not* be used; and forceful irrigation is *contraindicated.* (3) Should the catheter leak or break, the line should be clamped immediately with a cannula clamp and the repair procedure followed. The patient may be taught this procedure or to call for assistance.

Capped line procedure   1. Explain procedure to patient.
2. Wash hands.
3. Cleanse injection cap with povidone-iodine and allow to dry.
4. Attach syringe with needle.
5. Withdraw 8 ml of blood and discard with syringe and needle.
6. Attach syringe with needle for specimen.
7. Draw specimen(s). Transfer blood to appropriate collection tubes.
8. Flush with prescribed amount of heparin.
9. If there is difficulty in obtaining blood, and changing body position or taking deep breaths does not help, the following technique may be employed after clamping catheter with a cannula clamp: Remove infusion cap and attach syringe to catheter; remove clamp, draw blood, reclamp, apply new sterile infusion cap, and unclamp.

Continuous infusion procedure   1. Wash hands.

2. Clean connection with povidone-iodine.
3. Stop the infusion of IV fluid.
4. Attach syringe to stopcock.
5. Withdraw 8 ml of blood and discard.
6. Attach syringe(s) and withdraw specimens.
7. Flush with 10 ml normal saline.
8. Resume infusion.

The Centrasil, Intrasil, and other central lines require a stricter protocol for catheter maintenance. They have no extra protection as does the Hickman, which has a seal around the dacron cuff. Therefore, in order to significantly lower the septic complications from a contaminated catheter, sterile technique needs to be used for the dressing change. A suggested care plan for these access lines follows.

Central line dressing change: Supplies (often available as a kit) needed include (1) 3 povidone-iodine swab sticks; (2) 3 alcohol/acetone swab sticks; (3) Op-Site; (4) Skin-Prep; (5) 2 $\times$ 2-in. gauze; (6) gloves (optional).

Procedure 1. Explain procedure to patient.
2. Wash hands.
3. Remove old dressing slowly to prevent catheter dislodgement.
4. Observe catheter site for redness, irritation, or drainage.
5. Prepare supplies. Put on gloves (optional).
6. Clean area with alcohol/acetone swabs.
7. Clean area with povidone-iodine swab sticks.
8. Apply Skin-Prep to skin area.
9. Place 2 $\times$ 2-in. gauze over the exit site.
10. Apply Op-Site. Pinch the Op-Site together around the tubing where it exits from the dressing.

Supportive nursing management requires availability of resources if questions or complications occur. Emotional support while the patient learns the detailed procedures is important to development of comfort with these responsibilities. The patient cares for his catheter by performing the same procedures as the nursing staff. A written manual is very helpful to patients and family. These catheters are important factors in easing the administration of therapy, and the patient becomes dependent on being able to have the access line. When problems occur, patients worry that they will lose the central line. Nurses can alert patients to potential causes and symptoms of complications and the interventions to correct the problems, thus prolonging the life of the catheter and enabling the patient to have it for the duration of therapy.

INTRA-ARTERIAL CATHETERS

Arterial catheter placement is also a method used for access to administer cancer therapy. Arterial cannulation is performed for

TABLE 17–2

Nursing Protocol for Assessment of Patients with Central Venous Lines

Problem	Intervention
Preplacement Decision of best type catheter for the patient	Evaluate patient's mental status: Is he alert? Can he care for the catheter? Can he recognize reasons to call for help? Share this information with the physician. Assess availability of family members to assist in catheter care. Items to consider when assessing best type of catheter for use for that patient: Resources: Hickmans are surgically placed. Intrasil and Centrasil do not require an operating room but do need experienced persons to insert the catheters properly. Need for catheter: Hickmans are more permanent and can be used for longer time periods. Ability to handle dressing change: Once the site has healed, the Hickman requires less care than the others. Sterile technique is required for dressing change of the Intrasil and Centrasil. Activity level: The Hickman and Centrasil are placed within a major vein of the chest. The Intrasil is placed in an arm vein, decreasing mobility and ease of care. The Intrasil has the potential for fracture of the line with use. Use for blood drawing: Greater precaution needs to be taken if using the Centrasil or Intrasil for blood removal. They are made of a flexible material that breaks with increased pressure or can be displaced more easily than the Hickman.
Patient's need for information	Discuss procedure with the patient: why, how, expectations after insertion, care responsibilities, and potential problems.

Insertion Complications of catheter placement	Assess the patient for the following problems: Pneumothorax: cyanosis, dyspnea, chest pain, tachycardia, tachypnea, respiratory embarrassment. Pulmonary embolism: dyspnea, tachypnea, pleuritic pain, cyanosis, unexplained deterioration of the patient's condition, engorgement of neck veins. Pleural effusion: increasing dyspnea, minimal or absent breath sounds. Notify the physician if these symptoms occur. An x-ray will document the findings.
Postplacement Potential complications: Local	Evaluate for pain, bleeding, leakage of fluid, or hematoma. Assess for signs of infection such as redness, irritation, discharge from the catheter exit site or fever. If any of these occur, culture site to identify local sources of infection and blood to identify systemic sources. Periodically check the patient's dressing change procedure for compliance with the institution guidelines.
Mechanical (catheter function)	A thrombosis of the vein can occlude the catheter. The following signs and symptoms may indicate vein thrombosis: Fluid cannot be instilled through catheter; unable to withdraw fluid back through catheter; feeling of resistance when trying to flush the IV line; reddening or swelling along vein; tenderness along course of the catheter. If the catheter is not functioning, or other symptoms of occlusion are present, the catheter may need to be irrigated with streptokinase or urokinase by the physician. Removal of the catheter may be required if flow cannot be restored. Depending on the type of catheter, the line may be fractured by use or trauma. Some catheters can be repaired. The nurse will need to review individual catheter information to determine necessary precautions. A clamp should be provided to the patient if this risk is present. Displacement of a catheter can occur. X-ray or scan may be required to evaluate catheter position. There are no signs or symptoms to alert the nurse to this problem.

several reasons. An intra-arterial catheter can be used for continuous arterial blood sampling without frequent punctures; to provide a site for blood removal during fluid overload; and for diagnostic studies of cardiac output. Cancer patients may require an intra-arterial catheter for infusion of antineoplastic drugs. Arterial drug administration allows a high concentration of the drug to be delivered to tumor sites with decreased systemic toxicity. Tumors treated via this route are liver, colon, head, neck, or bone cancers. The major artery chosen for catheter placement depends on disease site; it could be the celiac, femoral, brachial, radial, or external or internal carotid artery. Drugs tested by arterial administration are floxuridine and 5-fluorouracil.

An arterial catheter can be placed surgically at the time of a laparotomy or by a radiologist. When the procedure is performed by a radiologist, the catheter is placed percutaneously using local anesthetic, and placement is checked by x-ray, as the catheter is radiopaque. Although surgical placement allows a more stable and permanent placement of the catheter, because it is sutured in place, this procedure requires general anesthesia. Intermittent flushing of the surgically placed catheter is possible. The percutaneous catheter is not sutured in place and usually needs continuous IV flushing. The percutaneous catheter is used more often for short-term therapy.

Assessment

The nurse should be thoroughly familiar with the two methods of arterial catheterization so that she can prepare the patient for arterial line insertion. Base-line information, such as color, temperature, and blanching time of the area around the proposed insertion site should be observed and noted. Table 17–3 discusses in detail the problems requiring assessment pre- and postplacement and appropriate nursing interventions.

Management

Medical care is directed toward decisions as to which type of catheter insertion method should be used and where catheter placement should occur and continues with follow-up for problems encountered during therapy (e.g., clotted catheter). The decision to remove the catheter or to try to remove the clot with urokinase is up to the medical team.

Nursing management focuses on patient preparation for insertion and on care of the catheter. The patient needs to be educated as to what to expect, potential problems, and preventive care of the exit site. Care will depend on routines of each individual institution but might use the following guidelines.

Guidelines for intra-arterial exit site care: The nurse or patient should note the color and temperature of the extremity q 6 hr. Assessment should be made for bleeding at the insertion site. Pressure should be applied to the site and maintained while the dressing is removed to look for bleeding or fluid around the connection pieces, to determine if there are any disconnections within the system. Care of the site should be performed daily. Supplies needed will include (1) povidone-iodine swabs; (2) povidone-iodine ointment; (3) acetone swab; (4) 2 × 2-in. gauze; (5) cotton applicators; (6) tape. *Strict sterile technique* must be maintained any time the catheter is manipulated. This includes insertion, blood drawing, changing the line components, and drug preparation.

Procedure 1. Remove old dressing. Check the site for signs of infection, such as redness, swelling, or discharge. If signs of infection are present, blood cultures should be drawn.

2. Clean exit site with acetone and then povidone-iodine.

3. With an applicator, apply ointment to the exit site.

4. Place 2 × 2-in. gauze over catheter and secure dressing.

Drawing blood from an arterial line: Supplies needed will include (1) 1 3-ml syringe for discard; (2) alcohol swabs; (3) syringes for blood specimens; (4) labeled collection tubes for blood specimens; (5) heparin per physician's order.

Procedure 1. Remove the cap from the stopcock and insert the 3-ml syringe. Turn stopcock to open, and blood will flow freely into the syringe. Withdraw 3 ml discard.

2. Close the stopcock halfway to stop blood flow and quickly remove discard syringe. Insert specimen syringe, turn stopcock to full open, and obtain blood specimens.

3. Turn stopcock to off position and remove the specimen syringe.

4. Transfer blood to collection tubes.

5. Immediately flush the line with heparin solution until the catheter is clear.

6. Clean the outside of the stopcock with the alcohol swab and replace cap.

Patients are often at home while chemotherapy is running through the arterial line via an infusion pump. Often the nurse will have started the drug therapy, but the patient monitors its administration. Resources must be available when questions or problems occur. A checklist could be used by the nurse to ensure that the patient is adequately prepared for intra-arterial chemotherapy.

Good teaching will assure greater patient self-confidence, cooperation in taking therapy and completing procedures, and an awareness of the signs and symptoms of problems or abnormal effects. Greater patient awareness will open communications with the staff so that early

TABLE 17–3

Nursing Protocol for Assessment of Patients with Intra-Arterial Lines

Problem	Intervention

Preplacement
Decision about best type of catheter for the patient
	Evaluate patient's needs. Can he care for the catheter? Can he recognize complications, precautions, and reasons to call for help? Share this information with the physician. Assess availability of family members to assist in catheter care.
	Items to consider when assessing the best type of catheter to use:
	   Resources: Percutaneous catheter can be placed by a radiologist or an anesthesiologist, but a surgically placed arterial catheter requires use of the operating room.
	   Need for catheter: The surgically placed catheter is sutured in place and is more permanent. The percutaneous catheter is more appropriate for short-term use.
	   Activity level: The surgically placed catheter can be capped and flushed intermittently with heparin, allowing greater mobility than the percutaneous catheter, which often requires continuous IV irrigation to prevent clotting.
	   Safety: Both types of intra-arterial lines present a tremendous danger from hemorrhage. If the patient or family members are unable to demonstrate safety measures necessary to stop bleeding, then this type of catheter should not be considered for that patient.

Patient's need for information	Discuss procedure with the patient: why, how, preparations for catheter placement, expectations postinsertion, care responsibilities, and potential problems.

Postplacement
Potential complications:
Local

Assess for bleeding at insertion site, hematoma development, or swelling. If present, apply direct pressure to the site. Whenever an arterial catheter is removed, pressure must be applied to the site for a full 5 min to prevent a hematoma.

Monitor for pain, redness, swelling, discharge around the arterial catheter, or fever that might signal infection.

Displacement of catheter

Teach patient to report excessive side effects of treatment. These might include nausea and vomiting, diarrhea, dyspepsia, stomach pain, twitching, paresthesia, or motor weakness.

Mechanical (catheter function)

Assess for decreased or absent pulse distal to the insertion site. This might be caused by an occluded catheter. Preventive treatment involves heparin flushing either q 4–6 hr and then q 24 hr for a surgically placed catheter or continuously for a percutaneous catheter. Intermittent flushes may occasionally be used, and if so, careful monitoring for backflow of blood between flushes is necessary. Pain or numbness in the extremity might signal a problem.

An arterial catheter can be broken by wear and tear or trauma. The patient needs to have a clamp available and be taught what to do if breakage should occur. Luer-Lok connectors need to be used with arterial infusions so that hemorrhage does not occur. If bleeding is noted, pressure or clamp should be applied immediately. Monitor for signs of hemorrhage, such as blood backup caused by a loose connection, leakage of fluid from site, or frank bleeding. Safety measures include evaluation of all connecting sites frequently, use of Luer-Lok connections, and use of a built-in alarm system to monitor pressure changes within the arterial line. If the patient is to go home, it is essential to teach him and his family to immediately apply pressure to the site and elevate the affected part should bleeding occur.

recognition of problems is possible. Nurses are valuable resources for patients should problems occur.

Management of intra-arterial drug infusion requires a high level of responsibility as well as technical skill. The nurse needs to know as much as possible about this method of drug administration so that patients are adequately prepared. Frequent supervision and opportunity to practice will enhance patient comfort with the procedures. Home care by the patient and family places demands on them because of the transfer of responsibility. The nurse is a source of support both during hospitalization and after discharge.

Because this method of drug therapy has become more popular, new implantable devices have been designed to decrease the incidence of complications and reduce patient responsibilities at the same time. The implantable system for drug delivery is now being tested for intra-arterial drug administration.

IMPLANTABLE DRUG DELIVERY SYSTEMS

Several drugs used in the treatment of cancer work best when the drug is infused into the bloodstream continuously. Therapeutic levels of drug can be maintained when a constant rate of drug delivery is achieved, and a continuous infusion directly into the bloodstream avoids the peak-and-valley effects of bolus injections. Adequate levels of drug needed to kill cancer cells are maintained and therefore a greater number of cells are affected. This constant infusion is made possible by an implantable device that has also been used for long-term heparin infusions or diabetic control with continuous insulin infusions. The ability of the pump to deliver drug to a specific target area is another feature that has made it attractive for the treatment of cancer. In cancers such as hepatoma or colon carcinoma, the blood supply is almost exclusively arterial. This pump can be implanted and will deliver chemotherapy by infusion directly into the hepatic artery. Because most of the drug passes through the liver, where it is metabolized, and not out into the systemic circulation, its systemic side effects are decreased.

There are available several types of implantable infusion pumps that are placed SC to deliver drugs continuously. The infusion rate can be adjusted to slowly deliver the drug to a selected body site. Safe and reliable use of the system requires knowledge of the pump used, the way it is implanted, how it works, its problems or limitations, and the need for follow-up care. The following discussion will address these issues for one type of these pumps called an Infusaid (Fig. 17-3), which is refilled by percutaneous injection. The pump is designed for long-term therapy in the ambulatory patient.

It is composed of a lightweight metal that encloses two chambers separated by a flexible metal bellows. The interior chamber holds the drug; the surrounding outer chamber holds a two-phase charging fluid, which is the power supply. The charging fluid is in either a vapor or liquid state, depending on a number of variables. Pressure differences between the two chambers activate the pump. The vapor pressure of the charging fluid exerts a constant pressure on the bellows, causing drug flow from the pump into the catheter and to the selected body site. When the pump is refilled, the increasing volume causes pressure on the charging fluid, which condenses from the vapor to liquid state. The liquid once again vaporizes, which provides the energy to move the bellows and deliver the desired drug flow. The flow rate is calibrated at the factory, but variations in body temperature or altitude may cause variation in the rate of pump flow, as these may change the rate at which the charging fluid is converted from liquid to vapor. These variations are predictable, and each pump is delivered with specific calibration curves defining the flow characteristics for the planned catheter placement site, hometown elevation, and drug to be used.

Attached to the pump is a silicone rubber catheter, which is placed in the vein, artery, or other body site. The refill septum, which is in the center of the pump, can be easily palpated. The pump also has a side port, which can be used to bypass the reservoir and administer bolus injections of medication through the catheter. The technique for using this side port is the same as for other, similar implantable access ports and is described below.

Assessment

Nursing assessment of the patient suitable for a totally implantable system involves the factors discussed in Table 17–4. Interventions presented need to be individualized.

Management

Nursing focus is primarily on patient education. Each pump has its own specific precautions. The Infusaid has several that the patient needs to know and understand. The nurse is an important resource in sharing this information with the patient and family, and teaching is enhanced by a patient booklet available from the manufacturers of the Infusaid. The booklet delineates several patient responsibilities. Instructions include avoiding rough physical activities, changes of altitudes (such as long airplane flights or scuba diving), long hot baths or saunas, which elevate pump temperature. In addition patients are advised to consult the physician during febrile illnesses or to report unusual signs or symptoms and to notify hospital personnel about the

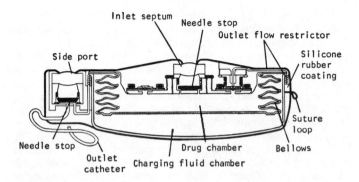

Figure 17–3. Infusaid pump.

pump if other medical procedures are planned. The pamphlet also encourages patients to return at the prescribed time for pump refill.

An identification card is provided for the patient with an Infusaid pump. This may be needed during emergencies, or if the patient is passing through an airport metal detector. The pump may be detected by the weapon surveillance machine, but performance of the pump will not be affected.

Surgical site care depends on the location of pump implantation, but it usually consists of keeping the area clean and dry. A delay of 3 to 7 days after implantation should be allowed for wound healing before beginning chemotherapy.

A potential nursing responsibility is drug administration. The Infusaid Corporation holds classes to teach the pump refill procedure. Refilling the Infusaid pump on schedule is important. The dose and volume should be calculated by the physician, considering the factory-set flow rate of the pump, drug concentration, and individual factors, such as hometown elevation. The pump refill procedure is as follows.

Infusaid pump refill procedure: Supplies needed will include (1) gloves; (2) 22-gauge special Infusaid needle; (3) medication syringe (prewarmed to 30–45°C); (4) stopcock; (5) anesthetizing agent; (6) sterile syringe; (7) povidone-iodine.

Procedure 1. Scrub the pump site with povidone-iodine.
2. Anesthetize the injection site.
3. Using sterile technique, feel the outer edges of the pump to locate the refill septum located in the pump center.
4. Attach a sterile stopcock (in open position) to an empty syringe barrel and needle. Puncture the skin and septum and allow the

TABLE 17–4

Nursing Protocol for Assessment of Patients with Implantable Pumps

Problem	Intervention
Preimplantation	
Examine any contraindications to having an implantable pump	Assess the patient for: severe emotional or psychologic disturbances that might indicate that he is unreliable; a small, thin body size that could not accommodate the weight of the pump; frequent travel, because altitude affects drug flow; or involvement in vigorous or rough occupations or activities, such as sports. Share this information with the physician.
Patient need for information	Utilize the teaching booklet supplied by the manufacturer of the Infusaid to supplement discussion of why, where, how, and patient responsibilities. Review instructions for contraindications, what to report, and the use of an identification card, especially in the airport, where the pump will set off the metal detector.
Postimplantation	Tailor wound care to the individual patient's needs. Review preimplantation instructions regarding precautions and what needs to be reported to the doctor or nurse. Emphasize the necessity of returning on time for pump refills.

pump's pressure to expel the infusate from the reservoir into the empty syringe. *Precaution:* The needle must be held securely against the needle stop. *Do not* put the needle at an angle within the septum.

5. When fluid has stopped returning, close the stopcock and remove the syringe barrel and stopcock from the needle. Air does not enter into the needle because of the pressurized system. Record the volume. *Precaution:* If no fluid returns into the syringe, the possibility is that the septum was not penetrated, the pump is empty, or there is a malfunction. Inject 5 ml of bacteriostatic water into the pump and then release the plunger. If fluid still does not return, repeat the procedure, beginning with

reinsertion of the needle. If you feel that you have penetrated the septum but have been unable to get return flow to the syringe, indications are that pump failure has occurred and the Infusaid Corporation needs to be notified.

6. Connect the prewarmed syringe of medication to the needle in the septum and slowly inject the contents. Remove syringe and needle when completed. *Precaution:* Make sure the needle point remains against the needle stop throughout the injection cycle.

7. The refill schedule should be planned several days before the end of the cycle to avoid an empty drug chamber.

IMPLANTABLE ACCESS PORTS

Other implantable access ports are available without a pump attached. These access ports allow repeated injections of cytotoxic drugs or frequent infusions of medications without repeated venous puncture. The first type of implantable port is called the Ommaya reservoir (Fig. 17-4). This device is used primarily in the treatment of meningeal carcinomatosis, the infiltration of the leptomeninges of the brain by cancer. Although the Ommaya has been used for chemotherapy of brain tumors, cystic tumor drainage, ventricular drainage, special diagnostic studies, and sampling of CSF, the reservoir is particularly useful for administration of intraventricular chemotherapy to leukemic patients. The Ommaya reservoir is a domed device with a catheter attached. The reservoir is usually positioned in the scalp SC, and the catheter then threads down into the lateral ventricle. The reservoir has a self-sealing membrane that allows repeated punctures, facilitating intraventricular chemotherapy. The most frequently reported chemotherapeutic agents used via this route are methotrexate, thiotepa, and ARA-C. Use of the Ommaya for drug administration produces optimal, consistant CSF levels in the area most needed. These same drugs given IV would not effectively cross the blood-brain barrier to provide optimal therapy for the disease.

Assessment

Assessment of the patient needing an Ommaya reservoir consists primarily of evaluation of the need for teaching. Factors that should be addressed are presented in Table 17-5.

Management

The Ommaya reservoir is placed surgically under local anesthesia by the medical team. Antibiotics are often given before and following Ommaya placement. Once the site is healed, the physician is often the

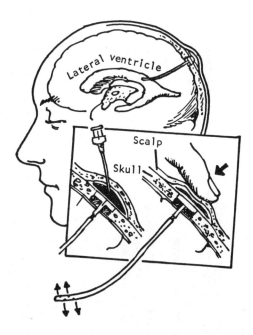

Figure 17–4. Placement of the Ommaya reservoir, an implantable access port used primarily to assist in the administration of intraventricular chemotherapy to leukemic patients or patients with meningeal carcinomatosis. Inset shows administration of medication into the dome of the Ommaya reservoir (left) followed by gentle pressure being applied, forcing the medication through the port into the lateral ventricle. *Reprinted with permission from* Ommaya, A., and R. Ratcheson. Experience with the subcutaneous CSF reservoir. *The New England Journal of Medicine* (November 7, 1968). p. 1026.

one who administers the drug through the reservoir. Strict practice of sterile technique during the tapping of this device helps decrease the incidence of infection. This complication or other problems with catheter function may necessitate Ommaya reservoir replacement.

Nursing management is primarily preventive. Infection is the primary complication of the Ommaya reservoir. Patient education should include preventive measures, such as care and observation of the surgical site as well as information about the drugs being used for treatment.

TABLE 17-5

Nursing Protocol for Assessment of Patients with Ommaya Reservoirs

Problem	Intervention
Preoperative	
Patient's ability to care for the reservoir	Evaluate ability to comprehend instructions. Determine if a family member is available for support and assistance. Share this information with physician.
Patient need for information on implantation procedure	Discuss rationale, preparations needed, why, where, how.
Teaching patient about responsibilities in maintaining the reservoir	Teach care for implantation site. Teach him to report signs of catheter infection. Advise him to prevent trauma to the site to avoid CNS injury; report signs of catheter malfunction, neurologic deficits, or exit site infection.
Postoperative	
Potential complications: Catheter malfunction	Assess patient for pain, failure to aspirate, or inflow obstruction. May necessitate catheter removal. A CAT scan or x-ray may be needed to check placement.
Neurologic deficits	Assess for changes in mental alertness or behavior, seizures, or headaches. Report any changes to the physician.
Infection at exit site	Assess site daily for redness, irritation, swelling, drainage, fever, or neck stiffness. Cultures may be needed if any of these signs are present.
Side effects of the drugs	These vary according to drug, dose, and schedule. Side effects experienced when drugs are given intraventricularly are similar to those with IV route. Provide patient with information about side effects.

The second type of implantable port (e.g., Port-a-Cath) is used primarily for vascular access. It is not used for any specific drug or type of cancer. It is implanted in the subcutaneous tissue in the area where access is easiest. This device also has a domed reservoir with a self-sealing membrane attached to a catheter. The catheter is threaded to the vein, artery, or organ where therapy is desired. This device helps decrease the trauma from multiple venipunctures while allowing easy access for delivery of drug to the patient.

The catheter can be implanted under local or general anesthesia. Management is similar to the Ommaya in that infection needs to be prevented. In addition, the complication of catheter occlusion is more prevalent in devices of this type than the Ommaya. The only symptom of occlusion is resistance when trying to inject fluid through the port. Irrigation is needed at least q 3 wk with 1 ml of the prescribed heparin solution to create a heparin lock in the catheter. No other dressing or exit site care is necessary. Use of the port for IV administration requires the nurse's attention to detail. A sterile field is established, and povidone-iodine is used to prepare the site for needle entry. The needles are special Huber-point needles, as are those used for implanted pumps. The needles should be inserted straight into the septum. If done at an angle, or with a twisting motion, the septum can be cut and leakage of fluid occur. Establishing blood return prior to drug administration through these ports will vary with the manufacturer's guidelines. Some of these ports can be used for blood drawings, though the nurse should refer to the manufacturer's guidelines before attempting this procedure.

INTRAPERITONEAL CATHETER

With the successful use of implantable access ports for local administration of drug therapy, a similar need was noted for treatment of peritoneal tumors. An intraperitoneal catheter for drug infusions theoretically presents an advantage over IV drug therapy because higher concentrations of drug can be delivered directly into the abdominal cavity. The abdominal cavity is often the site of tumor involvement in ovarian cancer. This treatment is intended to enhance the effectiveness of the chemotherapy because of the higher drug levels possible and the decrease of systemic toxicity. Because most of the drugs used via this route are cleared from the peritoneal cavity by the portal circulation and metabolized by the liver, only low levels of drug concentrations get into the systemic circulation. Therefore, side effects are fewer. This technique also enables treatment of colon cancer in instances where the liver is the major site of recurrence. The Tenckhoff catheter is an access device used by several treatment centers for peritoneal dialysis. Previously used for renal dialysis, this technique was adapted for intraperitoneal delivery of chemotherapeutic drugs for ovarian cancer. Drugs tested intraperitoneally thus far are methotrexate, 5-fluorouracil, adriamycin, cisplatin, ARA-C, and melphalan.

Assessment

Assessment of the patient requiring intraperitoneal chemotherapy includes evaluation of the need for information and for catheter monitoring. Variables to be evaluated are presented in Table 17–6.

Management

Medical management of these patients includes placement of the catheter and close follow-up in case problems occur. The Tenckhoff catheter implantation customarily takes place under local anesthesia but in an operating room because bowel perforation is a potential complication. Once the catheter is properly placed in the peritoneal cavity, it is threaded subcutaneously to exit thorugh a small incision ~5 to 7 cm from the initial incision. During healing, the cuff on the catheter causes proliferation of fibroblasts in the subcutaneous tunnel, creating a seal around the catheter and decreasing the possibility that infection will travel into the abdomen.

Nursing management consists of preventive measures against infection. Infection can occur around the exit site or within the peritoneal cavity. Patient education is essential because catheter function is directly related to quality of maintenance care performed by the patient. Sterile technique is observed in caring for the external catheter at all times. The catheter exit site should be completely healed ~2 to 4 wk following insertion, and no redness or tenderness should be present. For the duration of catheter implantation the dressing is changed daily. The prescribed procedure for care follows; the patient needs to be able to demonstrate proficiency in this procedure. A research study at the National Cancer Institute is currently comparing the standard dressing procedure, as presented here, with a modified procedure to determine the relative effectiveness in preventing the incidence of infection.

Tenckhoff catheter care: Supplies (often available as a kit) include (1) 1 sterile barrier disposable towel; (2) 10 packages sterile 4 × 4-in. gauze pads (2/package); (3) 1 package sterile applicators (2/package); (4) povidone-iodine solution; (5) hydrogen peroxide; (6) roll 2-in. paper tape; (7) masks; (8) sterile gloves.

Procedure   1. Wash hands. Assemble equipment at the bedside. Have all persons present including patient put on a mask.

TABLE 17-6

Nursing Protocol for Assessment of Patients with an Intraperitoneal Catheter

Problem	Intervention
Preplacement Patient's ability to care for catheter	Evaluate patient's mental status and ability to comprehend instructions and report complications. Share this information with physician. Assess availability of family members to assist in catheter care.
Patient need for information	Discuss the procedure with the patient — why, how, expectations after insertion, care responsibilities, and potential problems. Teach patient to report signs of infection. These include fever, chills, pain or discharge around catheter.
Postplacement Potential complications: Leakage of fluid	Leakage around the catheter is normal postoperatively because the seal is not tight until after 10–14 days. If leakage occurs during those first 2 wk, it is important to change the catheter dressing frequently to prevent infection.
Catheter malfunction	Assess the patient for pain with dialysis or problems with drainage. May need to irrigate catheter forcefully using sterile technique with 50 ml normal saline to remove blockage.
Infection	Evaluate the characteristics of dialysis fluid: the fluid will be bloody initially but should become clear. If the fluid becomes cloudy, or pain, redness, irritation, or drainage occurs around the exit site, peritoneal fluid and the exit site should be cultured.
Respiratory distress	If the patient has problems taking deep breaths when the dialysate is in the abdomen, the volume may need to be decreased.
Pain	Pain postoperatively is expected, and analgesics should be administered for relief. Pain caused by cold dialysate can be relieved by warming the fluid prior to administration. Pain caused by intraperitoneal infection is also accompanied by fever. Cultures should be obtained to determine the presence of an infectious organism. Pain related to chemotherapeutic agents is hard to distinguish from that pain caused by infections. It is related to drug, dose, and schedule. Analgesics should be administered for relief once a bacterial source has been ruled out.

2. Open barrier towel. Open and place on barrier towel contents of 10 packages of 4 × 4-in. pads. Pour povidone-iodine solution on 8 4 × 4-in. pads and hydrogen peroxide on 6 4 × 4's. Open and place applicators on barrier. Squeeze povidone-iodine ointment on barrier.

3. Remove old dressings and then put on sterile gloves.

4. Place saturated povidone-iodine 4 × 4-in. pad around exposed catheter and cap.

5. Wash area directly surrounding catheter exit site with hydrogen-peroxide-saturated 4 × 4's 3 times (until sutures are removed and area is healed). Note any inflammation at the exit site.

6. Scrub abdominal area with povidone-iodine-saturated 4 × 4-in. pads 3 times. Use a circular motion, working from the catheter exit site outwards.

7. Hold catheter by cap with povidone-iodine-saturated 4 × 4-in. pad. Clean cap using rotating motion. Cleanse entire length of exposed catheter with povidone-iodine-saturated 4 × 4's 3 times. Work from catheter exit site to catheter cap using a gentle rotating motion.

8. Apply povidone-iodine ointment around catheter exit site with applicator.

9. Redress with sterile 4 × 4-in. pads. Place one on abdomen under catheter. Two additional 4 × 4's are applied, overlapping, to completely cover catheter and exit site. Secure with paper tape.

10. Any time the dressing is opened to permit catheter connection or disconnection from the dialysis set, sterile technique is used, i.e., masks, sterile gloves, and the connector site is cleaned with povidone-iodine. This procedure is essential because it is very easy to introduce bacteria through the lumen of the catheter if precautions are not taken.

Nurses play a critical role in managing the care of patients receiving intraperitoneal therapy. They have the responsibility for managing catheter sterility, managing the dialysis treatments, and teaching patients to manage catheters independently.

INTRACAVITARY MANAGEMENT OF PLEURAL EFFUSIONS

Like the intraperitoneal administration of drugs, intracavitary injection of agents may be used to prevent reaccumulation of fluid caused by malignancy. The effectiveness of the treatment depends primarily on the drug's ability to sclerose the pleural tissue, rather than on its antineoplastic activity. Agents commonly used for this purpose are shown in Table 17–7. Dosage is generally the same as when drugs are administered systemically, but toxicity is less. This method of drug administration is achieved through thoracentesis.

A pleural effusion is an accumulation of fluid in the pleural space. The cause of the effusion may be congestive heart failure, pneumonia, a malignancy, or other pathologic conditions. Cancers most frequently associated with malignant effusions are breast, lung, ovary, and lymphoma.

A thoracentesis may help establish the diagnosis of a malignant effusion (Table 17–8), by analysis of pleural fluid removed during the procedure. Thoracentesis alone, either by means of a needle or a thoracotomy tube, cannot prevent reaccumulation of fluid in metastatic effusions. It does, however, help achieve the primary treatment goal, which is relief of symptoms by permitting greater lung expansion and making breathing easier.

Systemic chemotherapy may be effective in controlling malignant effusions if the primary disease is responsive to these treatments. Radiation may be helpful for some pleural effusions, but pneumonitis is a risk. Pleurectomy is an option, but it requires a thoracotomy.

Assessment

The nurse will often determine the need for a thoracentesis from her assessment of the patient's condition. Indications for pre- and postthoracentesis interventions are prescribed in Table 17–9, as is information that should be incorporated into patient teaching sessions.

TABLE 17–7
Sclerosing Agents for the Pleural Cavity

Class	Agent
Antineoplastic agents	Nitrogen mustard 5-Fluorouracil Thiotepa Bleomycin Adriamycin
Colloidal radioisotopes	Radiogold colloid Radioactive phosphorus
Antimicrobial agents	Tetracycline Quinacrine
Other	Talc

TABLE 17-8
Findings of Thoracentesis Fluid

Test	Finding
Gross appearance	Exudate or transudate may signal malignancy but are also associated with other causes such as TB, pneumonia, and congestive heart failure.
RBC count	Grossly bloody is suggestive of malignancy ($>100,000$ RBC/mm^3)
Total WBC count	Usually 4,000 cells/mm^3, but malignant pleural effusions have relatively low numbers of WBCs.
Differential WBC count	Lymphocytes predominate in a malignant pleural effusion. Predominance of neutrophils may be indicative of an inflammatory reaction.
Cytology	Positive in 60% of the effusions caused by malignancy.
Glucose	In 15% of malignant effusions this is <60 mg/100 ml.
Amylase	May be elevated with malignancy, pancreatitis, and esophageal rupture.
Fluid culture	May indicate infection.
CEA	>12 ng/ml suggestive of malignancy.
Absolute cell count	Acellular pleural fluid indicates obstruction. 50–1,000 cells/mm^3 indicates serosal surface tumor. 1,000–4,000 cells/mm^3 indicates free-growing tumor.

CEA, carcinoembryonic antigen; TB, tuberculosis.

Management

Nursing management of a patient having a thoracentesis is primarily supportive. During the procedure, which lasts from 15 to 30 min, a needle is inserted into the pleural space under a local anesthetic, fluid is removed, and a sclerosing agent is injected if necessary. Evaluation of pre- and posttreatment symptoms of restrictive lung is essential to measuring effectiveness of the drug injection. A chest x-ray

TABLE 17-9

Nursing Protocol for Assessment for Patients Undergoing Thoracentesis

Problem	Intervention
Pretreatment	
Symptoms indicating a pleural effusion	Evaluate patient for symptoms of a pleural effusion: increasing dyspnea, minimal or absent breath sounds, fatigue with exercise or minimal exertion. Report these findings to the physician.
Patient's need for information	Discuss thoracentesis with the patient.
	Explain nature and purpose of the procedure: indicated for removal of fluid in lungs; no special restrictions or diet prior to test; that patient must remain still during procedure.
	If a sclerosing agent is to be used, explain that a drug injection will be administered through the needle.
	Explain posttreatment expectations: A small pressure dressing will be applied; a chest x-ray will be done and vital signs monitored.
	Explain to patient that he may feel soreness at the puncture site. He should report any breathing difficulty to the nurse.
	If drug is to be instilled via thoracotomy tube:
	Explain nature and purpose of the procedure: that a tube will be inserted into the chest cavity and will remain in place for several days.
	Explain that body position needs to be changed frequently to assure maximum contact of pleural surfaces and the sclerosing agent.
	Explain that eventually the tube will be unclamped and drainage will be maintained for several days. Pain medication may be required.
Posttreatment	
Potential complications	Assess the patient for symptoms of pneumothorax: cyanosis, dyspnea, chest pain, tachycardia, tachypnea, respiratory embarrassment.
	Pain secondary to thoracentesis or presence of chest tube to drain effusion may require medication for relief.
Response to treatment	Evaluate patient for decrease or recurrence of symptoms of a pleural effusion. Frequency of thoracentesis depends on cause of effusion, effectiveness of the drug in sclerosing the cavity, and patient tolerance of fluid build-up.

is taken after the thoracentesis is completed. The nurse should check the patient's pulse, respirations, and BP. The patient may feel some soreness at the puncture site but should not experience any difficulty in breathing.

Thoracotomy tube instillation.   If the drug is to be instilled via a thoracotomy tube, hospitalization is necessary. The drainage tube is inserted under waterseal and the effusion evacuated. A premedication may be needed prior to injection of the sclerosing agent. The chest tube will then be clamped, and the patient should rotate through several positions to assure maximum contact between the pleural surfaces and the sclerosing agent. The tube will then be unclamped and drainage from the pleural space will be maintained for several days before the tube is removed.

A thoracentesis may be necessary quite often, depending on cause of the effusion, effectiveness of the drug in sclerosing the cavity, and patient tolerance of fluid build-up. Factors to be considered in an assessment of patients undergoing thoracentesis are presented in Table 17–9. Management is primarily supportive, with little chance of cure. Effectiveness of the treatment can be monitored by relief of symptoms.

Bibliography

1. Bubela, N. Technical and psychological problems and concerns arising from the outpatient treatment of cancer with direct intraarterial infusion. *Cancer Nursing* (August 1981). 305–309.

    Report of an exploratory study of four patients receiving intra-arterial infusion. Reviews four major areas of patient concern including technical problems and side effects, psychologic concerns, alteration in life-style, and communication.

2. Buchwald, H., T. Grage, P. Vassilopoulos, T. Rohde, R. Varco, and P. Blackshear. Intra-arterial infusion chemotherapy for hepatic carcinoma using a totally implantable infusion pump. *Cancer* (March 1980). 866–869.

    Describes the use of a totally implantable infusion pump used to treat five patients with liver cancer, including the method of and response to intra-arterial chemotherapy.

3. Ignoffo, R., and M. Friedman. Therapy of local toxicities caused by extravasation of cancer chemotherapeutic drugs. *Cancer Treatment Reviews* (March 1980). 17–27.

    Review of factors that increase the risk of extravasation of chemotherapy drugs. Discusses extravasation antidotes proposed in the literature.

4. Jenkins, J., P. Sugarbaker, F. Gianola, and C. Myers. Technical considerations in the use of intraperitoneal chemotherapy administration

by Tenckhoff catheter. *Surgery, Gynecology, and Obstetrics* (June 1982). 858–864.

Describes the rationale and method used for intraperitoneal chemotherapy and discusses catheter implantation procedure, postoperative care, dialysis technique, and catheter maintenance.

5. Johnston, S., and Y. Patt. Caring for the patient on intra-arterial chemotherapy. *Nursing 81* (November 1981). 108–112.

Intra-arterial chemotherapy is explained as a treatment alternative for cancer patients. Pros and cons of arterial catheters are reviewed, as is what to watch for after placement.

6. Lawson, M., K. McCredie, and J. Bottino. The use of silicone elastomer central venous catheters for intravenous therapy in patients with cancer. *National Intravenous Therapy Association* (November/December 1980). 245–248, 259.

Discusses silicone catheters, their care, use, and management. Complications of catheter function are reviewed.

7. Miller, S. Nursing actions in cancer chemotherapy administration. *Oncology Nursing Forum* (Fall 1980). 8–16.

Good review for the nurse preparing to administer chemotherapy. Outline form reviews checklist of things to do pretreatment, during administration, and posttreatment care including lists of dos and don'ts of IV therapy.

8. Oncology Nursing Society Task Force. Cancer Chemotherapy. Guidelines and Recommendations for Nursing Education and Practice. Oncology Nursing Society, Pittsburgh. 1984.

Excellent summary of information needed by chemotherapy nurses qualified to administer chemotherapy. Includes recommendations for an educational program (Part I) and suggestions for policies and procedures related to chemotherapy administration (Part II).

9. Sahn, S. Pleural effusion in lung cancer. *Clinics in Chest Medicine* (May 1982). 443–452.

Presents an overview of pleural effusions. Reviews the diagnostic approach, pathogenesis, and management of malignant effusions.

10. Wujcik, D. Meningeal carcinomatosis: diagnosis, treatment, and nursing care. *Oncology Nursing Forum* (Spring 1983). 35–40.

Excellent nursing review of central nervous system metastases, or meningeal carcinomatosis. Presents the pathology, treatment, and nursing care plan for a patient with an Ommaya reservoir.

CHAPTER 18

RADIATION THERAPY IMPLANTS

Hilary Ann Wood

Radiation therapy (RT) has been one of the standard methods of treatment for cancer for >40 yr. Treatment may take the form of external-beam ionizing radiation by photon, electron, or neutron beam, using the cobalt-60 teletherapy unit or linear accelerators. Alternatively, brachytherapy may be used.

Brachytherapy is a method of RT in which an encapsulated source is used to deliver beta or gamma radiation to local tissue, either by surface, intracavitary, or interstitial application. The radioactive source — either sealed or unsealed — can be placed directly at the site to be irradiated. Sealed sources may take the form of an applicator containing radioactive material that is placed in a cavitary space, or the applicator may be implanted directly into the tissue. Unsealed sources may be given in a liquid form taken PO, by IV injection, or instilled into an intracavitary space, such as the abdomen or pleural cavity. In this way, radiation is delivered directly to the region of the tumor to provide localized treatment for a prescribed length of time.

The choice of treatment method is dependent on the tumor type, disease stage, accessibility to treatment, and known response to therapy. Gynecologic and eye tumors, and cancers of the prostate, breast, and head and neck are treated with sealed sources. Unsealed sources are used for cancers of the thyroid and bladder, polycythemia, and abdominal ascites. Usually, this type of radiation is used in combination with surgery, external radiation, and chemotherapy. The goal of treatment may be the eradication of disease (cure), or the reduction of symptoms (palliation).

Nursing involvement in the care of patients undergoing brachytherapy may involve use of radiation safety principles, pre- and postsurgical nursing care and education of patient or family, and planning for discharge.

Radiation safety principles

Nurses must be familiar with radiation hazards and be able to minimize these risks in their daily practice. The nurse caring for a patient with an implanted radiation source must practice in a manner that will reduce her exposure to radiation. The intensity of radiation decreases by the square of the distance from the source of radiation, and this principle of radiation safety, known as the inverse square law, is utilized when engaging in patient care. The farther away the nurse is from the source, the smaller the dose of radiation she will be exposed to over a given time. For example, if the distance from the source is doubled, the radiation dose intensity will decrease to $(1/2)^2$, or $1/4$, of the dose intensity at the original point.

Personnel are provided with monitoring badges or dosimeter pencils, which measure the amount of radiation to which the worker is exposed. These devices are to be worn whenever there is potential exposure to radiation. The dose received is calculated monthly, with records kept of the cumulative dose. These records are available to staff at all times for review. Maximum permissible dose equivalents allowed by the Nuclear Regulatory Commission are noted in Table 18–1. Risks to workers abiding by safety principles are slight. If a staff person receives a dose exceeding the permissible amount, however, that person must be reassigned to an area where there is no radioactivity for a specified time period, usually ≥ 3 mo.

The radiation physicist, in conjunction with the physician, calculates the amount of time that the nurse may spend within 6 feet of the

TABLE 18–1
Maximum Permissible Radiation Dose Limits

Populations at risk	Area	Dose
Radiation workers	Whole body	5.0 rem in 1 year (over age 18).
Pregnant women	Whole body	0.5 rem in 1 year (during gestation period).
General public	Whole body	0.5 rem in 1 year.

rem, roentgen-equivalent-man, is the measure of an absorbed dose of ionizing radiation in terms of its biological effect. Rad, roentgen, and rem are interchangeable for practical purposes.
From National Council on Radiation Protection and Measurements. Radiation Protection for Medical and Allied Health Personnel (NCRP Report No. 48). National Council on Radiation Protection and Measurements, Washington, D. C. November 1977. p. 36.

patient in any one week. This calculation is based upon the type and amount of radioactive material and the strength (measured in milligram radium equivalents) of the sources being used. This time limit must be strictly adhered to. The nurse spends only as much time as is absolutely necessary at the bedside (Fig. 18–1). Copies of the instruction sheets are usually kept in the patient's chart, on the door to the patient's room, and in the radiation therapy department.

The door to the room must contain a radioactive warning sign. Patients are not permitted to leave the room or the hospital unless specifically allowed by the physician. Patient activity is dependent upon the site of the implant. For example, patients with ^{137}Cs cervical implants are kept on strict bed rest, lying in semi-Fowler's position, whereas patients with ^{192}Ir breast implants are free to move around the room. Patients are encouraged to do as much self-care as possible.

Additional protection is available, both to staff working with brachytherapy patients and to other patients on the patient care unit. Patients are assigned to private rooms that are specifically designed for brachytherapy treatments. The location of these rooms should preferably be in the corners of the unit, where only one wall connects to another patient's room. Mobile lead shields may also be placed at the bedside as additional protection for the nurse providing care.

Radiation detector devices, a lead container for dislodged sources, and long-handled forceps should be available on the patient care unit at all times. Personnel must *never* pick up a source with their hands. Long-handled forceps are used to place the sources in a lead container for removal from the unit. Each hospital has a radiation safety officer, usually the physicist, who is called immediately if a source is lost, spilled, or accidentally removed. In the event of an accidental spillage of a radioactive source, the following precautions will be taken by the radiation safety officer:

1. Close all windows and turn off air conditioners.
2. Drop absorbent material onto spills and put on waterproof gloves.
3. Clear all people from the room. The patient is placed in another prepared room and radiation safety procedures continued. Close and lock doors. Contaminated shoes are left in the room. No attempt should be made to clean up the spill.
4. Doors are sealed to prevent entry to the room (usually done for radium spills).
5. Test every staff member involved in the incident for radioactivity.
6. The radiation safety officer or other qualified expert will determine the length of time of closure of the room based on the type and half-life of the radioactive material, as well as the severity of the spill and the current activity of the sources. Once

BETHESDA HOSPITAL
RADIATION SAFETY INSTRUCTIONS

Room _____

Implant Date _____   Time _____

Isotope _____   Site _____

Total amount brought to floor _____

Total amount implanted _____

Total amount unused - Returned to dept. _____

Postadministration survey - dose rate:

Bedside _____mr/hr Foot of bed _____mr/hr Room doorway _____mr/hr

Restricted areas: L. sidewall _____mr/hr R. sidewall _____mr/hr

Nursing precautions:

Minutes/wk/person not to exceed:

Bedside _____ Foot of bed (1 meter) _____ Doorway _____

Nursing Instructions:

(Comply with checked items)

1. _____ Wear film badge
2. _____ Wear rubber gloves
3. _____ Precaution sign on patient's door
4. _____ Save laundry in linen bag for survey
5. _____ Housekeeping may not enter room
6. _____ Visitors' time permitted other than listed on patient's door
7. _____ Nursing safety instructions on chart
8. _____ Lead shields required
9. _____ Radiation precaution sticker on chart
10. _____ Other instructions: _____

_____   _____
Physicist   Physician

Removal instructions:

Date out _____   Time _____

Amount removed - Returned to dept.   _____

Dose rate: Patient surface _____mr/hr Linen bag _____mr/hr

Post-removal x-rays ordered: Patient   ___ yes ___ no ___ N/A
                              Applicators ___ yes ___ no ___ N/A

_____   _____
Physicist   Physician

Figure 18–1. Radiation safety instructions. mr, millirem; N/A, not applicable. *Reprinted with permission of* Bethesda Hospital Radiation Therapy Department, Cincinnati, Ohio.

the physicist declares the room safe, it can be cleaned and used normally again.

7. Restrict contaminated persons to a designated area and survey body and clothing with a Geiger counter. Decontamination, if needed, may consist of multiple bathings, especially orifices, nail beds, and body folds. A physician will recommend any further action, e.g., chest x-ray, CBC, urine collection, etc.

If a source is lost, all measures should be taken to find it. All linens must stay in the room until monitored for radioactivity and the radiation safety officer notified. Other specific radiation safety precautions are outlined in Table 18-2.

Unsealed sources

Colloidal radioactive gold (^{198}Au) or radioactive phosphorus (^{32}P). These two preparations may be used intracavitarily in the treatment of malignant pleural effusion or ascites. They may also be administered IV for polycythemia vera.

^{198}Au has a half-life (the time required for the radioactivity of the material to decrease by one-half) of 2.7 days and ^{32}P of 14 days. Patients undergo complete removal of fluid by thoracentesis or paracentesis. The liquid radioactive substance is then instilled into the cavitary area by the physican and will remain permanently in the cavity. Protective clothing is necessary for any involved staff.

Radiation safety precautions are primarily concerned with proper handling and disposal of dressing materials. Radioactive contamination of the dressing may be minimized by reducing leakage around the instillation site (e.g., using occlusive dressings and/or a pressure bandage). Sterile rubber gloves and long-handled forceps are used for all dressing changes. Dressings must be monitored for radioactivity before disposal. Contaminated dressings will be removed and disposed of by the radiation safety officer.

The patient will usually remain hospitalized for the duration of the half-life. As these patients tend to be very ill, attention needs to be given to pain control (*see* Chapter 7A), decubitus care (*see* Chapter 9C), and diet (*see* Chapter 8). Long-term effects may include some myelosuppression (*see* Chapter 9A). The patient may be rotated from side to side and from front to prone to ensure complete distribution of the radioactive source to all areas. Daily abdominal girth measurements are taken when ascites is being treated. Assessment of respiration should be documented, with special attention to excessive dyspnea, after instillation of agents for malignant pleural effusion. Symptomatic relief with these procedures is achieved in ~30 to 40% of patients.

TABLE 18-2

Classification and Special Precautions for Radioactive Sources

Type	Route	Use	Possible contaminants	Special orders
131I	PO or IV	Thyroid cancer	Urine, linens, clothing, food, utensils, skin	Monitor all urine, linens, etc., before disposal.
198Au 32P 90Y	IV or intracavitary	Malignant ascites, malignant pleural effusion	Intracavitary fluid drainage, dressings, excreta	Use gloves, long-handled forceps for dressings.
125I 192Ir	Permanent implant in tiny containers placed directly into tissues	Prostate cancer Breast cancer Bladder cancer	Patient emits gamma radiation for specific time period	Isolation, limit visitors, etc. for specified time period. No children on lap.
137Cs 226Ra 90Sr	Brachytherapy applicator to body orifice for specific period of time	Gynecologic implants, melanoma, eye cancers	Patient removal of applicator, packing	Isolation, limit visitors and staff. No linens to leave room without monitoring. No bed baths. No perineal care (gynecologic implants).

Radioactive iodine (^{131}I). ^{131}I is chiefly used to treat thyroid cancer. It has a half-life of 8.4 days. It is most effective against well-differentiated papillary or follicular cell types and is most commonly uses as ablative adjuvant therapy after thyroidectomy. Repeated doses every 3 mo may be used for patients with metastatic disease. Any thyroid medication should be held for 2 to 3 wk prior to hospitalization for administration of ^{131}I. Thyroid-stimulating hormone (TSH) may be given daily for the 3 days immediately prior to the administration of ^{131}I to increase uptake by the thyroid. The ^{131}I dose is usually given PO as a liquid or a capsule, or IV. As with other unsealed sources, strict isolation should be maintained for the ~8 to 9 days' duration of the half-life. Uptake of ^{131}I is almost exclusively limited to thyroid tissue, with elimination from the body in urine, sweat, and saliva. Absorbent paper may be placed around the toilet or catheter-drainage bag to soak up any possible spillage. No linens should be removed from the room without being monitored.

Side effects of treatment may include nausea and vomiting. All vomitus must be monitored for radioactivity before disposal, especially for patients who received the ^{131}I in an oral form.

Dentures and contact lenses should be rinsed under water daily. Careful hygiene, promoting self-care as far as possible, is emphasized. When entering the room, staff wear gowns, gloves, and shoe covers as protection from contamination.

Visiting is not normally allowed for at least 24 hr after administration of ^{131}I and is then restricted to immediate family only. Any visitors should be instructed not to touch either the patient or the linens in the room or to use the patient's bathroom. Nursing staff need to be sensitive to the patient's feelings of isolation during the long treatment period and help him through this difficult time with understanding.

When being discharged, the patient may be given special instructions about avoiding crowded public places, as well as keeping the telephone mouthpiece and commode clear of all secretions, which are potential contaminants. Discharge teaching should also include the importance of avoiding close contact with pregnant women and children for a specified length of time that is calculated by the physicist, usually 2 to 3 wk.

Sealed sources

Cesium-137 implants (^{137}Cs). Applicators containing ^{137}Cs are used for the treatment of cervical, vaginal, and uterine cancer in combination with hysterectomy and external beam radiation. Early detection for cervical cancer using the Pap smear has enabled physicians to treat those cancers with a high degree of success. The implants are usually used after hysterectomy, to deliver a high local dose to the site of tumor. The whole pelvis is then treated with external radiation for the eradication of any remaining regional disease.

Fletcher's afterloading applicators are most often used for carcinoma of the cervix and the body of the uterus (Figs. 18–2, 18–3). They consist of a hollow uterine tube and two vaginal ovoids. The applicators are surgically inserted and checked for placement by x-ray. The physician then loads the applicators with the radioactive source in the patient's room. The physicist or technologist prepares the sources according to the physician's prescription in the isotope lab. The prepared sources are transported to the patient's room in a lead pig (container). The physician takes the prepared sources from the pig, using long-handled forceps and, working from behind a lead shield, threads them into the afterloaders and then caps them in place. The applicators are maintained in place with the use of proflavine packing. This loading procedure minimizes the number of personnel exposed to radiation. The sources are left in place ~60 to 72 hr.

Simons afterloading capsules are used for carcinoma of the uterus. They consist of numerous small metal-and-plastic containers attached to plastic tubes, which are inserted into the uterus during surgery and, again, loaded with the sources in the patient's room (Figs. 18–4, 18–5).

Table 18–3 outlines the main nursing measures used for the treatment of these patients. In addition to all routine preoperative procedures, the patient usually receives specific bowel preparations and is restricted to a low-residue diet for several days. These preparatory procedures ensure an empty colon. Special concern for emotional well-being is a major consideration in the preoperative teaching and supportive preparation of the patient, especially with regard to issues of sexuality, perceived body image, and sterility (see Chapter 12).

On return from surgery, the patient is placed in semi-Fowler's position to maintain correct placement of the afterloaders and usually has an IV line and a Foley catheter in place. Special observations are made of the patient's temperature and perineal pad at least q 4 hr for the first 24 hr postoperatively to assess for infection. The patients are usually maintained on a low-residue diet while the implant is in place to prevent bowel movements, which might cause dislodgment of the implant.

The sources and applicators are usually removed by the physician on the patient care unit. The Foley catheter is also removed at this time. The patient may require an analgesic and/or sedation prior to this procedure. The physician may prescribe vaginal douches after removal of the implant. The radiation safety officer is responsible for all monitoring procedures for the room and the patient.

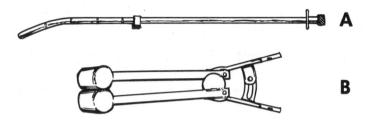

Figure 18–2. Fletcher's afterloading applicators. (A) Fletcher tandem. (B) Fletcher ovoids. The tandem is inserted into the uterine cavity and the ovoids against the outer walls of the cervix as in Figure 18–3. The sources are threaded through the ends of the tandem and ovoid.

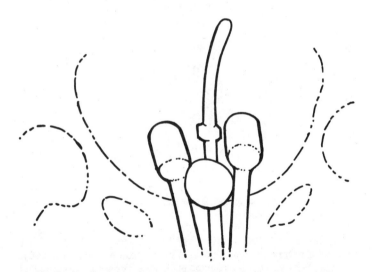

Figure 18–3. Fletcher's afterloading applicators in situ. Note the balloon of the Foley catheter in the central position.

Discharge from the hospital usually occurs on the day after removal of the implant. Some patients require a second implant, which may be done 2 to 3 wk later. Prior to discharge, the patient is advised to avoid sexual intercourse for at least 2 to 3 wk, as the treatment tends to dry the vaginal mucosa. At the first follow-up visit, the patient may be given vaginal dilators with a lubricant to gently stretch the area and prevent fibrosis (*see* Chapter 12).

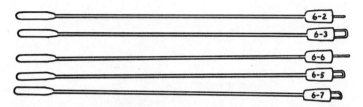

Figure 18–4. Simons afterloading capsules. These are loaded by pulling the metal end and inserting a wire containing the sources. The numbers enable counting to make sure none are lost; also, capsules may be placed in numerical order and removed in reverse order.

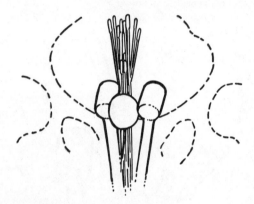

Figure 18–5. Simons afterloading capsules in situ in the uterus with Fletcher ovoids for ^{137}Cs implant.

Radioactive iodine-125 seeds (^{125}I).   Seeds containing ^{125}I are often used to treat prostatic cancer. This procedure is done surgically, using the Mick gun semi-automatic applicator. The seeds are contained in cartridges and advanced through previously placed trocars to the site of the tumor. The trocars are then removed, leaving the seeds in place. Iodine seeds implanted in this manner remain permanently in the prostate. There are no special preoperative preparations for patients undergoing ^{125}I implants. Postoperatively, the patient will have a Foley catheter in place and will be maintained on bed rest in the semi-Fowler's position for 4 to 5 days. Patients may experience burning and discomfort on micturition for ≤6 mo after the procedure. Other side effects are related to abdominal surgery, i.e., pain at the wound site and impotence. The patient is usually discharged on the fifth or sixth day following surgery. [125]I seeds have a relatively low strength, a low penetration to the surface of the skin and, therefore, the radioactivity emitted from the patient is low. The room, urinary drainage bag, and the patient are carefully monitored for radioactivity before discharge and the room rechecked when empty. Because children have a higher mitotic rate of cell growth, there is increased radiation risk with close contact. Sexual counseling may need to be made available to patients who have concerns about impotence or altered body image (*see* Chapter 12).

Iridium-192 seeds (^{192}Ir).   The use of ^{192}Ir seed implants with lumpectomy, axillary node dissection, and external beam RT is now chosen by many patients with stage I and II breast cancer as an alternative to the modified radical mastectomy offered as standard therapy by most surgeons. When implants are used, they are done once at initial surgery and repeated 2 to 3 wk later. Two layers of plastic tubes are threaded through the affected breast and held in place with buttons. After x-ray to ensure that tubes are properly placed, rows of ^{192}Ir seeds are threaded through the tubes and left in place for several days. After removal of the implants, the patient will usually receive external beam RT and/or chemotherapy to complete the treatment. In this way, the patient does not lose her breast and a good cosmetic effect is usually achieved (Figs. 18–6, 18–7).

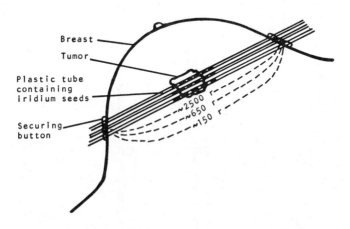

Figure 18–6.   Cross-section of the breast showing placement of ^{192}Ir seeds and approximate radiation dose.

TABLE 18–3

Nursing Protocol for the Management of Gynecologic Implants

Problem	Intervention
Patient/family anxiety related to lack of knowledge and understanding of radiation	Assess patient/family knowledge base and provide all support necessary to decrease anxiety prior to procedure. Provide instructions for any home-care precautions to be taken, based on patient/family understanding of radiation safety principles.
Potential depression related to fear of disease, loss of body image, loss of sexual function	Be alert to signs from patient/family related to body-image problems, etc. Help patient explore feelings. Provide instructions about when to resume sexual activity (usually 3–6 wk), the use of vaginal dilators and lubricants to prevent atrophy of the vaginal canal and painful, dry intercourse.
Reduced mobility and self-care ability while implant in site	Provide instructions including rationale prior to implantation to ensure patient cooperation. Reduce mobility to maintain implants in correct place and prevent potential for uterine or peritoneal perforation. Explain need for patient to perform as much self-care as possible while nursing staff limiting exposure to radiation. If patient is confused, raise bed rails and sedate, if necessary.
Pain related to procedure	Carry out full pain assessment. Assist patient to position of comfort and use decubitus-preventing bed equipment as necessary.

	Administer pain medication regularly during implantation period and assess effectiveness.
Possible dislodging of applicator and radiation source; possible uterine perforations	Prevent dislodgment by: providing low-residue diet; ensuring clean bowel prior to procedure and that patient has no bowel movements throughout procedure; regular administration of antidiarrheic agent; instructing patient to remain in position allowed; observe for compliance; instructing patient not to touch genital region, not to remove packing or applicators; observe for compliance.
Possible operative-site bleeding	Observe pads for bleeding or drainage. Save pads for physician estimate of blood loss. Notify physician promptly of unusual amounts of drainage.
Possible site infection	Monitor temperature only if fever suspected. Obtain culture if necessary.
Possible site breakdown	Observe irradiation site for erythema, dry or moist desquamation. Douche genital area with saline solution after procedure. Encourage good genital hygiene habits for home care. Teach patient to apply cortisone ointment if ordered.
Possible urinary tract infection	Carry out Foley catheter care every shift. Encourage fluid intake unless contraindicated by other medical conditions.

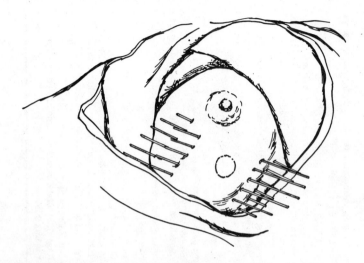

Figure 18–7. Needles in situ in breast during ^{192}Ir implant. Iridium seeds in a fine plastic tube are threaded through the needles, which are then removed, leaving the plastic tubes in situ.

There are no special nursing implications other than observation and assessment of the site and maintaining a dry, intact dressing. Edema may be present, but it usually will disappear after a few days. General nursing principles such as maintaining radiation safety procedures, patient and family education, physical hygiene, and emotional well-being are all important aspects of the nursing of these patients. Antibiotic creams may be needed if puncture wounds become superficially infected. The patient may be ambulatory in the room during the treatment.

Radium-226 implants (^{226}Ra). Recurrent vaginal or rectal cancer and neck tumors may be treated with radium-needle implants. Radium has a half-life of 1,600 years and a high radium milligram equivalent strength. When needles that contain the radioactive material are placed by surgery, there is an increased radiation safety risk to physician and operating room staff. Consequently, it is usually only used when other therapeutic measures to treat the tumor have failed. The needles have long, numbered strings that must be counted every shift to ensure that no needles are lost. The needles are inserted surgically and removed either in the operating room or in the patient's room, depending upon the level of difficulty in removal, anticipated pain, and patient preference. Often the patient will be premedicated with an analgesic, such as meperidine (Demerol), because this procedure usually causes much discomfort, both after placement and during removal. When tongue, mouth, or lip implants are anticipated, a dental consultation and teeth extractions may need to be performed. Temporary dentures may be fitted after 3 to 4 mo. Permanent dentures should not be fitted until all healing of the area is complete and all anticipated gum shrinkage known (usually ≥6 mo).

These patients are taught to perform oral hygiene measures to maintain as clean a field as possible without dislodgement of the sources. Frequent mouthwashes or irrigations with warm saline solutions are required. Liquid diet taken through a straw or nasogastric-tube feedings may be necessary. Highly seasoned foods should be avoided to prevent burning. Occasionally, antibiotics and/or steroids may be required to reduce infection and inflammation.

Lip, mouth, or neck swelling may cause distress and difficulty in swallowing or breathing. Excessive edema causing related problems may need to be treated with diuretics, although usually the swelling will disappear untreated after a few days. Although the needles will not cause lasting damage to the skin or mucosa, many of these patients experience severe body-image problems because of the disfiguring effects of previous surgeries, pigmentation from external RT, and disease proliferation. A great deal of understanding and encouragement to the patient should be provided by the nurse.

The needles are removed in reverse order of their numbers. The patient is discharged with oral care or genital hygiene instructions. The skin may be erythematous and swollen for several days, and steroid preparations may be sent home with the patient. Table 18–4 summarizes the features of sealed sources that are important to the proper understanding of RT implants. Table 18–5 contains a protocol for general nursing care of such patients.

Bibliography

1. Committee for Radiation Oncology Studies. Criteria for Radiation Oncology in Multidisciplinary Cancer Management. National Cancer Institute, Washington, D. C. 1981.

   This pamphlet is a useful guide for those involved in maintaining quality control for their RT departments. It was devised to set standards for RT departments.

2. National Council on Radiation Protection and Measurements. Protection Against Radiation from Brachytherapy Sources (NCRP Report No. 40).

TABLE 18-4
Sealed Sources of Radiation

Source	Half-life	Type of equipment	Irradiation emitted	Site	Duration	Typical dose administered
198Au	2.7 days	seeds	beta	Oral cavity, prostate	permanent implant	2,000 r 4,000 r
90Sr	28 yr	concave disc	beta	Eye cancers, melanoma	removed	15,000 r
137Cs	30 yr	Fletcher's afterloaders, Simons afterloading capsules	gamma	Cervix, uterus, vagina	removed, afterloading technique	3,000–4,000 r
192Ir	74 days	seeds	gamma	Breast, bladder, anal canal	removed	2,000 r
125I	60 days	seeds	beta	Prostate, head and neck	permanent	2,000–16,000 r
226Ra	1,600 yr	needles	gamma	Head and neck	removed	3,000 r

r. rad.

National Council on Radiation Protection and Measurements, Washington, D. C. March 1972.

3. National Council on Radiation Protection and Measurements. Radiation Protection for Medical and Allied Health Personnel (NCRP Report No. 48). National Council on Radiation Protection and Measurements, Washington, D. C. November. 1977.

These pamphlets are two of some 55 pamphlets available at low cost from the National Council on Radiation Protection and Measurements. They provide vital information on radiation protection regulations for nurses and other allied health personnel.

4. Tiffany, R., editor. Cancer Nursing, Radiotherapy. Faber & Faber, London. 1979.

This useful English text has a practical "hands on" approach to the nursing care of oncology patients receiving RT. Although some material does not apply in the USA, in general the authors give good basic information on radiation and important safety principles, as well as specific treatment modalities; particularly useful are the chapters by P. Barkes on unsealed sources (pp. 92–103) and S. Cox on sealed sources (pp. 104–123).

TABLE 18–5

Nursing Protocol for the Management of Radiation Implants

Problem	Intervention
Patient/family education	Ensure that patient/family understand rationale and aspects of care, throughout hospital stay and at home: include information about disease; treatment rationale, description of treatment, how patient will feel during it, side effects, and complications.
	Ensure that patient demonstrates knowledge and understanding *prior* to treatment.
	Explain why nurse can spend only limited time with patient.
	Use booklets, audiovisuals, demonstrations with instruments to be used and models.
	Reassure concerning fears of radiation.
	Stress importance of adhering to safety regulations and regulations governing visiting time and proximity to patient.
	Inform patient and spouse that use of sealed or unsealed sources may cause temporary or permanent sterility.
	See Chapter 5.
Psychologic issues	Provide support and comfort as much as possible with restrictions of radiation safety precautions.
	Avoid showing fear of radiation; avoid making patient feel "untouchable."
	Make time spent with patients "quality time" and focus complete attention on patient in this period.
	Assuage fears of altered body image, loss of sexual function, fear of death, and fear of rejection when patient returns to community through open communication with patient and family and specific sexual instructions (where appropriate). *See* Chapters 6, 12.
	Involve social worker, chaplain, and/or psychologic counsel as indicated.
	Refer to community services where appropriate.
Comfort Pain	Assess for pain: type, intensity, location.
	Treat:
	Use special mattresses in lieu of decubiti care.
	Assist patient to comfortable position.
	Provide self-administered minor anesthetic, e.g., 50% O_2:50% nitrous oxide, for procedures, e.g., removal of GYN implants.
	Monitor bowel movements.
	Alter diet.
	Obtain prescriptions from physician and monitor to be sure prescriptions adequate in relieving the pain experienced.
	Plan pain management incorporating psychologic, cultural, and spiritual factors that may influence pain (*see* Chapter 7A).
Sleep	Ensure that patients who have difficulty sleeping, because of pain or position required by implants, obtain sleep medications (*see* Chapter 7B).

Problem	Intervention
Dislodgment	Maintain semi-Fowler's position for those with GYN implants. Avoid vomiting, constipation, or diarrhea. If dislodgment occurs, notify radiation safety officer immediately; follow radiation safety procedures.
Side effects **Short-term** GI	Prevent nausea/vomiting wherever possible by use of antiemetics, administered ½ hr before meals. Minimize nausea/vomiting by appropriate diet, use of antiemetics as ordered, and pain medications. If vomiting occurs, monitor head and neck patients for dislodgment of radiation sources or aspiration of vomitus; monitor patients with cervical or uterine implants for dislodgment. Prevent bowel movements during implant (abdominal only) by use of low-residue diet. Ensure patient not constipated prior to return home (laxative may be needed) (*see* Chapter 11). Minimize dysphagia and mucositis through use of soft or liquid diet, pain medications or topical anesthetic as ordered and careful oral hygiene after removal of implant (*see* Chapter 9B). Ensure that diet is suited to minimize side effects: IV or tube feeding or liquid diet for patients with lip needle implants. Monitor for malnutrition, weight loss.
Skin	Monitor for erythema, moist or dry desquamation. Apply topical creams as ordered after implant removal, e.g., cortisone for GYN implants, A & D ointment to anal area.
Edema	Monitor for excessive edema and treat with diuretics if necessary.
Infection	Practice preventive care: Monitor temperature; assess dressing site; practice careful hygiene and/or dressing care after dressing removed. Be alert to possibility of infection in GU tract, oral cavity, and pelvis (cellulitis, abscess, or perforation of uterus [rare]). Be alert for complications caused by myelosuppression.
Bleeding/hemorrhage	Monitor blood loss on dressings; vital signs for increased pulse, decreased BP (*see* Chapter 9A).
GU	Minimize transient frequency and dysuria (GYN and prostatic implants) by increasing fluid intake, if not contraindicated.
Long-term Fibrosis, stricture, adhesions, dyspareunia	Head and neck: Provide saliva substitute and encourage consumption of fluids prior to eating. Gradually advance diet from liquid to soft to solid foods. GYN: Teach use of topical creams and lubricants to affected areas; teach use of vaginal dilators after implants. Inform patient of alternate sexual positions to decrease/eliminate painful penile penetration (*see* Chapter 12).

GYN, gynecologic.

APPENDIX A: TUMOR TYPE AND METASTATIC SPREAD

Primary disease	Common sites of metastases													
	Bone	Marrow	Skin	Lung	Liver	Bowel/rectum	Nodes	Spleen	Kidney/GU	Brain	Serosa	Other pelvic organs	Meninges	Adrenal glands
Bladder							X		X			X		
Brain	X												X	
Breast	X			X	X		X			X			X	
Cervix				X	X	X	X		X					
Colon				X	X		X							
Esophagus	X			X	X		X							X
Head/neck			X	X			X							
Hepatoma	X			X			X							
Kidney	X			X	X		X			X				

586

Lung	X	X	X	X		X	X	X
Melanoma	X		X	X	X	X	X	X
Mycosis fungoides		X	X		X			
Ovary			X	X	X	X	X	
Pancreas			X	X	X	X		
Prostate	X		X	X	X	X		
Sarcoma			X	X		X		
Stomach	X		X	X	X	X		
Testes	X		X	X	X	X		
Thyroid	X		X	X	X	X		
Uterus			X						X

APPENDIX B: TUMOR TYPE AND ONCOLOGIC EMERGENCY

Tumor type	Increased intracranial pressure	Spinal cord compression	Superior vena cava syndrome	Tracheal obstruction	Bowel obstruction	Hypercalcemia	Tumor lysis syndrome	Syndrome of inappropriate antidiuretic hormone	Sepsis†	Disseminated intravascular coagulation	Thrombosis	Hyperviscosity	Carotid artery rupture	Leukostasis	Other
*Bone		X				X									Pathologic fracture
Bladder					X										Renal failure
*Brain	X							X							
Breast		X				X									
Colon/rectum					X										Hemorrhage
Esophagus			X			X									Hemorrhage
Head/neck				X									X		

588

Site						Hyperglycemia	Renal failure
Kidney	X	X		X			
Lung	X	X	X	X	X		
Melanoma							
Ovary				X			
Pancreas	X			X	X	X	
Prostate	X		X		X	X	
Sarcoma							
Stomach							
Testes					X		
Thyroid							
Uterus		X					
Leukemia			X	X	X		X
Lymphoma	X	X	X	X	X		
Myeloma	X	X		X		X	

* Risk for oncologic emergency exists for patients with either primary or metastatic disease in these sites.

‡ Risk for oncologic emergency exists for any patient experiencing bone marrow depression from chemotherapy or radiotherapy.

APPENDIX C:
STAGING OF CANCER*

Proper classification and staging allow the physician to determine the appropriate treatment, to evaluate the results, and to compare statistics from various institutions.

The American Joint Committee on Cancer (AJCC), sponsored by the American College of Surgeons, the American College of Radiology, the College of American Pathologists, the American College of Physicians, the American Cancer Society, and the National Cancer Institute, developed a system of staging based on the premise that cancers of similar histology or site of origin share similar patterns of growth and extension. This committee, with the TNM committee of the International Union Against Cancer (UICC) and representatives from other specialty groups agreed upon the TNM staging system. Three significant events — tumor growth (T), spread to primary lymph nodes (N), and metastasis (M) — are used to indicate the degree of involvement of the cancer.

The T, plus the numbers 1 through 4, stands for the primary tumor and describes the size and/or level of invasion. The higher the number, the larger the size of the tumor and/or the depth or amount of involvement.

The N, plus numbers 1 through 4, indicates whether or not there is evidence that the tumor has spread to the regional lymph nodes and the size and number of nodes involved.

M, with numbers 0 or 1 indicates the absence or presence of distant metastases. Letters are sometimes added to the M to show other areas involved:

BRA	Brain
EYE	Eye
HEP	Hepatic
LYM	Lymph nodes
MAR	Bone marrow
OSS	Osseous
PLE	Pleura
PUL	Pulmonary
SKI	Skin
OTH	Other

---

*This appendix was compiled by Marion E. Morra, Assistant Director of the Yale Comprehensive Cancer Center, New Haven, Connecticut.

The following TNM symbols normally have the same meaning regardless of cancer site (and, unless there are other special explanations needed, are not repeated in the tables that follow):

TX Tumor cannot be assessed
T0 No evidence of primary tumor
TIS Carcinoma in situ
NX Regional lymph nodes cannot be assessed
N0 Regional lymph nodes not found to be abnormal
MX Metastasis cannot be assessed
M0 No known distant metastasis
M1 Distant metastasis present

Staging systems for the most common tumors are included alphabetically; in some cases more than one staging system is presented. Unless otherwise indicated, all tables have been based on material from American Joint Commission on Cancer. The Manual for Staging of Cancer. J. B. Lippincott Co., Philadelphia. 1983. Second edition.

BREAST CANCER

The most widely used staging classification, adopted by both the International Union Against Cancer and American Joint Committee on Cancer, is based on the TNM system.

Table 1: *Staging Classification for Breast Cancer*

TNM	Explanation
T1	Tumor 2 cm or less in greatest dimension.
T2	Tumor more than 2 cm but not more than 5 cm in its greatest dimension.
T3	Tumor more than 5 cm in its greatest dimension.
T4	Tumor of any size with direct extension to chest wall or skin.
N0	No palpable homolateral axillary nodes.
N1	Movable homolateral axillary nodes: a. nodes not considered to contain growth; b. nodes considered to contain growth.
N2	Homolateral axillary nodes containing growth and fixed to one another or to other structures.
N3	Homolateral supraclavicular or infraclavicular nodes containing growth or edema of the arm.

See Table 2 for Stage Groupings.

Table 2: *Stage Groupings for Breast Cancer*

Stage	TNM
Stage I	T1, N0, M0
Stage II	T0–T1, N1, M0 or T2, N0–N1, M0
Stage IIIA	T0–T2, N2, M0 or T3, N0–N2, M0
Stage IIIB	Any T, N3, M0 T4, or any N, M0
Stage IV	Any T, any N, M1

CERVICAL CANCER

The staging of cervical cancer is based on a system developed by FIGO (International Federation of Gynecology and Obstetrics). The International Union Against Cancer and the American Joint Committee on Cancer have adopted this system, which conforms to the TNM classification. Therefore, the FIGO nomenclature is the accepted terminology for staging cervical cancer.

Table 3: *TNM and FIGO Staging for Cervical Cancer*

FIGO	TNM	Explanation
Stage 0	TIS	Carcinoma in situ
Stage I	T1, N0, M0	The carcinoma is confined to the cervix.
Stage II	T2, N0, M0	The carcinoma extends beyond the cervix but has not extended to the pelvic wall. The carcinoma involves the vagina but does not extend as far as the lower third.
Stage III	T3, N0–N1, M0	The carcinoma has extended to the pelvic wall.
Stage IV	T4, NX-N1, M0 or any T, any N, M1	The carcinoma has extended beyond the true pelvis or has clinically involved the mucosa of the bladder or rectum.

COLON AND RECTAL CANCER

Colon and rectal cancer can be staged by the TNM system, by Dukes' system, or by the Astler-Coller modification of Dukes' system.

Table 4: *TMN Staging Classification for Colon and Rectal Cancer*

TNM	Explanation
T1	Confined to mucosa or submucosa.
T2	Limited to wall of colon or rectum but not beyond.
T3	Invading the bowel wall, including serosa, with or without extension to adjacent structures.
T4	Spread by direct extension beyond adjacent organs.
N1	1–3 involved nodes adjacent to primary tumor.
N2	Involved nodes extending to line of resection.
N3	Involved nodes, location not identified.

Table 5: *Staging Groupings for Colon and Rectal Cancer*

Stage	Dukes' (Astler-Coller modification)	TNM	Explanation
Stage IA	Dukes' A	T1, N0, M0	Tumor confined to mucosa or submucosa.
Stage IB	Dukes' B1	T2, N0, M0	Tumor involves muscularis propria but not beyond.
Stage II	Dukes' B2	T3, N0, M0	Tumor involves all layers of bowel wall, with or without invasion of immediately adjacent structures.
Stage III	Dukes' C	Any T, N1–N3, M0, or T4, N0, M0	Limited to wall of colon/rectum without serosal involvement (C1), or extension through the wall to the perirectal fat (C2) with regional node involvement.
Stage IV	Dukes' D	Any T, any N, M1	Any degree of regional disease involvement.

ENDOMETRIAL CANCER

There are two staging systems commonly used: one proposed by the International Federation of Gynecology and Obstetrics (FIGO) and the other by the American Joint Committee on Cancer. Both are contained in the following table.

Table 6: *TNM and FIGO Staging for Endometrial Cancer*

FIGO	TNM	Explanation
Stage 0	TIS	Carcinoma in situ.
Stage I	T1, N0, M0	Carcinoma confined to corpus.
IA	T1a, N0, M0	Uterine cavity 8 cm or less in length.
IB	T1b, N0, M0	Uterine cavity greater than 8 cm in length.

		Stage I subgrouped by histotogy as follows:
		    G1 — highly differentiated,
		    G2 — moderately differentiated,
		    G3 — undifferentiated.

Stage II	T2, N0, M0	Extension to cervix only.
Stage III	T3, N0, M0 T1–T3, N1, M0	Extension outside the uterus but confined to true pelvis.
Stage IV	T4, N0–N1, M0 or any T, any N, M1	Extension beyond true pelvis or invading bladder or rectum.

HODGKIN'S AND NON-HODGKIN'S LYMPHOMAS

The Ann Arbor Staging Classification, proposed in 1970, modified previous staging systems and is now the standard method for classification of the lymphomas. The TNM system is not used for staging these diseases because it is not possible to differentiate among possible sites of primary tumors (T), nodal (N), or metastatic (M) involvement.

Table 7: *Staging Classification for Hodgkin's Disease*

Stage*	Explanation
Stage I	Involvement of a single lymph node region (I) or a single extralymphatic organ or site (I_E).
Stage II	Involvement of two or more lymph node regions (II) or localized involvement of an extralymphatic organ or site (II_E), on the same side of the diaphragm.
Stage III	Involvement of lymph node regions (III) or localized involvement of an extralymphatic organ or site (III_E) on both sides of the diaphragm or spleen (III_S) or both (III_{SE}).
Stage IV	Diffuse or disseminated involvement of one or more extralymphatic organs, with or without associated lymph node involvement.

*Each stage is divided into an A or B category: A, asymptomatic; B, fever, sweats, weight loss >10% of body weight.

LUNG CANCER

Lung cancer is staged by a TNM staging system. The system can be applied to all histologic types of lung cancer (except oat cell).

Table 8: *Staging Classification for Lung Cancer*

TNM	Explanation
T1	A tumor 3.0 cm or less in greatest diameter.
T2	A tumor more than 3.0 cm in greatest diameter or that invades the pleura or has associated atelectasis or obstructive pneumonitis extending to the hilum.
T3	Any tumor that extends into an adjacent structure; or that involves a main bronchus less than 2.0 cm distal to the carina; or that is associated with atelectasis or obstructive pneumonitis of an entire lung, or pleural effusion.
N1	Involvement of lymph nodes in the peribronchial or the ipsilateral hilum, or both.
N2	Involvement of lymph nodes in the mediastinum.

Table 9: *Stage Groupings for Lung Cancer*

Stage	TNM	Explanation
Occult carcinoma	TX, N0, M0	An occult carcinoma with secretions containing malignant cells but without other evidence of the primary tumor or evidence of involvement of lymph nodes or metastasis.
Stage I	T1, N0–N1, M0 or T2, N0, M0	Carcinoma in situ. Tumor that can be classified T1 without any metastasis or with local lymph node involvement, or a tumor that can be classified T2 without any nodal involvement or metastasis.
Stage II	T2, N1, M0	A tumor classified as T2 with involvement of local lymph nodes.
Stage III	T3, any N, any M Any T, N2, any M Any T, any N, M1	Any tumor larger than T2, or any tumor with metastasis to the lymph nodes in the mediastinum, or any tumor with distant metastasis.

PROSTATE CANCER

Cancer of the prostate is staged according to the TNM classification.

Table 10: *Staging Classification for Prostate Cancer*

TNM	Explanation
T1	No palpable tumor.
T2a	Palpable nodule less than 1.5 cm in diameter.
T2b	Palpable nodule more than 1.5 cm in diameter or palpable evidence of disease in both lobes.
T3	Palpable tumor extending into or beyond the prostatic capsule.
T4	Tumor fixed or involving adjacent tissues.
N1	Involvement of a single lymph node on the same side.
N2	Involvement of multiple regional lymph nodes.
N3	A fixed mass on the pelvic wall without direct extension by tumor mass.
M1	Distant metastasis.

Table 11: *Stage Grouping for Prostate Cancer*

Stage	TNM
Stage I	T1–T2a, N0, M0
Stage II	T2b, N0, M0
Stage III	T3, N0, M0 Any T, N1, M0
Stage IV	T4, N0, M0 Any T, N2 or N3, M0 Any T, any N, M1

APPENDIX D:
AVAILABLE RESOURCES*

MAJOR CANCER AGENCIES

American Cancer Society
90 Park Avenue
New York, New York 10016
(212) 599-8200

The American Cancer Society (ACS) is a national voluntary organization. It offers a wide range of services to patients and their families and carries out programs of research and education. It also provides pamphlets, films, and reprints for patients and professionals. It is financed solely through donations from individuals and private groups. The ACS has 58 divisions located in every state, Washington, D.C., and Puerto Rico, and 3,000 local units, which function at the county level. The national headquarters of the ACS is responsible for overall planning and coordination. For local units, consult the white pages of your local phone directory.

National Cancer Institute
Bethesda, Maryland 20205
(301) 496-4000

The National Cancer Institute (NCI), part of the Department of Health and Human Services, National Institutes of Health, is responsible for federally funded cancer research and control programs.

Within the NCI, the Office of Cancer Communications is responsible for providing the public, cancer patients, and the news media with accurate, up-to-date responses to inquiries about cancer. Furthermore, the Office of Cancer Communications develops and distributes special information and education programs about cancer to health professionals, cancer patients, and the public.

---

*This appendix was compiled by Marion E. Morra, Assistant Director of the Yale Comprehensive Cancer Center, New Haven, Connecticut.

Cancer Information Clearinghouse
National Cancer Institute
Bethesda, Maryland 20205
(301) 496-6756
The Cancer Information Clearinghouse is an information service for organizations that use or develop materials for public and professional information and education. The Clearinghouse provides information exchange, either in the form of bibliographic services or in custom searches of its collection of 7,000 citations of cancer informational and educational materials and services.

Cancer Information Service
1-800-4-CANCER*
The Cancer Information Service (CIS) is a nationwide toll-free telephone program sponsored by the NCI. Trained information specialists are available to answer questions about cancer from the public, cancer patients and their families, and health professionals. By calling the toll-free number — 1-800-4-CANCER — you will be automatically connected to the CIS office serving your area. Booklets and brochures (single copies or orders for bulk shipment) are also available through this number.
*In Alaska call 1-800-638-6070; in Washington, D.C., and its suburbs in Maryland and Virginia, call 636-5700; on Oahu call 524-1234 (call collect from neighboring islands). Spanish-speaking staff members are available to callers from the following areas (daytime hours only): California (area codes 213, 619, 714, and 805), Florida, Georgia, Illinois, Northern New Jersey, New York, and Texas.

International Cancer Information Center
National Cancer Institute
Bethesda, Maryland 20205
(301) 496-7403
The International Cancer Information Center (ICIC) sponsors CANCERLINE, which includes (a) ~400,000 citations and abstracts of articles published since 1963 on all aspects of cancer, (b) descriptions of ~10,000 ongoing cancer research projects, and (c) ~4,500 summaries of clinical investigations of new anticancer agents and treatment modalities. The ICIC also sponsors Physician Data Query (PDQ), a user-friendly, physician-oriented data base that contains information about specific tumor types as well as abstracts of current research protocols.

SPECIAL INTEREST GROUPS

Candlelighters Foundation
2025 I Street N.W.
Washington, D.C. 20006
(202) 659-5136

The Candlelighters Foundation is an organization formed by parents of young cancer patients. Their goal is to help families of pediatric and adolescent cancer patients cope with the emotional stresses of their experience. Candlelighters hold regular meetings to discuss problems and exchange information. Candlelighters now includes some 175 parents' groups in 50 states and other countries throughout the world. Local information is available through American Cancer Society units or the Cancer Information Service.

CANSURMOUNT
C/O American Cancer Society
90 Park Avenue
New York, New York 10016
(212) 599-8200

CANSURMOUNT is a group that offers patient and family education and support; local information is available through American Cancer Society units.

Hospice Programs
National Hospice Organization
1901 North Fort Myer Drive - 4th Floor
Arlington, Virginia 22209
(703) 243-5900

The hospice concept is modeled after St. Christopher's Hospice in England. It focuses on quality of survival rather than length of survival. In most cases, to be admitted, patients must be referred by a physician and live in the area served by the hospice. The national organization, formed in 1978, aims at realizing the goal of hospice as individual programs and as a nationwide method of delivering health care. For hospices in your area, contact the national organization or the Cancer Information Service.

I Can Cope
C/O American Cancer Society
90 Park Avenue
New York, New York 10016
(212) 599-8200

I Can Cope is a course designed to address the educational and psychological needs of people with cancer. It is run locally, usually by nurses and social workers. Information about local courses is available through local American Cancer Society units.

International Association of Laryngectomees
C/O American Cancer Society
90 Park Avenue
New York, New York 10016
(212) 599-8200

The International Association of Laryngectomees (IAL) assists people who have lost their voices as a result of cancer. The IAL provides education in the skills needed by laryngectomees and works toward the total rehabilitation of the patient. The organization maintains a registry of post-laryngectomy speech instructors, publishes educational materials, and sponsors meetings and other activities. It is sponsored by the American Cancer Society (ACS). A local chapter may be listed in your telephone directory or you may contact your local ACS.

Leukemia Society of America, Inc.
733 Third Avenue
New York, New York 10017
(212) 573-8484

This is a national voluntary health agency that provides supplementary financial assistance to patients with leukemia, the lymphomas, and Hodgkin's disease, as well as referral services to other sources of help in the community. The program is administered through society chapters located throughout the USA. Payment can be made for drugs used in care, treatment and/or control of disease, transfusing of blood, x-ray treatment, and transportation to and from a doctor's office, hospital, or treatment center. There are chapters in most states. Call the Cancer Information Service.

Make Today Count, Inc.
P.O. Box 303
Burlington, Iowa 52601
(319) 753-6521

The organization Make Today Count provides psychological assistance to patients with cancer or any other life-threatening illness. A primary aim is to help these people live each day as fully and happily as possible. Activities include group meetings for the discussion of mutual problems, home visit programs, educational workshops for patients and health-care providers, newsletters, and the distribution of cancer-related materials. Founded in 1974, the organization has grown to some 300 chapters throughout the USA and in several foreign countries. A local chapter may be listed in your telephone directory.

MASTECTOMY PROGRAMS

Reach for Recovery
C/O American Cancer Society
90 Park Avenue
New York, New York 10016
(212) 599-8200

The American Cancer Society's "Reach For Recovery" offers
assistance to breast cancer patients. Trained volunteers who have had
breast cancer lend emotional support and furnish information to
women before and after breast surgery. Additional information about
this program can be obtained from a local chapter of the American
Cancer Society listed in the telephone directory.

Encore
YWCA
Encore Supervisor-National Board
135 West 50th Street
New York, New York 10020

The YWCA's "Encore" program offers discussion and exercise
programs for women who have had breast cancer surgery. The program
has been developed to help restore physical strength as well as
emotional well-being. "Encore" meetings include exercise to music,
water exercises, and a discussion period. Phone your local YWCA
branch for additional information.

OSTOMY PROGRAMS

Ostomy Rehabilitation Program
American Cancer Society
90 Park Avenue
New York, New York 10016
(212) 599-8200

The Ostomy Rehabilitation Program of the American Cancer
Society (ACS) furnishes services to ostomates. The ACS helps the
ostomate adjust to the everyday experiences of work, travel, and
recreation. Some ACS divisions sponsor their programs with the
United Ostomy Association. Call your local ACS unit listed in the
telephone directory for information.

United Ostomy Association, Inc.
2001 West Beverly Boulevard
Los Angeles, California 90057
(213) 413-5510

The United Ostomy Association, Inc. (UOA), organized and administered by ostomates, helps ostomy patients return to a normal life through mutual aid and emotional support. The UOA, which has over 652 local chapters, provides information to patients and the public and supports the improvement of ostomy equipment and supplies. In addition, the UOA sends volunteer ostomates to visit with new ostomy patients. It publishes the *Ostomy Quarterly* and other educational materials. You can get information about local activities through the address above or through the American Cancer Society.

CANCER CENTERS

COMPREHENSIVE CANCER CENTERS

There are 20 comprehensive cancer centers designated by the National Cancer Institute. These medical research centers investigate new methods of diagnosis and treatment of cancer patients and provide new scientific knowledge to physicians who are treating cancer patients. They must meet 10 specific criteria, which include basic and clinical research and patient care. Call 1-800-4-CANCER (the CIS) for the names and locations of these cancer centers.

NATIONAL INSTITUTES OF HEALTH CLINICAL CENTER

The National Cancer Institute conducts research programs to which patients are admitted at the Clinical Center of the National Institutes of Health (NIH) in Bethesda, Maryland. The Clinical Center, a research hospital, provides nursing and medical care without charge. When a physician wishes to refer a cancer patient for clinical study, he may send a complete medical history and an evaluation of the person's condition to the Deputy Clinical Director, National Cancer Institute, Bldg. 10, 6B15, Bethesda, Maryland 20205. The telephone number is (301) 496-4251. A pamphlet giving general information about the Clinical Center can be received by calling the Cancer Information Service.

CLINICAL AND LABORATORY CANCER CENTERS

Clinical and laboratory cancer centers are medical centers that have support from the National Cancer Institute for clinical programs to investigate promising new methods of cancer treatment or for laboratory research programs. For information about local centers, call the Cancer Information Service.

CLINICAL COOPERATIVE GROUPS

More than 4,000 cancer research physicians at hundreds of institutions in the USA and abroad are members of Cancer Clinical Cooperative Groups and Projects, supported in part by the National Cancer Institute (NCI). Each Cooperative program studies one or more kinds of cancer and assists the NCI in the clinical evaluation of new anticancer drugs and other investigational approaches to treatment. Patients admitted to these studies receive expert medical care from specially trained teams of physicians. Information about groups and protocol being investigated by clinical cooperative groups is available through PDQ or the Cancer Information Service.

COMMUNITY CLINICAL ONCOLOGY PROGRAM (CCOP)

The CCOP is an opportunity for community physicians to participate in cancer treatment research by means of clinical trials. Sponsored by the National Cancer Institute, CCOPs will be encouraging the affiliation of community physicians and their treatment facilities with clinical research resources. For names of local participants, call the Cancer Information Service.

PROFESSIONAL ASSOCIATIONS

American Society of Clinical Oncology, Inc. (ASCO)
Suite 1717
435 North Michigan Avenue
Chicago, Illinois 60611
(312) 644-0828
Promotes and fosters the exchange and diffusion of information and ideas relating to neoplastic diseases, with particular emphasis on human biology, diagnosis, and treatment.

Association of Pediatric Oncology Nurses (APON)
Department of Hematology-Oncology
The Children's Hospital
1601 6th Avenue South
Birmingham, Alabama 35233
(204) 250-9285
Establishes lines of communication among nurses caring for children with cancer.

European Oncology Nursing Society
Stewart House
Stewart's Grove
London SW3 6JT England
   Strives to improve the nursing care of people suffering from cancer by promoting and developing oncology nursing as a specialty in countries throughout Europe.

International Association for Enterostomal Therapy (IAET)
505 A. Tustan Avenue
Suite 282
Santa Ana, California 92705
(714) 972-1725
   Organizes enterostomal therapy nurses for the promotion of education to patients, nurses, physicians, and other allied health professionals in the biopsychosocial and sexual rehabilitation of persons with abdominal stomas, fistulas, draining wounds, incontinence, and pressure sores.

International Society of Nurses in Cancer Care
C/O Memorial Sloan-Kettering Cancer Center, M1929
1275 York Avenue
New York, New York 10021
(212) 794-6903
   Provides communications network to disseminate information (especially in countries where no national group exists), assists nurses to establish national oncology societies, and supports international organizations such as International Council of Nurses, the International Union Against Cancer (UICC), and World Health Organization on nursing issues. Membership includes a subscription to *Cancer Nursing*, published 6 times/yr.

Oncology Nursing Society (ONS)
3111 Banksville Road
Pittsburgh, Pennsylvania 15216
(412) 344-3899
   Promotes the highest professional standards of oncology nursing: to study research and exchange information, experiences, and ideas leading to improved nursing and to encourage nurses to specialize in the practice of oncology nursing. Membership includes a subscription to the *Oncology Nursing Forum*, published 6 times/yr. There are local chapters in many areas.

INDEX